Polycystic Ovary Syndrome

Polycystic Ovary Syndrome

Edited by

ROY HOMBURG, MB BS
Professor of Obstetrics and Gynaecology
Lis Maternity Hospital
Tel Aviv Sourasky Medical Centre

Emma Neiman Chair of Childbirth Research
Sackler School of Medicine
Tel Aviv University
Israel

MARTIN DUNITZ

© 2001 Martin Dunitz Ltd, a member of the Taylor & Francis group

First published in the United Kingdom in 2001
by Martin Dunitz Ltd, The Livery House, 7–9 Pratt Street, London
NW1 0AE

Tel.:   +44 (0) 20 7482 2202
Fax.:   +44 (0) 20 7267 0159
E-mail: info.dunitz@tandf.co.uk
Website: http://www.dunitz.co.uk

A CIP record for this book is available from the British Library.

ISBN 1-84184-016-5

Distributed in the United States by:
Blackwell Science Inc.
Commerce Place, 350 Main Street
Malden MA 02148
Tel.: 1-800-215-100

Distributed in Canada by:
Login Brothers Book Company
324 Salteaux Crescent
Winnipeg, Manitoba R3J 3T2
Tel.: 1-204-224-4068

Distributed in Brazil by:
Ernesto Reichmann Distribuidora de Livros, Ltda
Rua Coronel Marques 335
Tatuape 03440-000, Sao Paulo

Composition by Wearset, Boldon, Tyne and Wear
Printed and bound in Great Britain by Biddles Ltd, Guildford and
King's Lynn

Contents

Foreword

We have been witness to an enormous acceleration of interest in polycystic ovaries during the last ten years. Almost half the relevant original articles have been published since 1990; moreover, over 400 of the 564 relevant review articles were published during the same time period.

Although progress is increasingly palpable, the fundamentals of the etiology and pathophysiology of polycystic ovaries can seem as elusive as ever. Since we have crossed the millennial divide, it appears appropriate that an interim progress report be called. This compilation attempts to meet just such a goal. As such, it is an important contribution and must be viewed as an incremental step on the long road to elucidating the mysteries of this seemingly multifacted entity, the precise origins of which may continue to bedevil generations of investigators.

Eli Y Adashi

List of contributors

Eli Y Adashi
Department of Obstetrics and Gynecology
University of Utah Health Sciences Center,
Suite 23200
50 North Medical Drive
Salt Lake City, UT 84132
USA

Ghanim Almahbobi
Institute for Neuromuscular Research
Level 3, Clinical Sciences Building
The New Children Hospital
Hawkesbury Road
Westmead, NSW 2145
Australia

Adam Balen
Department of Obststrics and Gynaecology
General Infirmary
Leeds LS2 9NS, UK

Mary Birdsall
Fertility Associates
131 Remuera Road
Remuera
Auckland 5
New Zealand

Paul Devroey
Centre for Reproductive Medicine
Dutch-speaking Brussels Free University
Laarbeeklaan 101
1090 Brussels, Belgium

Margo R Fluker
Genesis Fertility Centre
Suite 550-555
West 12th Avenue
Vancouver, BC, Canada V5Z 3X7

Stephen Franks
Reproductive Endocrinology Group
Department of Obstetrics and Gynaecology
Imperial College School of Medicine
St Mary's Hospital
London W2 1PG, UK

Pilar Gaitán
IVI-Valencia
C/Guardia Civil 23
46020 Valencia
Spain

Juan A García-Velasco
IVI-Madrid
C/Santiago de Compostella, 88
28035 Madrid
Spain

Linda C Giudice
Division of Reproductive Endocrinology and
Infertility
Center for Research on Women's Health and
Reproductive Medicine
Department of Gynecology and Obstetrics
Stanford University Medical Center
Stanford, CA 94305-5317, USA

Vera Haitsma
Centre for Reproductive Medicine
Dutch-speaking Brussels Free University
Laarbeeklaan 101
1090 Brussels, Belgium

Roy Homburg
Obstetrics and Gynaecology
Lis Maternity Hospital
Tel Aviv Sourasky Medical Centre
Tel Aviv 64239, Israel

Peter GA Hompes
Department of Obstetrics and Gynecology
Academisch Ziekenhuis
Vrije Universiteit
Postbus 7057
Amsterdam, The Netherlands

Howard S Jacobs
Department of Medicine
Royal Free and University College London
Middlesex Hospital
Mortimer Street
London W1N 8AA, UK

Helen Mason
Department of Obstetrics and Gynaecology
St George's Hospital Medical School
London SW17 0RE, UK

Dror Meirow
Department of Obstetrics and Gynecology
Rabin Medical Centre
Campus Beilinson
Petah Tikva, Israel 49100

José Navarro
IVI–Sevilla
Avenida República Argentina, 58
41011 Seville
Spain

Antonio Pellicer
IVI–Valencia
C/Guardia Civil 23
Valencia, Spain

Peter Platteau
Centre for Reproductive Medicine
Dutch-speaking Brussels Free University
Laarbeeklaan 101
1090 Brussels, Belgium

Gordana M Prelevic
Department of Medicine
Royal Free & University College London
Medical School
Cobbold Laboratories
The Middlesex Hospital
Mortimer Street
London W1N 8AA, UK

José Remohí
IVI–Valencia
C/Guardia Civil 23
46020 Valencia, Spain

Robert L Rosenfield
The University of Chicago
Pritzker School of Medicine
University of Chicago Children's Hospital
5841 S Maryland Avenue, MC–5053
Chicago, USA

Joop Schoemaker
Institute for Endocrinology, Reproduction and
Metabolism
Division of Reproductive Endocrinology and
Fertility
Vrije Universiteit Medical Center, Amsterdam
Verwersweg 30
8437 PE Zorglied, The Netherlands

Carlos Simón
IVI–Valencia
C/Guardia Civil 23
Valencia, Spain

Alan O Trounson
Centre for Early Human Development
Monash Institute of Reproduction and
Development
Monash Medical Centre
27–31 Wright Street
Clayton, Vic 3168
Australia

1

Polycystic ovary syndrome: consensus and controversy

Roy Homburg

The diversity of ideas about the cause and treatment of polycystic ovary syndrome (PCOS) throughout the world can only be matched, in my experience, by life in Israel, a country with about 5 million people, each of whom has a different view on the problems of the country and how they should be solved. In this book, I have been fortunate enough to have been able to gather together the opinions of the leading researchers into PCOS. Despite the fact that even the name of this entity – not to mention its definition and diagnosis – has conjured up a deal of heated argument, contributors from as far apart as Australasia, Europe, the Middle East and North America have produced chapters on their particular area of expertise that make a great deal of consensus possible. From recent meetings, it has become obvious that it is not only the geographical divide of the Atlantic Ocean that separates the USA from Europe – so does the argument on the geographical features of the polycystic ovary. One of the main aims of this book is to allow the world experts to set out their stalls and present their evidence to help us close the gaps in our knowledge. What is certain is that the enthusiasm and drive of the authors to understand the pathophysiological mechanisms involved and the best method of treating the consequences is a recurrent and obvious feature throughout all of the chapters in this book. This has made the editing of this volume both a pleasure and a labour of love, and I thank the contributors very much indeed for their efforts.

A POTTED HISTORY

As early as 1844, Chereau described sclerocystic changes in the human ovary,[1] some 90 years before the classic paper of Stein and Leventhal in 1935.[2] Elevated luteinizing hormone (LH) concentrations were first reported in 1958, creating a criterion for diagnosis, and the introduction of radioimmunoassays in 1971 stimulated reliance on a biochemical diagnosis. Although it was clear as early as 1962 that there was a wide variety of clinical presentation, it was only in 1976 that the concept of PCOS with normal LH concentrations was developed.[3] A further milestone was the discovery of the association of PCOS and insulin resistance by Khan et al in 1976 and Burghen et al in 1980.[4,5] Swanson first described the ultrasound findings of women with PCOS in 1981, but only after Adams et al refined and critically defined diagnostic criteria in 1985 did the ultrasonographic diagnosis of PCO become accepted.[6,7] The familial traits of PCOS are now well recognized and progress into the era of molecular biology has brought with it a frantic search for the responsible gene defects. Abnormalities in the action of tens of growth factors are being cited as culprits of the dysfunctional mesh of interactions within the cell and follicular fluid.

On the therapeutic side, surgical treatment by bilateral wedge resection of the ovaries was first suggested by Stein and Leventhal.[2] In retrospect, this was an amazingly successful procedure whose principles are now being widely revived using ovarian cautery by means of lasers introduced through the laparoscope. Induction of ovulation was made possible by clomiphene citrate and furthered by the introduction of human menopausal gonadotrophins into the armamentarium. The latter treatment uncovered the realization that the PCO is particularly sensitive to gonadotrophins, demanding meticulous monitoring to avoid the all-too-familiar complications of ovarian hyperstimulation syndrome (OHSS) and multiple pregnancies. A modern answer to these problems is the chronic low-dose regimens of gonadotrophin administration. The advent of gonadotrophin releasing hormone (GnRH) agonists has been reported to reduce the high miscarriage rates – another disheartening aspect of treatment – and these agonists are expected to be replaced by GnRH antagonists in the near future, hopefully making life easier for patient and doctor alike. The coming of in vitro fertilization (IVF) added an important alternative for those not conceiving with gonadotrophins and has also given us greater access and opportunity to learn what is going on within the follicle, the oocyte and the early embryo. The emotional distress caused by the aesthetic blemishes of acne and hirsutism resulting from hyperandrogenism is unmeasurable but considerable, especially in younger women. These problems are now largely, if laboriously, being overcome by antiandrogen treatment. Disturbing long-term sequelae are now being uncovered and PCOS seems to promote a number of risk factors for cardiovascular disease in later life. Lately, emphasis on the treatment of the metabolic aspects of the syndrome, particularly the influence of hyperinsulinaemia, obesity and their treatment on the symptomatology of the syndrome, will carry a great deal of weight. All the treatments mentioned here are symptomatic, and further understanding of the basic pathogenic mechanisms is sorely needed.

WHERE DO WE STAND TODAY?

It is a well-nigh impossible task to attempt to construct a consensus from our present knowledge of PCOS; nevertheless, in the last few years, several important concepts have emerged which have received general agreement. First, the clinical entity often associated with the presence of polycystic ovaries is now much more regularly called a syndrome rather than a disease, and this seems to be a more accurate term. Second, in determining a diagnosis of any syndrome, I would have thought that two facts would be of great help: (a) the possibility of actually being able to visualize the affected organ and to examine its morphology, and (b) the determination of even one feature that is common to all those affected. For these reasons, the concept presented by Howard Jacobs that the typical ultrasonographic appearance of the polycystic ovary is the diagnostic *sine qua non* makes good sense and is being adopted by most clinicians, albeit tempered by antagonistic arguments that endocrine features must be incorporated into any definition of PCOS. While this typical ultrasound appearance may be seen in symptomless women, it is the one common feature of a wide variety of clinical and biochemical presentations. Further to Jacobs' concept is the possibility of transition of a symptomless young woman with PCO into a patient with PCOS by extraovarian factors such as the expression of insulin resistance and hyperinsulinaemia. Now that there are more solid criteria for the ultrasound diagnosis of PCO, the adoption of this definition of PCO according to these criteria and that of PCOS with the additional symptoms of menstrual disturbance and/or signs of hyperandrogenism, would seem to be eminently sensible but, alas, is still far from being universally accepted.

Adam Balen, carrying on this line of thinking, presents his own very large series of patients with ultrasonically detected PCO and the associated clinical and endocrine features. The concept of a wide spectrum of signs and symptoms, ranging from the single finding of polycystic ovarian morphology as detected by ultrasound, to obesity, hyperandrogenism, menstrual cycle disturbances and infertility, occurring singly or in combination, nicely encapsulates clinical reality. Anywhere along this line, metabolic disturbances involving increased levels of LH, insulin and androgens and dyslipidaemia are all in evidence and fertility potential disturbed.

We have long known about the familial clustering of PCOS, suggesting a major genetic component to its aetiology. The enormous progress in ability to identify specific genes has enabled us to start investigating the identity of the putatively malfunctioning genes. Rather than 'looking for a needle in a haystack', Steven Franks logically started his search by looking at the genes involved in androgen production and the secretion and action of insulin. The results of both linkage and association studies suggest the involvement of two key genes in the aetiology of PCOS; the steroid synthesis gene *CYP11a* and the insulin gene variable number tandem repeats (VNTR). Franks suggests that other genes are probably involved in a quantitative trait contributing, in addition to environmental factors, to the clinical and biochemical heterogeneity observed. The newest candidate suggested is the follistatin gene, found to have the strongest linkage with PCOS from 37 genes examined by Urbanek et al.[8] This finding has not been confirmed in an enlarged series; nevertheless, hyperactivity of follistatin would 'fit the bill', in keeping with the concept that PCOS is a syndrome of general hyperactivity interfering with normal follicle development, linked with a possible abnormal functioning of pancreatic insulin secretion.

The increased number of small follicles and

their abnormal growth pattern are undisputed features of the polycystic ovary. The reasons for these occurrences are being examined intensively and their consequences may well hold the key to explaining downstream events in PCOS. In the same painstaking fashion in which she counts, winkles out and examines individual small follicles, Helen Mason has scientifically set out the possible reasons for the increased follicular number and attenuated apoptosis and has linked these to increased ovarian steroidogenesis. The idea that the increased follicle numbers and their abnormal development are the 'root of all evil' in PCOS, first proposed by another of this book's contributors, Joop Schoemaker, is picking up some momentum.

Amongst the heterogeneous biochemical manifestations of PCOS, ovarian hyperandrogenism is the most common feature. The source of this ovarian hyperandrogenism is central to the understanding of the pathogenesis of the syndrome and its sequelae. In a series of carefully constructed experiments, Robert Rosenfield has revealed that patients with classic PCOS have a characteristic ovarian secretory response to gonadotrophin stimulation which differs from that expected from any known enzyme block and principally includes a hyper-response of androstenedione secretion. He proposes that a dysregulation of androgen secretion accounts for this abnormality, probably due to hyperactivity of an enzyme, cytochrome P450c17. Rosenfield goes on to suggest that PCOS may arise from either LH excess or an escape from desensitization (downregulation to LH stimulation). The latter possibility may be related to an excessive production of insulin or intraovarian growth factors. A single genetic defect enhancing serine phosphorylation, which would decrease the activity of the insulin receptor and selectively increase 17,20-lyase activity, could account for both the hyperandrogenism and the insulin resistance of PCOS.

Abnormal ovarian steroidogenesis is now an established fact in PCOS. While this may involve an intrinsic defect within the ovary itself, it is most definitely also influenced by extraovarian factors, in particular, hypersecretion of LH and of insulin. Hypersecretion of LH occurs in approximately 40% of women who have polycystic ovaries. Adam Balen has examined all the proposed theories for the aetiology of this phenomenon and has come up with the hypothesis that hypersecretion of LH follows a disturbance of non-steroidal ovarian-pituitary feedback. He speculates that women with PCOS who hypersecrete LH have deficient production of an ovarian non-steroidal factor, the mysterious and elusive gonadotrophin surge attenuating factor, which normally inhibits LH secretion. While the evidence is still scanty, it is a very attractive notion. What seems more certain is that high LH concentrations not only influence ovarian androgenic production but may well also have a deleterious effect on ovulation and the rate of miscarriage by a direct effect on oocyte maturation. Balen presents convincing evidence that tonic hypersecretion of LH is detrimental to reproductive health.

In addition to hyperfunctioning of the thecal compartment, the PCO has an accumulation of multiple, small antral follicles which are neither atretic nor apoptotic but are arrested in development. The mechanism of selection of a dominant, preovulatory follicle seems to have been lost. Linda Giudice has reviewed the potential contributions of insulin-like peptides to this enigmatic but central aspect of the pathophysiology of PCOS. Although not atretic, the arrested follicles in PCOS contain similar profiles of insulin-like growth factor binding proteins (IGFBP), lack of IGFBP proteases, and levels of insulin-like growth factor II as in the atretic follicles of normo-ovulatory women. Therefore, the question that still needs answering is: what are the other factors that probably interface with the IGF system that prevent the arrested follicle from becoming atretic? In addition to the IGF system, a number of other factors may possibly be involved in this and other ovarian dysfunctions in PCOS; they include sex hormone binding globulin (SHBG), plasminogen activator inhibitor type 1 (PAI-1) and leptin. What they have in common is that they are all affected by insulin status.

Dror Meirow highlights the central role of the changes in insulin sensitivity in PCOS. Not only does insulin stimulate ovarian androgen production but it also interferes with the transport of testosterone by decreasing SHBG concentrations. Obesity adds insult to injury by exacerbating these changes and the importance of the short-term and long-term benefits of control of insulin levels by both diet and drug therapy is indisputably emphasized by Meirow. Two relative newcomers may be part of the pathophysiological chain of events involving insulin: leptin and PAI-1. Their role is yet to be clearly defined. The use of insulin sensitizers has opened up a new channel of attack. Most experience has been gained with metformin which was closely followed by the now-defunct troglitazone and the up-and-coming rosiglitazone. Although these medications seem to achieve the same clinical results as loss of weight, for those who fail to lose weight, or who have a normal body weight but are insulin resistant, they may prevent the long-term effects of PCOS and give short-term help in fertility treatment.

Hirsutism, acne and irregular menstruation are usually the first presenting symptoms at the younger end of the age scale and it is important to appreciate the social and psychological impact of these disorders. They should be treated when PCOS is diagnosed. Gordana Prelevic has reviewed possible treatment regimens. Although imperfect, and of necessity laborious, treatment with antiandrogen drugs – in particular cyproterone acetate – has proved remarkably effective in eliminating or markedly diminishing the distressing stigmata of hirsutism and acne. Most clinicians share the opinion that the early initiation of this treatment may well also conserve fertility potential and maybe even prevent the long-term sequelae of the syndrome.

Clomiphene citrate (CC) is still the first-line treatment for anovulatory women with PCOS who desire pregnancy. The safety, simplicity and relatively good success rate of this drug have maintained its place at the forefront and we tend today to take it for granted. Margo Fluker reawakens us to its value by thoroughly reviewing the pros and cons of its use, with an emphasis on non-conventional protocols to improve efficiency and results. Fluker comes to the conclusion that an individualized treatment protocol and active management of ovulation induction can help anovulatory women achieve a satisfactory ovulatory response or progress to more complex forms of therapy in a safe, economical and timely fashion.

The next step following failure to conceive with CC (failure to ovulate on 150 mg per day or failure to conceive after six ovulatory cycles) is the chronic low-dose step-up protocol using follicle-stimulating hormone (FSH). Joop Schoemaker has immaculately set forth the physiology of follicular growth and the FSH threshold concept, providing exact information on why this mode of treatment should replace the conventional mode of gonadotrophin therapy in use for so long. By quoting his own and other groups' work, he clearly illustrates that by achieving monofollicular ovulation there is an impressive decrease in multiple pregnancy rate and almost complete elimination of OHSS. Schoemaker leaves us in no doubt that the low-dose step-up protocol has the highest effective/side effect ratio for the treatment of women with PCOS who fail to conceive with CC.

Two further main options remain open for induction of ovulation in PCOS: the use of GnRH analogues, and laparoscopic ovarian puncture. Peter Hompes deals with the mounting evidence that GnRH agonists suppress the excessive tonic levels during the follicular phase with gonadotrophin stimulation, suppress the premature LH surge and may have a possible direct effect on the ovum, so producing higher pregnancy rates and smaller pregnancy wastage than gonadotrophins alone. The logical step of combining GnRH agonist treatment with chronic low-dose FSH has proved difficult to handle and fails to produce monofollicular development in anything like the proportion of cycles that would make this combination safe and reliable. Obviously some refinement of this protocol is needed to improve efficiency. Combinations of GnRH agonist with pulsatile GnRH, with oral contraceptives or for triggering ovulation are discussed by Hompes, who

wisely concludes that the available data demand more research. Following the learning curve of the application of GnRH agonists in the treatment of PCOS, Platteau, Haitsma and Devroey have reviewed the advantages that the GnRH antagonists may confer. Based on the early results of clinical trials and intelligent hypothesis, several therapeutic approaches are presented, using the antagonist for induction of ovulation, superovulation for IVF, improvement of miscarriage rate and, in addition, the treatment of hirsutism in PCOS. The GnRH antagonists seem to have a number of advantages over the current treatment with agonists, which should make future therapy simpler, shorter, safer and more efficient.

Given that most of the modes for ovulation induction referred to above produce a more than acceptable pregnancy rate, the emphasis should now be placed on the avoidance of complications, in particular, multiple pregnancies and OHSS. Howard Jacobs sets out a forceful argument in this direction, for the use of laparoscopic ovarian puncture. In contrast to medical induction of ovulation, there is no increased risk of multiple pregnancy and no need for intensive monitoring. Jacobs finds the operation to be efficient and efficacious and recommends its use particularly in the slim, anovulatory woman with PCOS and raised LH concentrations.

Using the treatment modes detailed above, a large majority of infertile patients with PCOS should conceive. For those who do not, the last-resort treatment is in vitro fertilization and embryo transfer, for which excellent results have been reported. In view of the failure of these women to conceive by other means, it is interesting to speculate to what this success may be attributed: to an obscure mechanical defect or, more probably, to the fact that the ovaries have been stimulated in a more cavalier fashion than would be acceptable for ovulation induction. The team from Valencia describe their own and others' experiences and review the pros, cons and therapeutic pitfalls of the procedure.

The long-term sequelae of PCOS are a matter of importance, considering the wide prevalence of polycystic ovaries. Mary Birdsall deals valiantly with the limited data so far available, points the way ahead in the possible establishment of an association with cardiac risk factors, and offers sound advice on their avoidance. Ghanim Almahbobi and Alan Trounson were given the task of looking into the future of research into the aetiology of PCOS. Their guiding principle is the search for the reasons behind the hyperactivity of cell function and the interruption of normal regulatory mechanisms obviously involved in PCO. They describe their experiments in which they found that the granulosa cells hyperexpress functional FSH receptors and possess a strong aromatase enzyme which is inhibited, possibly by epidermal growth factor (EGF) and transforming growth factor alpha (TGFα), to which granulosa cells also expressed hypersensitivity. Whereas these aberrations could account for the excessive response to exogenous FSH stimulation and the production of high amounts of oestradiol both in vivo and in vitro, the hyperactivity of P450c17α enzymes in the thecal cells accounts for increased androgen production. The causes of this cell hyperactivity in the PCO – genetic, metabolic or endocrine – present the challenge for the next round of research.

SUGGESTIONS FOR A CONSENSUS

I have attempted to construct a brief statement regarding the aetiology and treatment of PCOS. As with most suggestions for a consensus, it will most probably serve as a basis for change, argument and correction, and is presented with this intention in mind.

Pathophysiology

The morphology of the polycystic ovary differs from that of the normal ovary in that it is larger, contains twice as many developing follicles, and has an increased stromal volume. The large number of follicles up to 10 mm in diameter that have been arrested in their development may be due to a number of factors: hyperfunc-

tion of EGF/TGFα, follistatin and inhibin B, all of which would interfere with the action of FSH; an increased number of LH receptors appearing earlier than usual and increasing the sensitivity to LH; excess insulin, excess androgens and maybe a deficiency of growth differentiating factor 9 (Figure 1.1). Contrary to expectations, a large proportion of these follicles do not become atretic and seem to exist in a viable state of attenuated atresia. This state hints at a disturbance of one or more of the genes affecting apoptosis or, more likely, some factor that influences the expression of these genes (Figure 1.1).

Increased numbers of FSH receptors on these follicles may account for the hypersensitivity to exogenous FSH despite the fact that endogenous FSH action is suppressed, possibly by excessive expression of EGF/TGFα and/or follistatin. A simpler explanation for the usual excessive response to gonadotrophin stimulation would be the much larger numbers of viable follicles 'lying in wait' for some FSH than are found in the normal ovary.

The abnormal ovarian steroidogenesis results in excessive production of androgens by PCO thecal cells which may originate from several possible sources, either alone or in combination: an intrinsic hyperfunction of *CYP11a* encoding for cholesterol side-chain cleavage, increased stimulation of enzyme P450c17α by LH mediated by insulin and IGF-I. Possible factors that may cause this accumulation of androgens in the polycystic ovary are presented in Figure 1.2.

A postreceptor genetic defect, unique to PCO, causing an abnormality of serine phosphorylation of the insulin receptor may be the source of insulin hypersecretion and resistance. Whatever the detailed cause, the resulting hyperinsulinaemia is responsible for increased androgen production, reduced transport of testosterone, menstrual irregularity, anovulation and, in the long run, factors for increased cardiovascular risk. All these effects are exacerbated by obesity.

Thus, PCOS may be conceived as a syndrome of ovarian hyperfunction, driven by genetic defects causing intrinsic ovarian dysfunction whose degree of symptomatology is

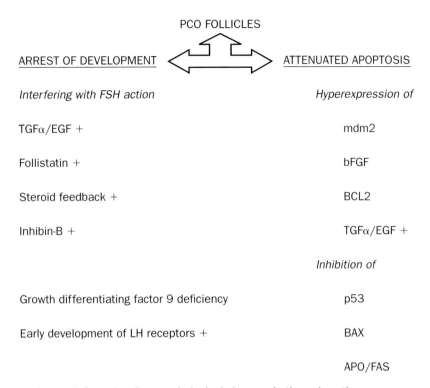

Figure 1.1 Possible factors influencing the morphological changes in the polycystic ovary.

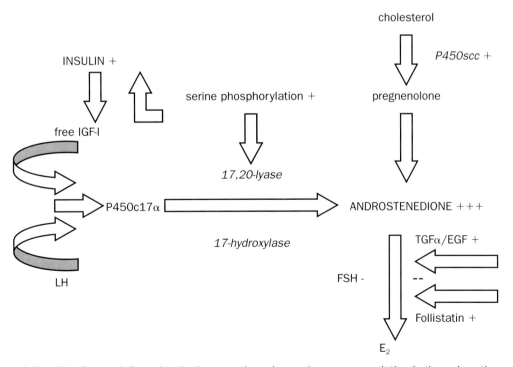

Figure 1.2 Possible factors influencing the increased ovarian androgen accumulation in the polycystic ovary.

largely influenced by extraovarian factors. The probably small number of causative genes involved have yet to be delineated and so the treatment of the syndrome remains symptomatic.

Treatment

Treatment depends on the symptoms expressed and whether the therapy is for aesthetic reasons in patients not desiring pregnancy, for infertility, or even for the prevention of late-onset risk factors for cardiovascular disease. Broadly, treatment is based on reduction of insulin levels, lowering of LH and androgen concentrations, and/or administration of FSH. In addition, antiandrogens (notably cyproterone acetate) are in wide use for the treatment of hirsutism and acne. Whatever the purpose of the treatment, loss of weight by the patient and the consequent decrease in insulin, androgen and LH concentrations are of prime importance. Drugs increasing insulin sensitivity, it seems, have identical effects and may also prove to be of value but it is too early to make a convincing statement to this effect.

For anovulation, clomiphene citrate followed by chronic low-dose administration of FSH if the former is unsuccessful, are at the forefront (Figure 1.3). More controversial is the use of GnRH agonists in ovulation induction protocols, which is probably best reserved for patients with particularly high tonic LH levels in whom it may confer the advantage of increased pregnancy and decreased miscarriage rates. The antagonists of GnRH can be expected to replace the agonists in the near future. Laparoscopic ovarian puncture is now emerging as a valuable addition to the armamentarium, especially in the normal-weight patient with high LH concentrations. In vitro fertilization has proved a successful last-resort therapy.

In summary, the contents of this book will pose as many questions as answers, and will hopefully serve as a stimulant for further research until this most intriguing of syndromes is shorn of its mystery.

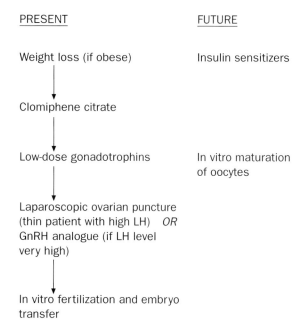

Figure 1.3 Suggested treatment plan for the infertile patient with polycystic ovary syndrome.

REFERENCES

1 Chereau A. *Mémoires Pour Servir a l'Étude des Maladies des Ovaries* (Fortin, Masson: Paris, 1844).
2 Stein IF, Leventhal ML. Amenorrhea associated with bilateral polycystic ovaries. *Am J Obstet Gynecol* (1935) **29**: 181–91.
3 Rebar R, Judd HL, Yen SCC, Vandenberg G, Naftolin F. Characterization of the inappropriate gonadotropin secretion in polycystic ovary syndrome. *J Clin Invest* (1976) **57**: 1320–9.
4 Khan CR, Flier JS, Bar RS, Archal JA, Gorden P. The syndromes of insulin resistance and acanthosis nigricans. *N Engl J Med* (1976) **294**: 739–45.
5 Burghen GA, Givens JR, Kitabchi AE. Correlation of hyperandrogenism with hyperinsulinism in polycystic ovarian disease. *J Clin Endocrinol Metab* (1980) **50**: 113–16.
6 Swanson M, Sauerbrie EE, Cooperberg PL. Medical implications of ultrasonically detected polycystic ovaries. *J Clin Ultrasound* (1981) **9**: 219–22.

7   Adams J, Franks S, Polson DW, Mason HD, Abdulwahid N, Jacobs HS. Multifollicular ovaries: clinical and endocrine features and response to pulsatile gonadotrophin releasing hormone. *Lancet* (1985) **ii**: 1375–8.

8   Urbanek M, Legro RS, Driscoll DA et al. Thirty-seven candidate genes for polycystic ovary syndrome: strongest evidence for a linkage is with follistatin. *Proc Natl Acad Sci USA* (1999) **96**: 8573–8.

2

Definition and diagnosis

Howard S Jacobs

Polycystic ovary syndrome, also known as Stein–Leventhal syndrome, is normally diagnosed in European countries on the basis of ovarian morphology, gleaned from ultrasound examination. Workers espousing this point of view therefore regard the appearance of the polycystic ovary on ultrasound scan as central to diagnosis and classification. In contrast, in the USA greater reliance is placed on biochemical features. In endocrine terms the most widely accepted characterization is that the patient with polycystic ovary syndrome has evidence of excessive secretion of androgen from the (polycystic) ovary.

I shall be proposing here that central to our understanding is a distinction between polycystic ovaries (PCO) and polycystic ovary *syndrome* (PCOS). Polycystic ovaries as the essential phenotype can be detected in all patients with PCOS, in many normal women, in many children and in a proportion of patients with hypogonadotrophic hypogonadism (see below). Frequently PCO is detected in members of the same family. Although it is common experience to detect the ovarian phenotype in, say, each of three sisters, usually only one of them will have symptoms. It is the development of PCOS that

is the focus of much contemporary research. In fact, it seems that one of the major factors resulting in the transition of a symptomless young woman with PCO into a patient with PCOS is the development of insulin resistance (see Chapter 9). It is essential to distinguish between the morphological appearance of PCO and its clinical expression.

Because of the widely accepted (although, it must be remarked, rarely defined) heterogeneity of the Stein–Leventhal polycystic ovary syndrome, there have been several attempts to provide a classification of the condition. In my experience, while a classification based on clinical and to some extent endocrine factors is possible, one based on ultrasound appearance is not – at any rate, not yet. The implication of this view is that the heterogeneity that must underlie any classification lies in the clinical and endocrine phenotype and the ovarian disturbance is the one common theme in all the different manifestations of the polycystic ovary syndrome.

MULTICYSTIC OR MULTIFOLLICULAR OVARIES?

Before describing our studies of women with polycystic ovaries, it is important to distinguish polycystic ovaries, by which I mean the kind of ovary found in women suffering from the Stein–Leventhal syndrome, from those we earlier labelled 'multicystic' ovaries.[1] By multicystic ovaries we referred to the ovarian ultrasound appearance of the normal pubertal girl, as described histologically in the classic studies of Hanna Peters in Denmark.[2] The striking ultrasound features are the follicles of various size scattered throughout an ovary which has no excess of medullary stroma (Figure 2.1).

This appearance is a feature of normal mid-puberty, and the studies of Richard Stanhope and Judy Adams suggested that it results from incomplete pulsatile gonadotrophic stimulation of the ovaries.[3] Thus when treating hypo-gonadotrophic children by application of pulsatile gonadotrophin releasing hormone (GnRH), these workers found that the normally immediately premenarchal ovarian appearance of multicystic ovaries could be reproduced by restricting application of the pulsatile GnRH to less than 24 hours per day. When the pulsatile infusion was maintained for the full 24 hours a single dominant follicle developed and there was then suppression of the cohort follicles. The results were most simply interpreted to indicate that the ovaries in these girls with delayed

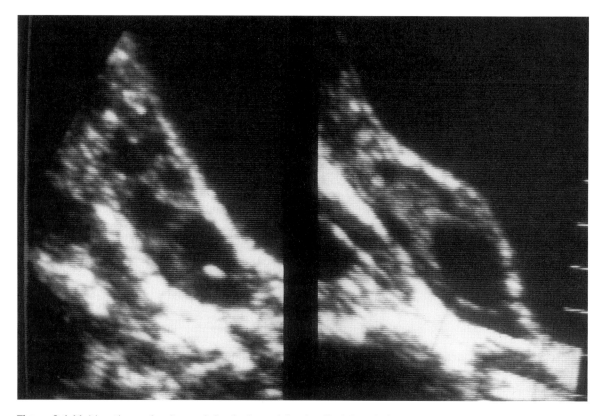

Figure 2.1 Multicystic ovaries (transabdominal scan) for detailed description, see text.

puberty were essentially normal and the genesis of the problem lay in incomplete pituitary control of ovarian follicular development. When normal pulsatile gonadotrophin stimulation of the ovary was attained physiologically or through treatment (i.e. gonadotrophin stimulation that was normal in amplitude, frequency and duration), the normal intraovarian regulation that underlies establishment of a single dominant follicle was established. The ovarian appearance then returned to normal.

The pathological version of this course of events occurs in two clinical situations. The first is during treatment of women with hypogonadotrophic hypogonadism in whom the amplitude or duration of the pulsatile stimulus, i.e. the dose of GnRH, is suboptimal. Occasionally this occurs with standard doses given subcutaneously, presumably because in these women absorption of GnRH is impaired. The ovarian appearance rapidly resolves when the same dose is given intravenously, or when the dose of subcutaneous GnRH is increased.

The second is in women recovering from a phase of suppression of endogenous GnRH activity – most commonly in our experience in women with partially recovered weight-loss-related amenorrhoea. The importance of the condition is that the ovaries are polyfollicular and have lost the external (i.e. pituitary) control which leads to unifollicular ovulation. This means that if they are exposed to ovarian stimulation there is a strong possibility, in the first cycle of treatment anyway, that they will have a multiple ovulation. At this stage therefore they are at risk of multiple conception.

POLYCYSTIC OVARIES

A useful distinction may be made between the presence of ultrasonographically detected polycystic ovaries and polycystic ovary syndrome.[4] The former situation occurs when characteristic ultrasound features are detected in a woman with a regular menstrual cycle in whom there are no symptoms or signs of hyperandrogenism. The latter exists when the ovarian ultrasound appearance is detected in a woman complaining of a menstrual irregularity (usually but not exclusively oligomenorrhoea), symptoms arising from hyperandrogenism and obesity. It is the former situation, the presence of polycystic ovaries, that is so common (20% or thereabouts in several series now). When this ovarian appearance occurs in a woman with hypogonadotrophic amenorrhoea[5] or in a woman undergoing assisted conception therapy,[6] the response to ovarian stimulation is excessive and similar to the response characteristically seen in polycystic ovary syndrome. The exaggerated response that these patients make to gonadotrophin stimulation must be caused by a primary ovarian abnormality rather than one conditioned by endogenous hormone levels.

High-definition computerized transvaginal ultrasound has been used to investigate polycystic ovaries. With the Kretz Combiscanner ultrasound data accumulate over an 8-second period from an immobilized intravaginal probe. The data are transferred to a computer and can then be analysed at leisure. For example, measurements can be made from an image that has been reconstructed in any plane, or a three-dimensional image can be created. Figure 2.2 shows the highly echodense central stroma with the cysts clearly arrayed in a 'necklace' around the cortex of the ovary. Reconstruction in different planes, however, shows that the cysts are also distributed throughout the ovary.

Using this type of ultrasound equipment, Dr Amma Kyei-Mensah studied 100 women undergoing infertility treatment by in vitro fertilization and embryo transfer.[7] The ovaries were classified as normal in 50 women; they were polycystic in the other 50 women, of whom 26 were regarded as suffering from the polycystic ovary syndrome, while 24 women had polycystic ovaries but no evidence of the syndrome. While Dr Kyei-Mensah found that the dimensions of the polycystic ovaries in the two latter groups were similar, they were some two and a half times larger than the 'normal' ovaries. The difference in ovarian size was entirely accounted for by differences in stromal volume, there being no differences in cyst

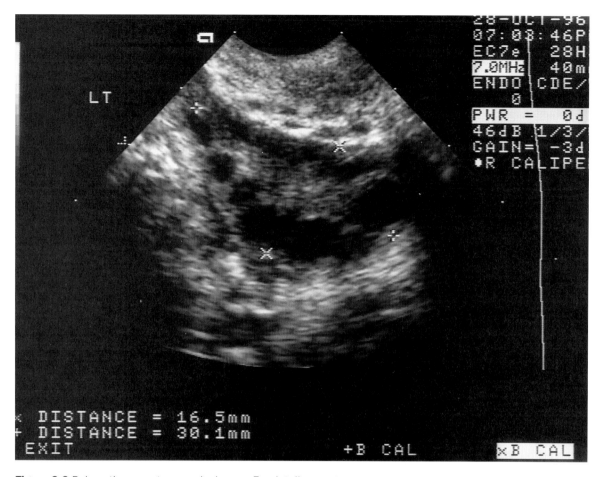

Figure 2.2 Polycystic ovary, transvaginal scan. For details, see text.

volume between normal and polycystic ovaries. On the other hand, the hormone concentrations in the women with normal ovaries were strikingly different from those with polycystic ovary syndrome, but indistinguishable from those with polycystic ovaries but normal menstrual cycles and no clinical signs of hyperandrogenism. Clearly, the ovarian ultrasound appearance cannot be used to predict which women will show clinical expression of the syndrome.

When a similar data set was analysed using colour Doppler ultrasonography, Jamal Zaidi and colleagues[8] found that polycystic ovaries were associated with a large and statistically significant increase in ovarian stromal blood flow (but no change in resistance to flow, as assessed by measurement of the pulsatility index). In this case too there was no difference between the findings in women with polycystic ovaries and those with the fully expressed syndrome. These results, which suggest considerable neovascularization of the ovarian stroma in women with polycystic ovaries, provide us with a background for understanding the exaggerated response to gonadotrophin stimulation, which occurs in women with polycystic ovaries as well as those with polycystic ovary syndrome.[5]

Dr Rina Agrawal and colleagues have found that women with PCO and PCOS have basal serum concentrations of vascular endothelial growth factor (VEGF) that are higher than those in women with ultrasonically normal ovaries.[9] The levels of VEGF remained higher even after downregulation by treatment with a super-active analogue of GnRH,[10] suggesting the difference is constitutive rather than regulated by luteinizing hormone (LH). We therefore incline to the view that defective regulation of VEGF gene expression may be one of the primary abnormalities of the polycystic ovary. Perhaps high intraovarian VEGF concentrations disturb the regulation of intraovarian blood flow and so underlie the failure of the autoregulatory process which is thought to cause selection of a dominant follicle (thereby ensuring unifollicular ovulation). Normal diversion of blood towards the dominant follicle may be prevented by the excessive VEGF-mediated intraovarian neovascularization, resulting in persistence of multiple follicles, so characteristic a feature of the polycystic ovary.

Returning to clinical matters, the polycystic ovary is one that on ultrasound scanning is usually expanded by a highly vascular and echodense stroma around which numerous cysts are scattered. The exact number that can be detected depends – not surprisingly – on the resolution of the equipment, itself to some extent dependent on the position of the probe. Resolution is more precise when the probe is placed close to the ovary, as with transvaginal rather than transabdominal scanning through a full bladder. Most authorities seem to accept the diagnostic criterion of Adams et al[1] of 10 cysts or more in the former case and 15 or more in the latter. However, it is the increase in stroma that is important rather than the exact number of cysts that can be resolved. This approach is supported by the finding that, in women with polycystic ovary syndrome, serum androgen concentrations correlate with stromal rather than cyst volume.[7]

CLASSIFICATION OF POLYCYSTIC OVARIES

So far as I can see there is as yet no suggestion in the literature of important – by which I mean predictive – variations in ovarian morphology in the ultrasound images obtained in women with polycystic ovary syndrome. Variations have been described, by Takahashi et al[11] amongst others, according to the exact distribution (one or two layers) of cysts, but I suspect that differences are outweighed by similarities between the so-called subgroups. If this conclusion is accepted, the first implication is that you cannot have the polycystic ovary syndrome without polycystic ovaries, so terms such as 'polycystic-appearing ovaries' are best abandoned.

The second implication is that the varying clinical phenotype is the basis for classification. For example, it is well known that many women with polycystic ovary syndrome are hyperinsulinaemic. A striking relationship exists between insulin secretion, menstrual disturbances and androgen levels.[12] I propose that one subgroup of women with polycystic ovary syndrome is composed of women with hyperinsulinaemia. These women would be predicted to have oligomenorrhoea and so, to the extent that their rate of ovulation is decreased, they would be expected to complain of infertility. Since obesity is such a profound regulator of insulin secretion I would expect the more severe cases to be obese. A combination of obesity-mediated and PCOS-mediated hyperinsulinism is likely to make them severely hyperandrogenized, and so I would predict a high prevalence of hirsutism, acne and seborrhoea in this subgroup. These are the patients who are likely to feature in reports of the association of coronary risk factors with polycystic ovary syndrome.

A second subgroup of women with polycystic ovary syndrome that I would like to propose comprises those with hypersecretion of LH. There appears to be little correlation of serum insulin levels with LH concentrations and indeed the physical characteristics of women with hypersecretion of LH seem to be different from the group described above – i.e. they tend to be slim women with regular menstrual cycles. There is a striking association of hypersecretion of LH with both infertility and the rate of miscarriage, even in a study in which one of the entry criteria was a regular menstrual cycle with a variation of less than 2 weeks.[13]

There must be other subgroups because this initial classification accounts for fewer than 85% of the patients with polycystic ovary syndrome seen in the author's department.[14] Even though it is incomplete, however, it provides a way of producing subsets of patients with homogeneous characteristics. The advantage of this process of 'splitting' is both clinical (for example it is immediately obvious that patients in the first group would be unlikely to benefit from the types of treatment considered appropriate for those in the second group) and investigative. Thus studies exploring hypersecretion of insulin and those exploring hypersecretion of LH need to be concentrated in groups 1 and 2 respectively. It seems to me on *a priori* grounds alone that the rate at which the LH pulse generator fires will in large part be genetically determined, but that the forces determining insulin secretion will have other genetic influences. This therefore is an argument for analysing the genetics of the polycystic ovary syndrome on a phenotypic basis, accepting the importance of clinical and endocrine phenotypic heterogeneity and not attempting a single overarching classification that has, in my opinion, been more Procrustean than profitable.

To summarize, I propose that the ultrasonographic appearance of polycystic ovaries is regarded as the diagnostic *sine qua non* of the polycystic ovary syndrome and that the syndrome's heterogeneity is embraced for its clinical and investigative value. I anticipate that genetic studies of the various subgroups will reveal various patterns of inheritance of genes involved in different aspects of the condition.

REFERENCES

1 Adams J, Franks S, Polson DW et al. Multifollicular ovaries: clinical and endocrine features and response to pulsatile gonadotropin releasing hormone. *Lancet* (1985) **ii**: 1375–9.

2 Peters H, Byskov AG, Grinsted J. The development of the ovary during childhood in health and disease. In: Coutts JRT, ed., *Functional Morphology of the Human Ovary* (MTP Press: Lancaster, 1981) 26–34.

3 Stanhope R, Adams J, Jacobs HS, Brook CGD. Ovarian ultrasound assessment in normal children, idiopathic precocious puberty and during low dose pulsatile gonadotrophin releasing hormone treatment of hypogonadotrophic hypogonadism. *Arch Dis Child* (1985) **60**: 116–19.

4 Jacobs HS. Polycystic ovaries and polycystic ovary syndrome. *Gynecol Endocrinol* (1987) **1**: 113–31.

5 Shoham Z, Conway GS, Patel A, Jacobs HS. Polycystic ovaries in patients with hypogonadotropic hypogonadism: similarity of ovarian response to gonadotropin stimulation in patients with polycystic ovarian syndrome. *Fertil Steril* (1992) **58**: 37–47.

6 MacDougal MJ, Tan SL, Balen AH, Jacobs HS. A controlled study comparing patients with and without polycystic ovaries undergoing in vitro fertilisation. *Hum Reprod* (1993) **8**: 233–7.

7 Kyei-Mensah AA, LinTan S, Zaidi J, Jacobs HS. Relationship of ovarian stromal volume to serum androgen concentrations in patients with polycystic ovary syndrome. *Hum Reprod* (1998) **13**: 1437–41.

8 Zaidi J, Campbell S, Pittrof R, Kyei-Mensah A, Jacobs HS, Tan SL. Ovarian stromal blood flow changes in women with polycystic ovaries. A possible new marker for ultrasound diagnosis? *Hum Reprod* (1995) **10**: 1992–6.

9 Agrawal R, Sladkevicius P, Engmann L et al. Serum vascular endothelial growth factor concentrations and ovarian stromal blood flow are increased in women with polycystic ovaries. *Hum Reprod* (1998) **13**: 651–5.

10 Agrawal R, Conway G, Sladkevicius P et al. Serum vascular endothelial growth factor and Doppler blood flow velocities in in vitro fertilization: relevance to ovarian hyperstimulation syndrome and polycystic ovaries. *Fertil Steril* (1998) **70**: 651–8.

11 Takahashi K, Ozaki T, Okada M, Uchida A, Kitao M. Relationship between ultrasonography

and histopathological changes in polycystic ovarian syndrome. *Hum Reprod* (1994) **9**: 2255–8.

12 Conway GS, Jacobs HS. Clinical implications of hyperinsulinaemia in women. *Clin Endocrinol* (1993) **39**: 623–32.

13 Regan L, Owen EJ, Jacobs HS. Hypersecretion of LH, infertility and spontaneous abortion. *Lancet* (1990) **336**: 1141–2.

14 Balen AH, Conway GS, Kaltsas G et al. Polycystic ovary syndrome: the spectrum of the disorder in 1741 patients. *Hum Reprod* (1995) **10**: 2107–11.

3

Clinical expression

Adam Balen

The polycystic ovary syndrome (PCOS) is one of the most common endocrine disorders, although its aetiology remains unknown.[1] This heterogeneous disorder may present, at one end of the spectrum, with the single finding of polycystic ovarian morphology as detected by pelvic ultrasonography. At the other end of the spectrum symptoms such as obesity, hyperandrogenism, menstrual cycle disturbance and infertility may occur either singly or in combination (Table 3.1). Metabolic disturbances such as elevated serum concentrations of luteinizing

Table 3.1 The spectrum of clinical manifestations of heterogeneous polycystic ovary syndrome

Symptoms (% patients affected)	Associated endocrine manifestations	Possible late sequelae
Obesity (38%)	↑Androgens (testosterone and androstenedione)	Diabetes mellitus (11%)
Menstrual disturbance (66%)		Cardiovascular disease
Hyperandrogenism (48%)	↑Luteinizing hormone	Hyperinsulinaemia
Infertility (73% of anovulatory infertility)	↑LH : FSH ratio	High LDL
	↑Free oestradiol	Endometrial carcinoma
Asymptomatic (20%)	↑Fasting insulin	Hypertension
	↑Prolactin	
	↓Sex hormone binding globulin	

FSH, follicle-stimulating hormone; LDL, low-density lipoprotein; LH, luteinizing hormone.

hormone (LH), testosterone, insulin and pro-lactin are common and may have profound implications on the long-term health of women with PCOS. The syndrome is a familial condition and a number of candidate genes have been implicated (see Chapter 4). The syndrome appears to have its origins during adolescence and is thought to be associated with increased weight gain during puberty.[2] However, the polycystic ovary gene or genes have not yet been identified and the effect of environmental influences such as weight changes and circulating hormone concentrations, and the age at which these occur, is unknown.

One of the problems with comparing studies of PCOS is the lack of consensus over definition. The European view generally is that the syndrome encompasses any of the above-mentioned signs, symptoms or endocrine abnormalities (elevated serum androgen and/or LH concentrations).[3,4] In North America, the consensus is that the syndrome is denoted by the combination of hyperandrogenism and ovulatory dysfunction, in the absence of non-classical adrenal hyperplasia, without necessarily having to identify the presence of polycystic ovaries by ultrasound scan.[5] The European definition, which we have designated PCO1, is broader than that of the USA (designated PCO2). There is considerable heterogeneity of symptoms and signs amongst women with PCOS[2] and for an individual these may change over time. The syndrome is familial[6] and various aspects may be differentially inherited. Polycystic ovaries can exist without clinical signs of the *syndrome*, which may then become expressed over time.

There are a number of interlinking factors that affect expression of PCOS. A gain in weight is associated with a worsening of symptoms, while weight loss will ameliorate the endocrine and metabolic profile and symptomatology.[7] Women with PCOS are more prone to eating disorders and herein may lie a link with leptin, which is now known to affect hypothalamic pulsatility of gonadotrophin releasing hormone with important effects on reproduction.[8] Feedback from the polycystic ovary to both the pituitary and the hypothalamus appears to be disturbed owing to abnormalities in the secretion of ovarian steroid hormones and – probably more important – of non-steroidal hormones, for example inhibin and related proteins.[9,10]

CLINICAL EXPRESSION OF PCOS DURING PUBERTY AND ADOLESCENCE

High-resolution ultrasound scanning has made an accurate estimate of the prevalence of polycystic ovaries possible. Several studies have estimated this prevalence in 'normal adult' women and have found rates of approximately 20%,[11–14] but it is not known at what age this condition first appears. If the genetic 'programming' for the PCOS is present from birth, when can polycystic ovaries first be detected? The ultrasound visualization of polycystic ovaries in girls depends upon a number of factors, not least of which being the detection of the ovary by transabdominal scanning and the resolution of the image. In a study by Fox et al transabdominal scanning failed to detect 30% of polycystic ovaries, compared with a 100% detection rate by transvaginal scan.[15] Bridges et al performed 428 ovarian scans in girls aged between 3 years and 18 years and found polycystic ovaries in 101 girls (24% of the total).[16] The rate of detection of polycystic ovaries was 6% in 6-year-old girls, rising to 18% in those aged 10 years and 26% in those aged 15 years. The implication of this study is that polycystic ovaries are present before puberty and are more easy to detect in older girls as the ovaries increase in size.

Prior to puberty, there appear to be two periods of increased ovarian growth. The first is at adrenarche in response to increased concentrations of circulating androgens, and the second occurs just before and during puberty due to rising gonadotrophin levels and the actions of growth hormone and insulin-like growth factor I (IGF-I) and insulin on the ovary.

Sampaolo et al reported a study of 49 obese girls at different stages of puberty comparing their pelvic ultrasound features and endocrine profiles with 35 control participants matched for age and pubertal stage.[17] Obesity was found to be associated with a significant increase in uterine and ovarian volume, and obese postmenarchal girls with polycystic ovaries had larger uterine and ovarian volumes than obese postmenarchal girls with normal ovaries. Sampaolo concluded that obesity leads to hyperinsulinism, which causes both hyperandrogenaemia and raised IGF-I levels, which augments the ovarian response to gonadotrophins. This implies that obesity may be important in the pathogenesis of polycystic ovaries, but further study is required to evaluate this. It is known that obesity is not a prerequisite for the polycystic ovary syndrome. Indeed, in a series of 1741 women with polycystic ovaries in a study by Balen et al, only 38.4% of patients were overweight (body mass index greater than $25 \, kg/m^2$).[18] Larger studies with both cross-sectional and longitudinal components are needed to answer the important questions about the evolution of the endocrine and metabolic disturbances of the PCOS and how they relate to changing ovarian morphology during the peripubertal years.

Weight changes during puberty may be associated with an increased risk of PCOS, which can then have a profound effect on the individual's long-term health – even beyond her reproductive years. In a study of 224 normal female volunteers aged 18–25 years polycystic ovaries were identified using ultrasound in 33% of participants.[19] Fifty per cent of the participants were using some form of hormonal contraception, but the prevalence rates of polycystic ovaries in users and non-users of hormonal contraception were identical. Polycystic ovaries in the non-users of hormonal contraception were associated with irregular menstrual cycles and significantly higher serum testosterone concentrations when compared with women with normal ovaries, but only a small proportion of women with polycystic ovaries (15%) had 'elevated' serum testosterone concentrations outside the normal range. Interestingly, there were no significant differences in acne, hirsutism, body mass index (BMI) or body fat percentage between women with polycystic and normal ovaries, and hyperinsulinism and reduced insulin sensitivity were not associated with polycystic ovaries in this group. Also, no significant differences were identified for B cell function between the groups, unlike other studies which have shown pancreatic β cell dysfunction in women with PCOS when compared with controls.[20]

In this study the prevalence of PCOS was as low as 8% using the American definition for PCOS, or as high as 26% if the broader European criteria were applied. However, features included in the European criteria (menstrual irregularity, acne, hirsutism, BMI > $25 \, kg/m^2$, raised serum testosterone, raised LH) were found to occur frequently in women without polycystic ovaries, and 75% of women with normal ovaries had one or more of these attributes.[19] Subgroup analyses of women according to the presence of normal ovaries, polycystic ovaries alone, or polycystic ovaries and features of PCOS, revealed greater mean BMI in women with PCOS, but also indicated *lower* fasting insulin concentrations and *greater* insulin sensitivity in polycystic ovary and PCOS groups when compared with women with normal ovaries, which is in contrast to studies of older women.[21,22] These interesting findings were difficult to interpret in the light of current understanding of PCOS, but forced us to consider the possibility that this young, mainly non-overweight population might represent women early in the natural history of the development of PCOS, and that abnormalities of insulin metabolism might evolve following weight gain in later life.

In the same study genotype frequencies were determined for the insulin gene minisatellite (INS VNTR) which has been linked to anovulatory PCOS.[19] Genotype frequency distributions were found to be similar in women with polycystic ovaries and those with normal ovaries. However, subdivision of the group with polycystic ovaries according to the 'severity' of PCOS (polycystic ovaries alone; polycystic ovaries and PCOS by European criteria; polycystic ovaries and PCOS by American criteria) revealed increasing frequency of the III/III genotype with increasing severity of the PCOS phenotype. This could suggest that the INS

VNTR locus may determine clinical severity of PCOS in women with polycystic ovaries, although larger studies would be necessary to determine this conclusively.

Many women with polycystic ovaries detected by ultrasound do not have overt symptoms of PCOS, although symptoms may develop later, after a gain in weight for example. Ovarian morphology using the criteria described by Adams et al (10 or more cysts, 2–8 mm in diameter, arranged around an echodense stroma) appears to be the most sensitive diagnostic marker for polycystic ovaries.[23] The classical features of oligo/amenorrhoea, obesity and/or clinical symptoms of hyperandrogenism in addition to the ultrasound features of the polycystic ovary are diagnostic of the polycystic ovary syndrome. Polycystic ovaries may be associated with several endocrinopathies. Studies comparing women with polycystic ovaries with normal controls have shown elevations of concentration of LH, LH : FSH ratio, and fasting insulin testosterone and androstenedione levels, and a reduction in concentration of sex hormone binding globulin (SHBG). However, the classical hormone changes are not seen in all patients. Indeed, Fox et al found that isolated measurements of serum concentrations of androgens, oestradiol, gonadotrophins and LH : FSH ratio confirmed the finding in only 75% of women with ultrasonographically identified polycystic ovaries and oligo/amenorrhoea.[15] Single hormone measurements may be unreliable because serum hormone concentrations vary with time. For example, sampling LH every 20 minutes over a 6-hour period gives a variability of 38% in the follicular phase and 92% in the luteal phase of normal women.

HETEROGENEITY OF PCOS

An initial report on 556 patients who attended the endocrine clinic at the Middlesex Hospital, London, described the heterogeneity of PCOS and clarified the significance of three endocrine patterns (raised concentrations of LH, testosterone and prolactin) and identified five clinical subgroups (hirsutism, infertility, obesity, alopecia and acanthosis nigricans).[24] The study was extended to describe what was believed to be the largest series of patients with ultrasound-detected polycystic ovaries in order to provide a reference for the spectrum of this disorder and to highlight the features of ultrasound morphology with endocrine parameters.[18] The findings of this large series of more than 1800 women with polycystic ovaries detected by ultrasound scan are summarized in Table 3.2.

The initial baseline ultrasound scan was performed transabdominally. Ovarian morphology and volume were recorded, together with uterine cross-sectional area (UXA) and endometrial thickness. The criterion of 10 or more cysts, 2–8 mm in diameter, arranged around an echodense central stroma, as described by Adams et al,[23] was used to diagnose the presence of polycystic ovaries. Although transvaginal ultrasonography is now the preferred technique in the gynaecology and infertility clinic, it is less appropriate as an initial investigation in patients attending an endocrine clinic with symptoms that are often unrelated – at least in the patient's mind – to the pelvic organs.

A full clinical history was taken and the patients were examined. The clinical data included age, body mass index (weight in kilograms divided by height in metres squared) and the presence of acne and hirsutism, which was defined using the Ferriman and Gallway score.[25] Acanthosis nigricans was diagnosed by clinical appearance. The menstrual cycle was described as being either regular, oligomenorrhoeic (a cycle interval of longer than 35 days but less than 6 months) or amenorrhoeic (no menstruation for more than 6 months). The fertility status was classified as 'proven fertile' (those with a previous pregnancy and no subsequent infertility), 'fertility untested' (those who had never tried to conceive) or 'primary/ secondary infertility' of at least 1 year's duration.

Serum was collected for measurement of LH, follicle-stimulating hormone (FSH), testosterone, prolactin and thyroid function. Sex hormone binding globulin was not measured routinely

Table 3.2 Characteristics of 1741 women with ultrasonographically detected polycystic ovaries

Characteristic	Mean	5–95 percentiles
Age (years)	31.5	14–50
Ovarian volume (cm^3)	11.7	4.6–22.3
UXA (cm^2)	27.5	15.2–46.3
Endometrial thickness (mm)	7.5	4.0–13.0
BMI (kg/m^2) [19–25]*	25.4	19.0–38.6
FSH (IU/l) [1–10]*	4.5	1.4–7.5
LH (IU/l) [1–10]*	10.9	2.0–27.0
Testosterone (nmol/l) [0.5–2.5]*	2.6	1.1–4.8
Prolactin [<350 mu/l]*	342	87–917

* Normal range values are shown in brackets.
BMI, body mass index; FSH, follicle-stimulating hormone; LH, luteinizing hormone; UXA, uterine cross-sectional area.

owing to financial constraints on the laboratory. Details of the radioimmunoassays were described by Conway et al.[11] In particular, the Chelsea radioimmunoassay kit (London, UK) for measurement of LH (which employs polyclonal antiserum F87 and NIBSC 68/40 International Reference Preparation) was used and a value of 10 IU/l was 2 standard deviations above the mean for normal women in the follicular phase. The hormone measurements were usually performed in the follicular phase of the menstrual cycle and were excluded from the analysis if FSH concentration was elevated (>10 IU/l), which suggested the presence of either a midcycle surge or a perimenopausal state.

The variables BMI, serum LH and prolactin concentrations and ovarian volume were log-transformed before parametric analysis and geometric means were presented for these variables. Group means were compared by analysis of variance with Duncan's procedure for multiple comparisons. Grouped variables (BMI and LH) and discrete data were tested with χ^2 and associations between continuous variables were sought with Pearson's correlation coefficients.

Multiple regression analysis was performed using the stepwise method with a probability threshold for inclusion of $P < 0.05$.

A total of 1871 women who attended the clinic were identified as having polycystic ovaries. Of these, 130 (6.9%) were excluded from the analysis because they were additionally found to be menopausal (13) or also had weight-related amenorrhoea (46), pituitary disease (27), a prolactinoma (25) or congenital adrenal hyperplasia (19). There were no patients with abnormal thyroid function tests or androgen-secreting tumours. The characteristics of the remaining 1741 patients are recorded in Table 3.2 and in Figures 3.1 and 3.2.

In this group 38.4% of patients were overweight (BMI > 25 kg/m^2), 39.8% had an elevated serum concentration of LH (>10 IU/l) and 28.9% had an elevated serum testosterone concentration (>2.5 nmol/l). With respect to menstrual history, 47.0% had oligomenorrhoea, 29.7% had a normal menstrual cycle, 19.2% had amenorrhoea, 2.7% had polymenorrhoea and 1.4% had menorrhagia. Hirsutism was observed in 66.2% of patients, and assessed as

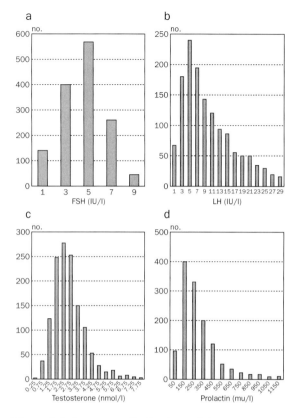

Figure 3.1 Frequency distributions of the characteristics of 1741 women with polycystic ovary syndrome: serum concentrations of (a) follicle-stimulating hormone (FSH), (b) luteinizing hormone (LH), (c) testosterone and (d) prolactin. From Balen et al,[18] with permission.

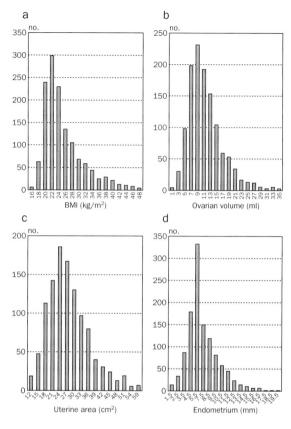

Figure 3.2 Frequency distribution of the characteristics of 1741 women with polycystic ovary syndrome: (a) body mass index, (b) ovarian volume, (c) uterine cross-sectional area and (d) endometrial thickness. From Balen et al,[18] with permission.

mild (20.6%), moderate (40.7%) or severe (4.9%). Acne was present in 34.7% of patients and 2.5% had acanthosis nigricans.

Using Pearson's correlation coefficient the patients' body mass index correlated significantly with ovarian volume (r 0.11; $P < 0.0005$) and UXA (r 0.15, $P < 0.0005$). A higher BMI was associated with a rise in serum testosterone concentration (r 0.254, $P < 0.0005$) and the prevalence of hirsutism ($P = 0.0002$) (Figure 3.3). Obesity was also associated with an increased rate of infertility and cycle disturbances. The rates of primary (15%) and sec-

ondary (8%) infertility were fairly constant with BMIs of 20–30 kg/m^2 but rose to 26% and 14%, respectively, when the BMI was greater than 30 kg/m^2 ($P < 0.00005$). Similarly the percentage of women with a regular menstrual cycle fell from approximately 32% to 22% when the BMI exceeded 30 kg/m^2 ($P = 0.032$).

With respect to fertility, 804 of a total of 1269 (63.4%) women had not yet tested their fertility. Of the remaining 465 women, 228 (49%) had primary infertility, 121 (26%) had secondary infertility and 116 (25%) had proved fertility. The LH concentrations related to fertility are

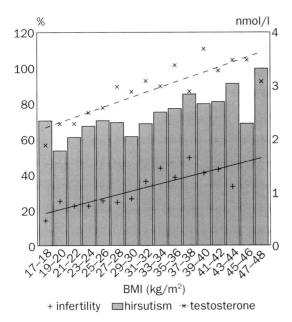

Figure 3.3 The relationship between body mass index and the rates of hirsutism (shaded bars) and serum testosterone concentration (x). From Balen et al,[18] with permission.

recorded in Table 3.3. The serum LH concentration of those with primary infertility was significantly higher than that of women with secondary infertility and both were higher than the LH concentration of those with proved infertility ($P < 0.00\,001$). The rate of infertility increased if the serum LH concentration was greater than $10\,\mathrm{IU/l}$ (x^2 58.72, df 12, $P < 0.00\,001$). There was also a significant increase in the rate of cycle disturbance with LH concentrations greater than $10\,\mathrm{IU/l}$ (x^2 68.96, df 24, $P < 0.00\,001$) (Figure 3.4).

The ovarian volume was significantly correlated with serum concentrations of LH (r 0.24, $P < 0.0005$), testosterone (r 0.16, $P < 0.0005$) and the BMI (r 0.11, $P < 0.0005$). These variables were independent of each other when tested with multiple regression analysis. A rising serum concentration of testosterone was associated with an increased risk of hirsutism ($P < 0.0005$), infertility ($P = 0.0225$) and cycle disturbance ($P = 0.0007$).

Ovarian morphology appears to be the most sensitive marker of PCOS, compared with the classical endocrine features of raised serum LH

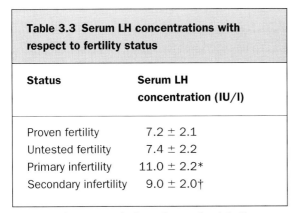

Table 3.3 Serum LH concentrations with respect to fertility status	
Status	**Serum LH concentration (IU/l)**
Proven fertility	7.2 ± 2.1
Untested fertility	7.4 ± 2.2
Primary infertility	11.0 ± 2.2*
Secondary infertility	9.0 ± 2.0†

* Different from proven fertile and secondary infertile groups.
† Different from proven fertile group.

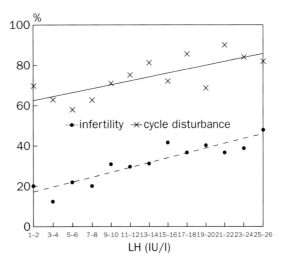

Figure 3.4 The relationship between serum LH concentration and the rates of infertility (●) and cycle disturbance (x). From Balen et al,[18] with permission.

and testosterone levels, which were found in only 39.8% and 28.9% of patients respectively in this study.

PCOS IN OLDER WOMEN

The polycystic ovary syndrome is one of the most common endocrine disorders.

It is a familial condition and appears to have its origins during adolescence when it is thought to be associated with increased weight gain during puberty. At the other end of reproductive life it has been shown that women with oligomenorrhoeic or amenorrhoeic PCOS appear to gain regular menstrual cycles as they get older.[26] In a study of 205 women aged 30 years or older there was a highly significant linear trend for a shorter menstrual cycle with age. The hypothesis is that this phenomenon is due both to the decline in follicle cohort with age and a new balance between inhibin-B and FSH in the early follicular phase of the cycle.[26] The findings of this study have implications for the continued use of agents such as the oral contraceptive pill, which carries increased cardiovascular risks for women over the age of 35 years. It is prudent therefore to consider stopping artificial methods of cycle control for short periods to see if there has been a natural resolution of the problem.

REFERENCES

1 Balen AH. The pathogenesis of polycystic ovary syndrome: the enigma unravels. *Lancet* (1999) **354**: 966–7.

2 Balen AH, Dunger D. Pubertal maturation of the internal genitalia (commentary). *Ultrasound Obstet Gynaecol* (1995) **6**: 164–5.

3 Balen AH, Conway GS, Kaltsas G et al. Polycystic ovary syndrome: the spectrum of the disorder in 1741 patients. *Hum Reprod* (1995) **10**: 2705–12.

4 Homburg R. Polycystic ovary syndrome – from gynaecological curiosity to multisystem endocrinopathy. *Hum Reprod* (1996) **10**: 29–39.

5 Dunaif A. Insulin resistance and the polycystic ovary syndrome: mechanisms and implication for pathogenesis. *Endocr Rev* (1997) **18**: 774–800.

6 Franks S, Gharani N, Waterworth D et al. The genetic basis of polycystic ovary syndrome. *Hum Reprod* (1997) **12**: 2641–8.

7 Clark AM, Ledger W, Galletly C et al. Weight loss results in significant improvement in pregnancy and ovulation rates in anovulatory obese women. *Hum Reprod* (1995) **10**: 2705–12.

8 Jacobs HS, Conway GS. Leptin, polycystic ovaries and polycystic ovary syndrome. *Hum Reprod Update* (1999) **5**: 166–71.

9 Balen AH, Tan SL, Jacobs HS. Hypersecretion of luteinizing hormone: a significant cause of infertility and miscarriage. *Br J Obstet Gynaecol* (1993) **100**: 1082–9.

10 Lockwood GM, Muttukrishna S, Groome NP, Matthews DR, Ledger WL. Mid-follicular phase pulses of inhibin B are absent in polycystic ovary syndrome and are initiated by successful laparoscopic ovarian diathermy: a possible mechanism for the emergence of the dominant follicle. *J Clin Endocrinol Metab* (1998) **83**: 1730–5.

11 Polson DW, Wadsworth J, Adams J, Franks S. Polycystic ovaries: a common finding in normal women. *Lancet* (1988) **ii**: 870–2.

12 Tayob Y, Robinson G, Adams J et al. Ultrasound appearance of the ovaries during the pill-free interval. *Br J Fam Plan* (1990) **16**: 94–6.

13 Clayton RN, Ogden V, Hodgekinson J et al. How common are polycystic ovaries in normal women and what is their significance for the fertility of the population? *Clin Endocrinol* (1992) **37**: 127–34.

14 Farquhar CM, Birdsall M, Manning P, Mitchell JM. Transabdominal versus transvaginal ultrasound in the diagnosis of polycystic ovaries on ultrasound scanning in a population of randomly selected women. *Ultrasound Obstet Gynaecol* (1994) **4**: 54–9.

15 Fox R, Corrigan E, Thomas PA, Hull MGR. The diagnosis of polycystic ovaries in women with oligo-amenorrhoea: predictive power of endocrine tests. *Clin Endocrinol* (1991) **34**: 127–31.

16 Bridges NA, Cooke A, Healy MJR, Hindmarsh PC, Brook CGD. Standards for ovarian volume in childhood and puberty. *Fertil Steril* (1993) **60**: 456–60.

17 Sampaolo P, Livien C, Montanari L, Paganelli A, Salesi A, Lorini R. Precocious signs of polycystic ovaries in obese girls. *Ultrasound Obstet Gynaecol* (1994) **4**: 1–6.

18 Balen AH, Conway GS, Kaltsas G et al. Polycystic ovary syndrome: the spectrum of the

disorder in 1741 patients. *Hum Reprod* (1995) **10**: 2705–12

19 Michelmore KF, Balen AH, Dunger DB, Vessey MP. Polycystic ovaries and associated clinical and biochemical features in young women. *Clin Endocrinol (Oxf)* (1999) **51**: 779–86.

20 Ehrmann DA, Sturis J, Byrne MM, Karrison T, Rosenfield RL, Polonsky KS. Insulin secretory defects in polycystic ovary syndrome. Relationship to insulin sensitivity and family history of non-insulin-dependent diabetes mellitus. *J Clin Invest* (1995) **96**: 520–7.

21 Dunaif A. Insulin resistance and the polycystic ovary syndrome: mechanism and implications for pathogenesis. *Endocr Rev* (1997) **18**: 774–800.

22 Conway GS, Clark PM, Wong D. Hyperinsulinaemia in the polycystic ovary syndrome confirmed with a specific immunoradiometric assay for insulin. *Clin Endocrinol (Oxf)* (1993) **38**: 219–22.

23 Adams J, Franks S, Polson DW et al. Multifollicular ovaries: clinical and endocrine features and response to pulsatile gonadotrophin releasing hormone. *Lancet* (1985) **ii**: 1375–8.

24 Conway GS, Honour JW, Jacobs HS. Heterogeneity of the polycystic ovary syndrome: clinical, endocrine and ultrasound features in 556 patients. *Clin Endocrinol* (1989) **30**: 459–70.

25 Ferriman D, Gallway JD. Clinical assessment of body hair growth in women. *J Clin Endocrinol Metab* (1961) **21**: 1440–7.

26 Elting MW, Korsen TJM, Rekers-Mombarg LTM, Schoemaker J. Women with polycystic ovary syndrome gain regular menstrual cycles when ageing. *Hum Reprod* (2000) **15**: 24–8.

4

Genetic factors in the aetiology

Stephen Franks

Polycystic ovary syndrome (PCOS) is the most common cause of anovulatory infertility and hirsutism.[1,2] Polycystic ovary syndrome has been defined as the association of menstrual disturbance with clinical or biochemical evidence of androgen excess,[3] but the validity of this definition is questionable.[4-6] Using ultrasonographic criteria, the majority of hirsute women with regular menses have been found to have polycystic ovaries[5,7] and the estimated prevalence of the polycystic ovaries in a normal (volunteer) population has been found to be over 20%.[8,9]

It has been suggested that PCOS represents a wide range of disorders rather than a single entity. Although it seems likely that there is more than one cause of the syndrome, there are, nevertheless, certain biochemical features that are common to all groups of subjects with ultrasonographic evidence of polycystic ovaries, irrespective of the clinical presentation. Hyperandrogenism is, however, the most consistent endocrine feature in women with polycystic ovaries, whether the mode of presentation is as the 'classic' syndrome or as an incidental finding on ultrasound examination.[10] The ovary, rather than the adrenal gland, is the major source of excess androgen[6] and data both from clinical investigations and from studies of isolated human theca cells implicate a primary ovarian abnormality rather than a 'downstream' effect of elevated serum luteinizing hormone levels.[11-13]

Polycystic ovary syndrome is also characterized by significant metabolic abnormalities which include fasting and glucose-stimulated hyperinsulinaemia, peripheral insulin resistance, abnormalities of energy expenditure and dyslipidaemia (for reviews see references 6, 14, 15). The syndrome represents a major risk factor for development of type 2 (non-insulin-dependent) diabetes mellitus. The prevalence of impaired glucose tolerance or frank diabetes in obese young women with PCOS is estimated to be between 11% and 38%, depending on the population studied.[14-17] The prevalence of type 2 diabetes in a long-term follow-up study of postmenopausal women with a previous history of PCOS was found to be 13% compared with less than 2% in the reference population.[18] These patients may also be at greater risk of developing cardiovascular disease in the future.[19]

Familial clustering of cases suggests a major

genetic component to the aetiology of PCOS. Although it seems unlikely that there is a single cause of the syndrome, much of the clinical and biochemical variability within PCOS can possibly be explained by the interaction of environmental (notably nutritional) factors with a small number of major causative genes which include those involved in androgen production and the secretion and/or action of insulin.

Genetic studies of polycystic ovary syndrome are difficult to perform.[20,21] The heterogeneity and the lack of universally acceptable clinical or biochemical diagnostic criteria have already been discussed. Another major problem is that this disorder primarily affects women of reproductive age, and it is therefore difficult for segregation studies to span more than one generation. In addition, as discussed below, there is no commonly accepted male phenotype. Lastly, the high prevalence of polycystic ovaries in the population means that large pedigrees may include subjects with polycystic ovaries arising from a different genotype from that of the proband. Nevertheless, given modern methods of genetic modelling and molecular genotyping, these problems can be overcome.

FAMILIAL POLYCYSTIC OVARY SYNDROME

Familial aggregation of cases of PCOS is well recognized.[20–27] Not surprisingly, the criteria used to identify probands and affected family members vary considerably between studies. Furthermore, identification of affected family members was made by direct clinical observation in some studies, by questionnaire alone in some, and by a combination of the two in others. In one of the largest studies[24] no attempt was made to identify a male phenotype. In three others, premature balding was suggested as the likely manifestation of affected status in men but this was based, in two of the three, on evidence from questionnaires,[23,26] and, in the other, on a combination of data from direct observation, telephone interview and questionnaires.[27]

There has been no general agreement about the mode of inheritance in PCOS. In four of six studies, segregation analysis gave results that were consistent with autosomal dominant inheritance;[22,23,26,27] one study suggested an X-linked mode,[25] and in the other, the prevalence of polycystic ovaries among siblings was too high to be explained by a simple dominant model.[24] It is advisable, therefore, to make no definite assumptions about the mode of inheritance when performing linkage studies, as suggested below.

Studies at St Mary's Hospital focused, initially, on segregation analysis in 10 well-characterized, multiply affected families with polycystic ovaries.[27] It differed from those previously published in that it relied principally on direct interview and observation of relatives rather than on indirect evidence from questionnaires. Results from 50 women of reproductive age and 22 men were analysed. Affected status was assigned on the basis of ultrasonographic evidence of polycystic ovaries in the women and premature onset (before age 30 years) of frontoparietal balding in men.

Despite the fact that the diagnosis of polycystic ovaries was made ultrasonographically, 92% of affected female family members had at least one clinical feature (hirsutism, acne, menstrual disturbance) or biochemical feature (raised concentration of serum testosterone or LH) of polycystic ovary *syndrome*. The segregation ratio – expressed as the percentage of affected subjects in each generation (excluding the proband to avoid ascertainment bias) – was calculated including data from the men and was found to be 51%, i.e. consistent with an autosomal dominant mode of inheritance. These initial results suggested a single gene effect.

Some of the existing pedigrees have been enlarged and new ones have been added so that the number of families now includes 23 informative pedigrees. The larger database reveals a more complex picture and traditional segregation analysis has proved difficult. This is well illustrated by the pedigree in Figure 4.1. The proband (6) presented with anovulation but was non-hirsute, whereas her affected sister (5) was hirsute but had regular menses. She had two sisters with normal ovaries (4, 7) who had regular cycles and were non-hirsute, and a

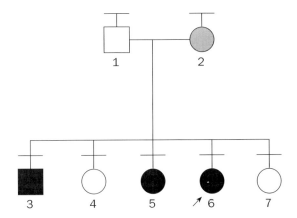

Figure 4.1 A pedigree with familial polycystic ovary syndrome (see text). Proband is arrowed; ■, affected male; □ unaffected male; ● affected female; ○, unaffected female; ◉, female, status unknown.

using a single-gene autosomal dominant model, we have used a linkage analysis programme which makes no assumption about the mode of inheritance. In the following section the results of association and linkage studies applied to examination of the role of possible candidate genes are discussed. Given the biochemical phenotype characteristic of women with polycystic ovaries, we focused on genes coding for steroidogenic enzymes in the androgen biosynthetic pathway and those involved in the secretion and action of insulin.

GENES ENCODING ENZYMES IN THE ANDROGEN BIOSYNTHETIC PATHWAY

The 17-hydroxylase/17,20-lyase gene (*CYP17*)

Our initial investigations focused on the possible role of *CYP17* (the gene encoding P450c17α) because clinical studies pointed to abnormal regulation of 17-hydroxylase/17,20-lyase (a known rate-limiting step in androgen biosynthesis).[28,29] A 459 base pair fragment in the 5′ regulatory region of *CYP17* was amplified by polymerase chain reaction (PCR). A single base change (a T to C substitution at −34 base pairs from the starting point of translation) was found.[30] This variant allele includes a restriction site for the enzyme *Msp*-1, thus allowing a simple method of screening DNA by restriction fragment length polymorphism (RFLP) analysis.

brother (3) with premature balding. Her mother (2) was postmenopausal and although she had no history of menstrual disturbance or hirsutism it was not possible to assess, accurately, her ovarian morphology. Her father (1) had no history of premature balding.

This pedigree exemplifies two points: (a) the symptomatic heterogeneity between the proband and her sisters; and (b) the problems associated with assigning definite affected status to more than one generation because of questions about the reliability of data from postmenopausal women. The results are certainly compatible with an autosomal dominant model but it would be unwise to consider this mode of inheritance to the exclusion of all others. In this context, the suggestion by Simpson[20] that PCOS should be treated as a quantitative trait disorder has considerable merit. This does not necessarily imply a truly polygenic aetiology because it would be possible to explain the variable phenotype on the basis of a small number of causative genes (an 'oligogenic' basis for disease). A candidate gene approach therefore remains valid; but rather than performing linkage studies

Linkage studies in PCOS families using polymorphic markers close to the gene made it possible to exclude *CYP17* as a major causative gene. Nevertheless, using RFLP screening of the −34 allele, preliminary case–control data suggested an association between a variant allele at *CYP17* and PCOS.[30] These findings were, however, based on a relatively small population of subjects (71 patients and 33 controls) and other studies have failed to confirm these results.[31–34] Significantly, in none of these studies was any relationship found between the *CYP17* variant and serum androgen levels.

The cholesterol side-chain cleavage gene, *CYP11A*

Studies of ovarian theca cells in culture have demonstrated that PCO theca cells produce an excess of progesterone as well as 17-hydroxy-progesterone and androstenedione.[11,35] The gene *CYP11a* (encoding P450 side-chain cleavage, P450scc) was therefore a possible candidate gene for abnormal steroidogenesis.[36] The segregation of *CYP11a* was examined in 20 families and association studies were performed in consecutively recruited, premenopausal, European women with polycystic ovaries on ultrasound and matched control women (with normal ovaries) from a similar ethnic background. Participants included 97 women with symptomatic PCOS, 51 women with polycystic ovaries and no symptoms, and 59 women with normal ovaries.

Genotype analysis was performed after PCR amplification, using an informative, microsatellite marker in the promoter region of *CYP11a*. In the case–control study, subjects were allocated to one of two groups according to the presence or absence of the most common polymorphism. Individuals were therefore designated as 216+ (at least one copy) or 216− (no 216 allele). Our results showed that variation at the *CYP11a* gene was associated with both PCOS and serum testosterone concentrations[36] (Figure 4.2).

In addition, we carried out non-parametric linkage analysis using the GENEHUNTER (multipoint linkage) program.[37] We found evidence for excess allele sharing (i.e. linkage) at the *CYP11a* locus, generating a maximum non-parametric log likelihood ratio (LOD, NPL) score of 3.03 ($P = 0.003$). The data from both association and linkage studies suggest that *CYP11a* is a major genetic susceptibility locus for PCOS.

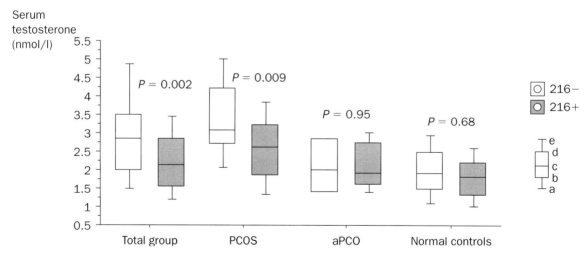

Figure 4.2 Relationship between serum testosterone level and alleles of *CYP11a* in a case–control data set. Serum testosterone concentrations in women with polycystic or normal ovaries are grouped according to genotype at the promoter region of *CYP11a*. The 216+ individuals are those with at least one 216 allele, 216− are subjects with no 216 allele. PCOS, subjects with polycystic ovary syndrome; aPCO, asymptomatic subjects with polycystic ovaries on ultrasound. The 'box and whisker' plots show 10th, 25th, 50th, 75th and 90th centiles (a, b, c, d and e, respectively). Groups were compared by the Mann–Whitney test. From Gharani et al,[36] with permission.

GENES RELATED TO SECRETION AND ACTION OF INSULIN

Numerous metabolic studies have revealed abnormalities of both insulin secretion and action in women with PCOS (for reviews, see references 14, 15). There is an interaction between body weight and PCOS, so that individuals with PCOS are more insulin-resistant than control subjects, after correcting for the effects of obesity. The results of such studies raise the possibility that genes implicated in the secretion and action of insulin may have a role in the aetiology of PCOS.

The insulin receptor gene

The demonstration of impaired sensitivity to insulin action in vivo and in vitro naturally led to the hypothesis that genetic abnormalities of the insulin receptor and/or postreceptor signalling were involved in the pathogenesis of familial PCOS. Although there have been sporadic reports of a PCOS-like phenotype occurring in patients with severe insulin resistance associated with defects of the insulin receptor gene,[38] an analysis of subjects with PCOS and insulin resistance showed no consistent abnormalities of the insulin receptor gene.[39] Molecular scanning of the entire coding region of the insulin receptor gene was carried out on DNA samples from 24 well-characterized women with PCOS. Common polymorphisms were detected, especially in the intron 5′ to exon 3, but no missense or nonsense mutations (i.e. those that would be expected to result in marked impairment of receptor function) were found. The authors concluded that mutations of the insulin receptor gene were rare in women with PCOS.

As far as postreceptor signalling is concerned, it remains to be determined whether there is a genetic basis for the putative abnormality of serine–threonine phosphorylation which characterizes a significant proportion of women with typical PCOS.[40]

The insulin gene

Abnormalities of insulin secretion have been reported in studies of women with PCOS, with and without a family history of type 2 diabetes mellitus.[17,41–44] The Imperial College's team therefore investigated the role of the insulin gene in the aetiology of PCOS. We evaluated the VNTR (variable number tandem repeats) minisatellite which lies 5′ to the insulin gene on chromosome 11p15.5, because variation at this element has been directly implicated in the regulation of insulin secretion, in susceptibility to type 2 diabetes,[45] and in hyperinsulinaemia related to central obesity.[46] At this locus there is a bimodal distribution of repeats, class I alleles being short (average 40 repeats) and class III alleles much longer (average 157 repeats).

Linkage of PCOS to the 11p15.5 locus was examined in 17 families with PCOS and male pattern balding. We also looked for an association between the insulin gene VNTR (particularly class I and class III alleles) and polycystic ovaries in two additional populations of women (all of European origin) presenting with symptoms of PCOS at two different endocrine centres.[47] The odds ratios for insulin VNTR genotypes were calculated either by using a conventional case–control approach or by the use of affected family-based controls (AFBAC).

The AFBAC approach and a related technique, the transmission disequilibrium test (TDT), are applicable if DNA is available from one proband and both parents.[48] These methods compare alleles transmitted from parents to affected offspring with those not so transmitted. The latter generate 'control' genotypes or alleles which are matched for ethnicity to those in the sample from the affected 'case'. It was found that class III alleles were associated with PCOS in each of the three populations. An important additional finding was that insulin VNTR class III alleles were most strongly associated with *anovulatory* PCOS. This is in keeping with the observation that hyperinsulinaemia is a more prominent feature in women with polycystic ovaries who have anovulatory menses (or amenorrhoea) than in equally hyperandrogenaemic subjects with regular menses.[16,49]

Another intriguing finding emerged from TDT analysis of the Middlesex Hospital population and of the 17 families with PCOS. Class III alleles were transmitted significantly more often from fathers than from mothers.[50] This parent-of-origin effect suggests genetic imprinting, as has previously been described for 11p15.5 in relation to type 1 (insulin-dependent) diabetes.[51]

In the families, non-parametric linkage analysis was performed with the aid of five polymorphic markers in the region of 11p15.5, using the GENEHUNTER program. There was evidence for excess allele sharing at the insulin gene VNTR locus, giving a maximum NPL score of 3.250 ($P = 0.002$). Using parametric analysis, it was estimated that approximately 60% of families showed linkage to this locus. When data were assigned from families according to linkage score, the geometric mean of fasting specific insulin levels was higher in those families with a positive lod score than those with a negative score[47] (Figure 4.3).

In summary, in three different populations, there was strong evidence for both linkage and association between alleles at the VNTR 5′ to the insulin gene and PCOS. These data suggest that the VNTR of the insulin gene is a major susceptibility locus for PCOS, particularly anovulatory PCOS, and may contribute to the mechanism of hyperinsulinaemia and to the high risk of type 2 diabetes in women with PCOS.

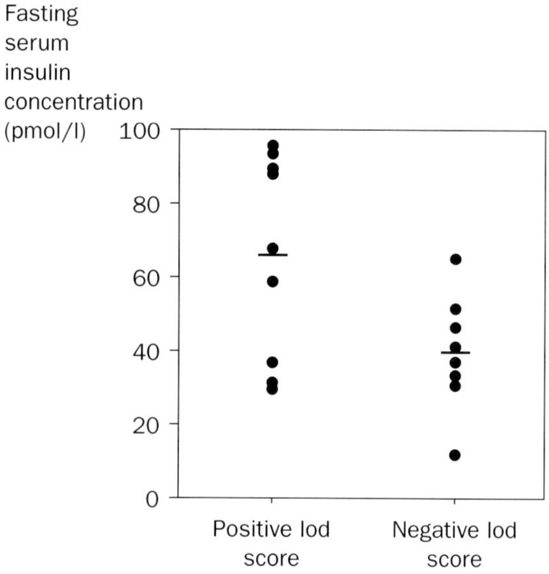

Figure 4.3 Geometric means of fasting serum insulin concentrations, measured by specific immunoradiometric assay, in families linked to insulin gene VNTR (positive lod) and in those not showing linkage (negative lod). The means of the groups are significantly different, $P = 0.033$. From Waterworth et al,[47] with permission.

GENES INVOLVED IN DEVELOPMENT OF OVARIAN FOLLICLES

The follistatin gene

Urbanek et al examined the follistatin locus on chromosome 5 as part of a panel of candidate genes related to gonadotrophin action.[52] Somewhat unexpectedly, they found the strongest evidence for linkage with PCOS of any of the 37 candidate genes they had chosen. In their affected sibling-pair analysis 72% of sisters were concordant for the follistatin genotype and this remained significant after correction for multiple testing. This intriguing finding remains to be confirmed in other populations but the possibility arises that this and other genes implicated in folliculogenesis may have a causal role in this disorder which is, after all, characterized by disordered follicle development.[52]

CONCLUSION

There is evidence for the involvement of two key genes in the aetiology of PCOS. The results of both linkage and association studies suggest that the steroid synthesis gene *CYP11a* and the insulin VNTR regulatory polymorphism are important factors in the genetic basis of PCOS and may explain, in part, the heterogeneity of the syndrome. Thus, differences in expression of *CYP11a* could account for variation in androgen production in women who have polycystic ovaries. Women carrying class III alleles at the insulin gene VNTR locus may be more likely to be hyperinsulinaemic and to suffer from menstrual disturbances.

These findings remain to be confirmed in larger studies and in other populations; whatever the outcome of such studies, it is unlikely that these are the only genes to be involved in the aetiology of PCOS. Recent results lend weight to the idea that PCOS represents a quantitative trait in which several genes – but perhaps a relatively small number of key genes – contribute, in conjuction with environmental (particularly nutritional) factors, to the observed clinical and biochemical heterogeneity. This does not necessarily imply that, as has been suggested by some, PCOS represents several different diseases or disorders.

It is proposed that the underlying problem is the development of the polycystic ovarian morphology with an implicit disorder of folliculogenesis. This predisposes the subject to the development of polycystic ovary syndrome. The gene or genes determining the development of this distinct ovarian morphology remain unknown. Both *CYP11a* and insulin gene VNTR may act independently or in concert to determine abnormalities of ovarian function and (in the case of insulin) metabolism. Environmental factors can alter the clinical and biochemical presentation in those with a genetic predisposition to PCOS. This is illustrated by the effect of obesity (or, conversely, dietary energy restriction) on serum insulin levels, insulin sensitivity and menstrual function.[16,44,53]

Acknowledgments

I thank Dr AH Carey, Dr S Batty, Dr M McCarthy, Dr CM-T Gilling-Smith, Dr DM White and Ms R Joseph-Horne (St Mary's Hospital, London), Dr GS Conway (The Middlesex Hospital, London), Professor R Williamson, Dr D Waterworth, Ms N Gharani and Mr S Hague (Department of Biochemistry and Molecular Genetics, Imperial College School of Medicine at St Mary's, London), Dr ST Bennett and Professor JA Todd (Wellcome Trust Centre for Human Genetics, University of Oxford) for their invaluable contributions to these studies. I am grateful for grant support from the Medical Research Council (studentship for DW and ROPA award to SF and RW) and from the research department of Unilever, UK.

REFERENCES

1 Adams J, Polson DW, Franks S. Prevalence of polycystic ovaries in women with anovulation and idiopathic hirsutism. (1986) *Br Med J* **293**: 355–9.

2 Hull MG. Epidemiology of infertility and polycystic ovarian disease: endocrinological and demographic studies. *Gynecol Endocrinol* (1987) **1**: 235–45.

3 Zawadzki JK, Dunaif A. Diagnostic criteria for polycystic ovary syndrome: towards a rational approach. In: Dunaif A, Givens JR, Haseltine FP, Merriam GR, eds, *Polycystic Ovary Syndrome* (Blackwell: Oxford, 1992) 377–84.

4 Conway GS, Honour JW, Jacobs HS. Heterogeneity of the polycystic ovary syndrome: clinical, endocrine and ultrasound features in 556 patients. *Clin Endocrinol* (1989) **30**: 459–7.

5 Franks S. Polycystic ovary syndrome: a changing perspective. *Clin Endocrinol* (1989) **31**: 87–120.

6 Franks S. Medical progress article: polycystic ovary syndrome. *N Engl J Med* (1995) **333**: 853–61.

7 O'Driscoll JB, Mamtora H, Higginson J, Pollock A, Kane J, Anderson DC. A prospective study of the incidence of clear-cut endocrine disorders and polycystic ovaries in 350 patients with hirsutism or androgenic alopecia. *Clin Endocrinol* (1994) **41**: 231–6.

8 Polson DW, Adams J, Wadsworth J, Franks S. Polycystic ovaries – a common finding in normal women. *Lancet* (1988) **1**(8590): 870–2.

9 Clayton RC, Ogden V, Hodgkinson J et al. How common are polycystic ovaries in normal women and what is their significance for fertility in the general population? *Clin Endocrinol* (1992) **37**: 127–34.

10 Franks S. The ubiquitous polycystic ovary. *J Endocrinol* (1991) **129**: 317–19.

11 Gilling-Smith C, Willis DS, Beard RW, Franks S. Hypersecretion of androstenedione by isolated

theca cells from polycystic ovaries. *J Clin Endocrinol Metab* (1994) **79**: 1158–65.

12 Gilling-Smith C, Story EH, Franks S. Evidence for a primary abnormality of thecal cell steroidogenesis in the polycystic ovary syndrome. *Clin Endocrinol* (1997) **47**: 93–9.

13 Ibanez L, Hall JE, Potau N, Carrascosa A, Prat A, Taylor AE. Ovarian 17-hydroxyprogesterone hyperresponsiveness to gonadotropin-releasing hormone (GnRH) agonist challenge in women with polycystic ovary syndrome is not mediated by luteinizing hormone hypersecretion: evidence from GnRH agonist and human chorionic gonadotropin stimulation testing. *J Clin Endocrinol Metab* (1996) **81**: 4103–7.

14 Dunaif A. Insulin resistance and ovarian dysfunction. In: Moller D, ed., *Insulin Resistance* (John Wiley: New York, 1993) 301–25.

15 Holte J. Disturbances in insulin secretion and sensitivity in women with the polycystic ovary syndrome. *Baillière's Clinical Endocrinology and Metabolism* (1996) **10**: 221–47.

16 Dunaif A, Graf M, Mandeli J, Laumas V, Dobrjansky A. Characterization of groups of hyperandrogenic women with acanthosis nigricans, impaired glucose tolerance, and/or hyperinsulinemia. *J Clin Endocrinol Metab* (1987) **65**: 499–507.

17 Dunaif A, Finegood DT. Beta cell dysfunction independent of obesity in the polycystic ovary syndrome. *J Clin Endocrinol Metab* (1996) **81**: 942–7.

18 Dahlgren E, Johannson S, Lindstedt G et al. Women with polycystic ovary syndrome wedge resected in 1956 to 1965: a long term follow up focusing on natural history and circulating hormones. *Fertil Steril* (1992) **57**: 505–13.

19 Dahlgren E, Janson PO, Johansson S et al. Polycystic ovary syndrome and risk for myocardial infarction: evaluated from a risk factor model based on a prospective study of women. *Acta Obstet Gynecol Scand* (1992) **71**: 599–604.

20 Simpson J L. Elucidating the genetics of polycystic ovary syndrome. In: Dunaif A, Givens JR, Haseltine FP, Merriam GR, eds, *Polycystic Ovary Syndrome* (Blackwell: Oxford, 1992) 59–77.

21 Legro RS. The genetics of polycystic ovary syndrome. *Am J Med* (1995) **98**(suppl. 1A): 9S-16S.

22 Cooper H, Spellacy W, Prem K, Cohen W. Hereditary factors in the Stein–Leventhal syndrome. *Am J Obstet Gynecol* (1968) **100**: 371–87.

23 Ferriman D, Purdie AW. The inheritance of polycystic ovarian disease and a possible relationship to premature balding. *Clin Endocrinol* (1979) **11**: 291–300.

24 Hague WM, Adams J, Reeders ST, Peto TE, Jacobs HS. Familial polycystic ovaries: a genetic disease? *Clin Endocrinol* (1988) **29**: 593–605.

25 Givens JR. Familial polycystic ovarian disease. *Endocrinol Metab Clin North Am* (1988) **17**: 771–83.

26 Lunde O, Magnus P, Sandvik L, Hoglo S. Familial clustering in the polycystic ovarian syndrome. *Gynecol Obstet Invest* (1989) **28**: 23–30.

27 Carey AH, Chan KL, Short F, White DM, Williamson R, Franks S. Evidence for a single gene effect in polycystic ovaries and male pattern baldness. *Clin Endocrinol* (1993) **38**: 653–8.

28 Barnes RB, Rosenfield RL, Burstein S, Ehrmann DA. Pituitary-ovarian responses to nafarelin testing in the polycystic ovary syndrome. *N Engl J Med* (1989) **320**: 559–65.

29 Rosenfield RL, Barnes RB, Cara JF, Lucky AW. Dysregulation of cytochrome P450c 17 alpha as the cause of polycystic ovarian syndrome. *Fertil Steril* (1990) **53**: 785–91.

30 Carey AH, Waterworth D, Patel K et al. Polycystic ovaries and premature male pattern baldness are associated with one allele of the steroid metabolism gene CYP17. *Hum Mol Genet* (1994) **3**: 1873–6.

31 Gharani N, Waterworth DM, Williamson R, Franks S. 5′ polymorphism of the CYP17 gene is not associated with serum testosterone levels in women with polycystic ovaries [letter]. *J Clin Endocrinol Metab* (1996) **81**: 4174.

32 Pugeat M, Nicolas MH, Cousin P et al. Polymorphism in the 5′ promoter of the human gene encoding P450c17a and adrenal androgen secretion in hirsute women. Programme of 10th International Congress of Endocrinology, San Francisco, June 1996. The Endocrine Society, abstract P2–626, 1996.

33 Tetchatraisak K, Conway GS, Rumsby G. Frequency of a polymorphism in the regulatory region of the 17a-hydroxylase-17,20 lyase (CYP17) gene in hyperandrogenic states. *Clin Endocrinol* (1997) **46**: 131–4.

34 Franks S. The 17α-hydroxylase-17,20-lyase gene (CYP17) and polycystic ovary syndrome [commentary]. *Clin Endocrinol* (1997) **46**: 135–6.

35 Franks S, Willis D, Mason H, Gilling-Smith C. Comparative androgen production from theca cells of normal women and women with polycystic ovaries. In: Chang RJ, ed., *Polycystic Ovary Syndrome* (Springer: New York, 1996) 154–64.

36 Gharani N, Waterworth DM, Batty S et al.

Association of the steroid synthesis gene CYP11a with polycystic ovary syndrome and hyperandrogenism. *Hum Mol Genet* (1997) **6**: 397–402.

37 Kruglyak L, Daly MJ, Reeve-Daly MP et al. Parametric and non-parametric linkage analysis: a unified multipoint approach. *Am J Hum Genet* (1996) **58**: 1347–63.

38 Moller DE, Flier JS. Detection of an alteration in the insulin receptor gene in a patient with insulin resistance, acanthosis nigricans and the polycystic ovary syndrome. *N Engl J Med* (1988) **319**: 1526–9.

39 Talbot JA, Bicknell EJ, Rajkhowa M, Krook A, O'Rahilly S, Clayton RN. Molecular scanning of the insulin receptor gene in women with polycystic ovary syndrome. *J Clin Endocrinol Metab* (1996) **81**: 1979–83.

40 Dunaif A, Xia J, Book CB, Schenker E, Tang Z. Excessive insulin receptor phosphorylation in cultured fibroblasts and in skeletal muscle. *J Clin Invest* (1995) **96**: 801–10.

41 O'Meara N, Blackman JD, Ehrmann DA et al. Defects in B-cell function in functional ovarian hyperandrogenism. *J Clin Endocrinol Metab* (1993) **76**: 1241–7.

42 Ehrmann D, Sturis J, Byrne M, Karrison T, Rosenfield R, Polonsky K. Insulin secretory defects in polycystic ovary syndrome: relationship to insulin sensitivity and family history of non-insulin-dependent diabetes mellitus. *J Clin Invest* (1995) **96**: 520–7.

43 Holte J, Bergh T, Berne C, Berglund L, Lithell H. Enhanced early insulin response to glucose in relation to insulin resistance in women with polycystic ovary syndrome and normal glucose tolerance. *J Clin Endocrinol Metab* (1994) **78**: 1052–8.

44 Holte J, Bergh T, Berne C et al. Restored insulin sensitivity but persistently increased early insulin secretion after weight loss in obese women with polycystic ovary syndrome. *J Clin Endocrinol Metab* (1995) **80**: 2586–93.

45 Bennett ST, Lucassen AM, Gough SCL et al. Susceptibility to human type 1 diabetes at IDDM2 is determined by tandem repeat variation at the insulin gene minisatellite locus. *Nature Genet* (1995) **9**: 284–92.

46 Weaver JU, Kopelman PG, Hitman GA. Central obesity and hyperinsulinaemia in women are associated with polymorphism in the 5' flanking region of the human insulin gene. *Eur J Clin Invest* (1992) **22**: 265–70.

47 Waterworth DM, Bennett ST, Gharani N et al. Linkage and association of insulin gene VNTR regulatory polymorphism with polycystic ovary syndrome. *Lancet* (1997) **349**: 986–9.

48 Spielman RS, Ewens WJ. The TDT and other family-based tests for linkage disequilibrium and association. *Am J Hum Genet* (1996) **59**: 983–9.

49 Robinson S, Kiddy D, Gelding SV et al. The relationship of insulin sensitivity to menstrual pattern in women with hyperandrogenism and polycystic ovaries. *Clin Endocrinol* (1993) **39**: 351–5.

50 Bennett ST, Todd JA, Waterworth DM, Franks S, McCarthy M. Letter. *Lancet* (1997) **349**: 986–90.

51 Bennett ST, Todd JA. Human type 1 diabetes and the insulin gene: principles of mapping polygenes. *Ann Rev Genet* (1996) **30**: 343–70.

52 Urbanek M, Legro RS, Driscoll DA et al. Thirty-seven candidate genes for polycystic ovary syndrome: strongest evidence for linkage is with follistatin. *Proc Natl Acad Sci USA* (1999) **96**: 8573–8.

53 Franks S, Mason HD, Willis DS (2000) Follicular dynamics in the polycystic ovary syndrome. *Mol Cell Endocrinol* (2000) **163**: 49–52.

5

Follicular growth and function

Helen Mason

Substantial research efforts focused on the aetiology and function of the polycystic ovary (PCO) have improved our knowledge of the associated endocrine disturbances, but little progress has been made in defining the changes in the growth patterns or function of the follicles in these ovaries. Analysis of the abnormalities in polycystic ovaries reveals several distinct aspects to the problem.

The first and most obvious abnormality, and the defining feature of the condition, is the increase in the number of follicles compared with normal ovaries. The second abnormality is the overproduction of steroids, particularly androgens, which is a common feature of PCO and is evident across the spectrum of presentation. The final aspect is the anovulation that occurs in a subgroup of women with polycystic ovary syndrome. Although these processes are not necessarily independent, it is helpful to consider them separately in the first instance.

There are few data regarding the mechanism of the increase in follicle numbers; however, it is useful to re-examine the available information. As there is still debate as to the definition of PCOS, and as PCO can be present with or without the syndrome, it is important to define the terms used. The following definitions are used in this chapter:

- anovulatory PCO (anovPCO) – ovaries fulfilling the criteria of Adams et al[1] on ultrasonographic findings in women with oligomenorrhoea or amenorrhoea
- ovulatory polycystic ovaries (ovPCO) – those fitting the Adams criteria, but present in women reporting regular cycles and showing evidence of a dominant follicle or corpus luteum.

There is clearly a spectrum of cycle regularity in PCOS and a true division between the two groups is difficult to make without a detailed cycle history and visualization of the ovary. Polycystic ovary syndrome is considered to be present when the appearance of PCO is accompanied by one or more of the clinical manifestations of the syndrome such as hirsutism, raised androgen levels or obesity.

Most of the studies reported here were performed on ovaries that were microscopically dissected. Morphological distinctions are more easily made during this process. For the in vitro studies discussed below ovaries were classified into three groups according to menstrual cycle history and macroscopic morphological features at the time of dissection.[2] A polycystic ovary had at least three of the following criteria: increased volume (>9 ml), 10 or more follicles 2–8 mm in diameter, an increase in the amount and density of stroma, and thickening of the tunica. Cases where patients had a history of anovulatory infertility and/or oligomenorrhoea or amenorrhoea and no evidence of recent corpora lutea were designated anovPCO; cases where ovaries from women reporting regular cycles met the above morphological criteria but contained a dominant follicle and/or a recent corpus luteum were designated ovPCO. Normal morphology was assigned when the ovary was of normal size with soft, pliable stroma and contained no more than five follicles exceeding 2 mm in diameter in a woman with regular menstrual cycles.

FOLLICLE GROWTH

Histological and morphological data of follicle size distribution

The only extensive morphological study to address the issue of the increase in follicle number was performed in the 1960s and 1970s by a pathologist, Hughesden.[3] Hughesden counted all stages of follicles in a large number of sections of normal and polycystic ovaries. There were similar numbers of primordial follicles in each type of ovary, but approximately twice as many of all of the growing and atretic stages of follicles in the PCO. Atresia is the fate of all follicles that are not selected to ovulate – which, by definition, is the majority of follicles in the ovary. It is characterized by increased intrafollicular androgen levels, decreased granulosa cell numbers and gradual disappearance of the follicle by apoptotic and other degenerative processes.[4,5]

Hughesden hypothesized that over-recruitment of follicles into the growing phases with an increase in follicle turnover was the likely cause of the appearance of PCO. It is possible that the raised intrafollicular androgen level stimulates the initiation of follicle growth, but there is no evidence as yet to support or refute Hughesden's hypothesis in the PCO.

An alternative explanation for the increase in follicle number in PCO is that it is due to anovulation itself and there is a common misconception that the follicles accumulate because they do not reach ovulatory sizes. This cannot be so because, by definition, there is also an increase in follicle number in women with PCO and regular cycles. In Hughesden's study the primary complaint of the patients was cycle irregularity, suggesting that the ovaries studied were predominantly from anovulatory women. Interestingly, the presence of recent or regressed luteal tissue was reported in many of the sections despite this. One problem in stating that the increase in follicle number cannot be due to anovulation alone is that there are no precise data on the frequency of ovulation in women diagnosed as having ovPCO. It is not clear whether women with ovPCO truly have regular ovulatory cycles or whether the increase in follicle number is also due to a higher than expected number of anovulatory cycles in these women. Patient-reported cycle-to-cycle variation is notoriously unreliable; for example in a recent study, a wide range of cycle length was found despite the subjects having reported regular cycles,[6] and in a study of the prevalence of PCO in the normal population, 75% of women with PCO were found to have irregular cycles on close questioning, despite no self-perceived problem.[7]

If follicle number was related to anovulation then it might be expected that numbers would increase with age and subsequent accumulated periods of anovulation. Extracting the data from Hughesden's paper shows that there is indeed a significant correlation between the number of tertiary follicles in the ovary and the age of the patient (Figure 5.1). A similar correlation was not seen in the data from normal ovaries. It is not known whether follicle numbers are lower in women with PCO having more regular cycles than in women with anovPCO, but in our department we have consistently noticed lower numbers of follicles by dissection in ovPCO than in those with chronic anovulation.

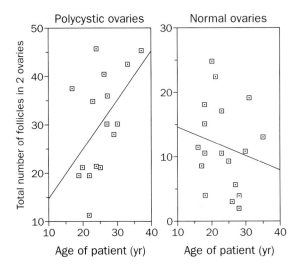

Figure 5.1 Relationship of follicle number (total number of tertiary and small dislocated follicles in both ovaries in each patient) with age in patients with PCOS or normal ovaries; data from Hughesden.[3] There was a significant correlation with age in the PCOS group ($P < 0.05$) which was not seen in normal ovaries.

It is generally considered that the follicles grow normally to a certain size in PCO and then development is arrested. It is clear, however, that the pattern of follicle growth is different even before growth ceases. Hughesden demonstrated increased numbers of all growing sizes of follicle in PCO indicating that early follicle growth is abnormal. It was suggested that follicle turnover was increased, but similar figures would be obtained if recruitment of follicles into the growing phases was increased but then subsequent growth impeded. Distinguishing between these possibilities is important if the mechanism of the increase is to be determined, but as yet there is no evidence for either hypothesis.

Clearly there must be some follicular turnover even in anovulatory PCO, as follicle numbers do not increase perpetually. Currently there is no mechanism for assessing the length of time that follicles have been in the ovary, and

reliably tracking the growth of follicles in a polycystic ovary by ultrasonography is difficult. For these reasons it is still not clear when the follicles stop growing and whether these follicles are similar to healthy or atretic follicles from normal ovaries, either at the time of cessation of growth or subsequently.

Health and atresia

One of the enduring debates regarding the polycystic ovary is whether the structures contained therein are follicles or cysts. Part of the reason for this is that there is no absolute dividing line between the two. The results of the earliest studies on PCO concluded that the follicular structures were cystic owing to their apparent inability to aromatize androgens.[8,9] This concept was explored further in studies in which the concentration of androgens in follicular fluid was found to be much higher in PCO than in follicles from normal ovaries.[10] One of the main problems with this series of studies was that the sensitivity of the assays at the time necessitated pooling of follicular fluid, masking the spectrum of results in different follicles. Also, only a limited number of follicles were studied. A clear answer to the question of follicle health and atresia in the PCO remained elusive.

During the 1970s McNatty et al collected and studied large numbers of follicles dissected intact from normal ovaries and established the criteria for follicle health.[11] In these studies the health of the oocyte and the number of granulosa cells in individual follicles were used to determine follicle health. It was found that a healthy follicle always had a ratio of androstenedione to oestrogen in the follicular fluid of less than 4, and this value has subsequently been used as the 'gold standard'.[4] McNatty also attempted to answer the question of follicle status in PCO. In contrast to the earlier work a large number of normal follicles was studied, and comparison with fluid from individual follicles from PCO led McNatty to conclude that the level of oestrogen in the latter was closer to that in healthy follicles from normal ovaries than the level in atretic follicles.[12]

One problem in this study was the assignment of ovarian morphology, in that the possibility of ovulatory PCO had not then been considered. A similar problem may have occurred in a later study by Pache et al in which the control group included results from several pairs of ovaries containing 11 or more follicles.[13] Even by dissection of whole ovaries we have never found this many follicles in normal ovaries and therefore conclude that the Pache study may contain results from women who have ovPCO. Despite this they also found no differences in androgen or oestrogen levels between the two groups.

In a study performed with the benefit of the subclassification of PCO morphology into ovulatory or anovulatory forms and by division of follicles into groups of more or less than 5 mm in diameter (Table 5.1),[2] there were no significant differences in the median or distribution of oestradiol concentration between groups of size-matched follicles from different types of ovarian morphology. If preovulatory follicles (>12 mm) were excluded from analyses, there was no correlation of oestradiol with follicle size in any type of ovary. This supports the concept that the proportion of atretic follicles in polycystic ovaries is no higher than in normal ovaries. Interestingly, androstenedione levels were similar in all small follicles but significantly higher in 5–11 mm diameter follicles from ovPCO than in either of the other morphologies, indicating an increase in the proportion of atretic follicles in this subgroup.

Androgens other than androstenedione and testosterone may be more important in the pathophysiology of PCO, in that the concentration of 5α-reduced androgens was higher in follicular fluid and serum from this group.[14] This is important because 5α-androstane-3,17-dione has been demonstrated to be a competitive inhibitor of aromatase.[15] In whole follicle studies the total 5α-reductase activity was approximately four times higher in PCOS than in

Table 5.1 Steroid levels in follicular fluid

Follicle size (mm)	Normal (ng/ml)	AnovPCO (ng/ml)	OvPCO (ng/ml)
Oestradiol			
<5	57 [2.5–1613] ($n = 15$)	24 [2–3272] (26)	31 [3.3–772] (42)
5–10	63 [1–4505] (52)	34 [1–4116] (42)	39 [1–6066] (91)
Androstenedione			
<5	3121 [300–7400] (10)	1381 [97–16 000] (19)	1961 [327–26 521] (21)
5–10	1019 [15–6900][a] (44)	1606 [203–8674][b] (43)	3033 [65–18 720][c] (93)

Follicular fluid steroid concentrations in ng/ml, given as median [range] (number), in three groups of ovaries. AnovPCO, anovulatory polycystic ovaries; OvPCO, ovulatory PCO. Results are shown in follicles grouped according to size, with preovulatory follicles excluded to allow comparisons between ovulatory and anovulatory groups. There were no significant differences in the median or distribution of oestradiol results in either size group between follicles from ovaries of different morphology.
[a–c] Androstenedione was significantly higher in larger follicles from ovPCO than either normal ovaries or anovPCO (c vs a, $P < 0.0001$, c vs b, $P = 0.02$), but this difference was not seen in small follicles. There were no significant differences in androstenedione between normal and anovPCO.
From Mason et al,[2] by kind permission of the Endocrine Society.

follicles from normal ovaries.[16] It is possible therefore that the alteration in the endocrine milieu in follicles in PCO is more complex than originally thought. It is likely, however, that follicles that have ceased growing will differ in some respects from both healthy and atretic follicles in normal ovaries. Only a study in which the status of the majority of follicles in several pairs of polycystic ovaries is ascertained will be able to give the definitive answer.

Granulosa cell proliferation

There have been remarkably few studies of other indices of follicle health in PCO. Those that have been performed include investigations of cell proliferation and markers of apoptosis. Takayama et al found no difference in the proliferation rate of cells between normal and polycystic ovaries.[17] This finding is paradoxical in the light of the apparent lack of growth of these follicles. These data do, however, reinforce the idea that these structures are not atretic follicles, at least by standard criteria. One study found that the proportion of apoptotic granulosa cells was no different in follicles from ovulatory PCO from that in normal ovaries.[18] It is clear from earlier work that normal ovaries contain a preponderance of atretic follicles and that follicles from ovPCO are different in some respects to those from anovPCO.[2] Again, only by studying individual follicles will the true picture of cellular health and proliferation rate in these follicles be revealed.

THE STEROIDOGENIC DEFECT

Thecal cells

Increased circulating androgen is one of the cardinal features of polycystic ovary syndrome[19] and is present in both ovulatory and anovulatory women.[20,21] As the adrenal gland and ovary contribute similar amounts of androgen to the circulation there has been considerable debate as to the origin of these androgens. In both glands the majority of the androgen is in the form of androstenedione, with testosterone being secreted in lesser amounts and approximately 50% of the circulating testosterone being derived from peripheral conversion of androstenedione.[22,23] A number of studies have addressed the issue of the site of overproduction of androgens and although there is evidence for dysregulation of adrenal production in some women,[24] the weight of evidence points to the ovary being the primary site.[25–27] Symptoms related to excess androgen are one of the main reasons for presentation[28] and the increase in androgens has been implicated in the mechanism of anovulation. In the ovary theca cell production of progesterone and androgen from cholesterol is primarily under the control of luteinizing hormone (LH) and levels of LH have been shown to be elevated in PCOS. For this reason, it was considered that LH may be responsible for increased thecal androgen output. However, many women with PCOS do not have abnormal LH secretion,[21] indicating that although LH may be a contributing factor it is not the primary cause.

Insulin is also known to increase thecal secretion of androgens[29] and it was therefore suggested that the hyperinsulinaemia of PCO may be causing hyperandrogenism.[30] However, the finding of elevated androgen concentrations in women with ovPCO,[20,21] a group in whom insulin sensitivity tends to be normal, indicates that (as for LH) insulin-stimulated androgen production adds to the hyperandrogenism, but is not the primary cause.

It is possible that the increase in ovarian androgens seen in women with polycystic ovary syndrome is simply due to the increased number of follicles in these ovaries and the presence of thecal hyperplasia. Preliminary studies of androgen production by thecae from normal or polycystic ovaries incubated as explants indicated that the production of androstenedione was higher per milligram of tissue. In order to make valid comparisons between equal numbers of thecal cells isolated from normal or polycystic ovaries a method of primary theca-cell monolayer culture was developed.[31] This enzymatic dispersion of the tissue into single cells overcame the problems of well-to-well variation seen with the explants and also allowed the comparative effects of LH on these cells to be studied.

Tissue from size-matched pools of follicles from nine pairs of PCO and five pairs of normal ovaries was dispersed and cultured with or without LH. Comparison of the results demonstrated that accumulation of androstenedione was approximately 20 times higher in the thecae from PCO than in the normal group. Production of 17α-hydroxyprogesterone (17-OHP) was also significantly higher than normal (median 7-fold) suggesting increased activity of both 17α-hydroxylase and 17,20-lyase. These studies confirmed clinical data showing increased androgen production in women with PCO and regular cycles, in that thecal androgen production was also increased above normal in this group. This finding is important because it indicates that raised androgen levels cannot be the primary cause of anovulation. Responses to LH were of similar magnitude in all of the theca cultures. Thus, increased 17α-hydroxylase/17,20-lyase activity appears to be an intrinsic characteristic of thecal cells from polycystic ovaries.

These results explain those obtained in vivo[32,33] and support the hypothesis that there is abnormal regulation of key steroidogenic enzymes in PCO. Investigation of steroid enzyme gene expression in thecae from normal and polycystic ovaries has confirmed that increased CYP11a (cholesterol side-chain cleavage enzyme) and CYP17 (17α-hydroxylase/17,20-lyase) messengerRNA expression are intrinsic properties of thecal cells from anovulatory PCO.[34] Both LH and insulin will cause thecal androgen production to be further raised in women with these biochemical abnormalities, creating a spectrum of raised androgen levels in serum.

Genetic studies have indicated that there may be a link between CYP11a and some women with PCO,[35] but CYP17 as a causative gene has been ruled out.[36] Further candidate genes need to be investigated using large, well-characterized families if the genetics of this condition are to be unravelled, but it appears that the final expression of the syndrome may be the result of a combination of several gene defects and external influences.

Stromal cells

As the stroma in polycystic ovaries is also a source of androgen and the volume of stroma is greatly increased, this will be a further contributing factor. Interestingly, the ubiquitous effects of insulin on ovarian function even extend to this tissue. Enzymatic dispersion of stromal tissue into single cells was performed to investigate the mechanism of this increase in stromal volume. Physiological levels of insulin were found to increase cell proliferation and the effect was dose-dependent.[37] Androstenedione production by stromal cells in culture also increased in response to insulin. These results, in combination with those seen in thecal cells, illustrate how hyperinsulinaemia in PCOS contributes to abnormal ovarian function and emphasize the importance of minimizing insulin resistance in these women.

Granulosa cells

In conjunction with studies on follicular health, there have been a number of investigations of the steroidogenic capacity of granulosa cells from polycystic ovaries.[38,39] These studies have often been limited by the lack of availability of such tissue, but were generally conducted to reveal the developmental stage of the follicles and to gain insight into the possible mechanism of anovulation. Our interest stemmed primarily from the latter and the possibility that there was an intrinsic defect in the ability of granulosa cells from polycystic ovaries to respond to follicle-stimulating hormone (FSH).[40] Experiments were performed in granulosa cells pooled from follicles from each of 11 pairs of normal ovaries and 7 pairs of anovulatory polycystic ovaries. The ages of the patients and the sizes of the follicles in each pool were matched, with all follicles larger than 11 mm being excluded. Measurement of oestradiol accumulation in the

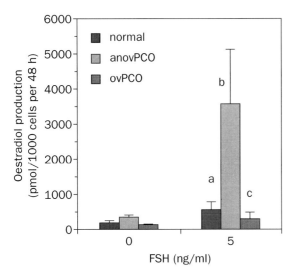

Figure 5.2 Oestradiol production in response to testosterone alone or with the addition of 5 ng/ml FSH by granulosa cells pooled from follicles of less than 12 mm in diameter from individual patients. Normal $n = 15$, anovPCO $n = 7$, ovPCO $n = 9$. There was a significant increase above normal and ovPCO in oestradiol production in response to FSH by cells from anovPCO. The response by ovPCO was generally lower than that of normal ovaries, although this did not reach significance: a vs b, $P = 0.03$; b vs c, $P = 0.01$; a vs c, $P = 0.09$.

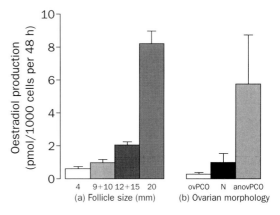

Figure 5.3 Oestradiol response to FSH by granulosa cells. (a) In individual or pooled follicles of similar size from normal ovaries. Each bar represents the mean and standard error (SE) of triplicate wells. (b) In follicles of less than 10 mm in diameter from ovaries of the three morphologies. Bars represent the mean SE of experiments in individual pools of cells from ovPCO ($n = 9$), normal ($n = 15$) and anovPCO ($n = 7$).

medium revealed that cells from anovPCO were in fact hyperresponsive to FSH compared with cells from normal ovaries, with 6–10 times more oestradiol being produced across the dose response (Figure 5.2).[2] The magnitude of this response was similar to that found in cells from preovulatory follicles from normal ovaries (Figure 5.3). In contrast, the response by granulosa cells from ovPCO ($n = 9$) was much reduced and resembled responses found in cells from atretic follicles. It became clear when the follicular fluid steroid content was analysed that the follicles in the latter were indeed primarily atretic. These experiments were the first indication that follicular function may be different in ovulatory and anovulatory PCO and that further

investigation of these differences may be helpful in elucidating the mechanism of anovulation.

Subsequent genetic studies revealed that there is no intrinsic defect in the aromatase gene in these women,[36] and so attention once again focused on insulin. Interestingly, it is primarily women with anovulation who are the most insulin-resistant and therefore have the highest levels of serum insulin to compensate.[20] Granulosa cells respond to insulin by increasing steroidogenesis[29] and (at least in terms of steroid output) granulosa cells from polycystic ovaries appeared to be spared the insulin resistance seen in other tissues in these women.[41] The effects of hyperinsulinaemia on the granulosa cell could therefore contribute to the paradoxical increase in response to FSH by granulosa cells from the anovulatory group.

A study which investigated these results in more detail has shed some light on the findings. Almahbobi et al[18] performed FSH-binding studies on granulosa cells collected as a by-product of the process of follicular aspiration for oocyte maturation. Ovarian morphology was assigned in the same way as in our study, enabling direct comparisons to be drawn. Interestingly, the cells from anovPCO showed increased FSH binding compared with both ovPCO and normal cells. It was not determined whether this was due to increased receptor number or increased binding affinity. The reason for the apparent increase is unknown.

MECHANISM OF ANOVULATION

The role of FSH

Although the levels of FSH in anovPCO are slightly lower than normal early to mid-follicular phase levels, they do not appear to be low enough to cause failure of follicle selection. Erickson suggested that the passage of FSH into the follicle may be impeded by the basal lamina in these follicles.[42] Measurement of follicular fluid levels of FSH has not shown convincing differences, but these studies are open to the criticism that follicular fluid was pooled or the assays lacked sensitivity.[2,43] The structure of the basal lamina in PCOS has not been studied in a systematic way, but it could be postulated that thickening occurs in response to the increased androgens or the hyperinsulinaemia. It is clear that raising the serum level of FSH in these women can induce follicle growth, but the exact role of FSH in anovulation in PCOS requires further investigation.

The role of paracrine factors

There seemed to be something of a paradox in the finding that granulosa cells from anovPCO were very responsive to FSH and yet in vivo the follicles did not grow to preovulatory sizes. It appeared likely that an endogenous inhibitor of aromatase was present, the effect of which was removed when the cells were placed in culture. The presence and production of a wide range of other endocrine and paracrine factors has been investigated in an attempt to explain the abnormal steroidogenesis and failure of ovulation seen in PCO.[40] The possible involve-

ment of these factors is discussed in a review by Giudice et al[44] and in Chapter 8. Although clear differences in a number of factors can be seen between healthy, oestrogen-dominant follicles and follicles from polycystic ovaries, it is difficult to determine if these changes could be responsible for the apparent cessation of follicle growth, or occur because the follicle has stopped growing.

The role of follistatin

A report concerning the activin binding protein follistatin has renewed interest in the role of paracrine factors in PCOS.[45] A multicentred group investigated 37 candidate genes for linkage with PCOS in 150 families and found the strongest link to be with the follistatin gene. As follistatin had previously been on the list of suspects for the failure of follicle growth in PCOS, a number of previous studies had investigated the levels and expression patterns in the ovary. Intriguingly, follistatin is involved in ovarian steroid, pancreatic insulin and pituitary FSH production[46] and so could have a causative role in all of the defects associated with PCOS. Although there is ample evidence of a role for activin and follistatin as paracrine modulators of ovarian function,[47] no differences in the levels of follistatin were found in follicular fluid from healthy, atretic or polycystic ovaries[48] and no changes were found in circulating levels through the menstrual cycle.[49] Even in granulosa cells aspirated from follicles from normal ovaries there was no relationship between follicle size and follistatin mRNA.[50] Interestingly, follistatin mRNA was entirely absent from sections of PCO examined by in situ hybridization compared with normal ovaries.[51] Further work is required to elucidate the activin/follistatin system in the normal ovary to reliably assess changes in this system in the polycystic ovary.

The 'premature luteinization' theory

In the morphologic study by Hughesden there was a suggestion that 'some factor possibly promotes early follicle ripening'. The data showing oestradiol responses to FSH similar to those in dominant follicles in combination with cessation of follicle growth indicate that follicles in anovPCO could be undergoing premature luteinization. A series of experiments by Willis et al provided some direct evidence that this may be the case. In these experiments granulosa cells were exposed to the levels of insulin found in women with PCOS and insulin resistance. It is known that both compartments of the follicle respond to insulin by increasing steroid output and – unlike other tissues in the anovPCO – the ovary does not appear to be insulin-resistant, at least in terms of steroidogenesis. Although preincubation with insulin slightly increased the sensitivity of these cells to FSH, the response to LH was significantly increased.[41] The mechanism of this differential sensitization is unknown.

Further experiments performed in granulosa cells collected from a series of individual follicles revealed that whereas granulosa cells from normal ovaries did not respond to FSH until the follicle was 9.5 mm in diameter, granulosa cells from anovPCO were LH-responsive in follicles of 4 mm.[52] This might have the effect of prematurely initiating events seen normally at the time of the mid-cycle LH surge, namely increased progesterone production and cessation of follicle growth. It was suggested that raised intrafollicular levels of insulin, in combination with the often raised circulating levels of LH in these patients, caused this premature luteinization of the follicles. The demonstration by Almahbobi et al[18] that there was increased FSH binding in the granulosa cells from anovPCO, however, may mean that they were more likely to acquire LH receptors during the 48 hours of culture. The presence of LH receptors in granulosa cells in small follicles from PCOS has not yet been demonstrated.

CONCLUSION

The mechanism of the increase in follicle number in polycystic ovaries remains elusive, but the majority of data indicate that follicle growth is abnormal from the earliest stages. An additional disturbance may be involved in increasing follicle numbers further in anovPCO than in ovPCO because retarded growth is combined with arrested development, possibly preventing the normal process of atresia. This idea is supported by evidence that the preponderance of structures in anovPCO are functional follicles rather than atretic cysts, whereas follicles in ovPCO are primarily atretic, analogous to the situation in the normal ovary. There is an intrinsic defect in the expression of the genes encoding for steroidogenic enzymes, in particular *CYP17*, in thecae from both ovPCO and anovPCO, but the serum levels of androgen tend to be higher in anovulatory women, suggesting that there may be a link between the intraovarian concentration and anovulation. The mechanism of anovulation is still a matter of debate. Granulosa cells from anovPCO were hyperresponsive to FSH and this, in combination with the finding of LH responsiveness in small follicles from anovPCO, has led to the suggestion that these follicles are prematurely luteinized. The finding that follistatin gene regulation may be abnormal in women with PCOS may provide a new insight into the function of these ovaries. Elucidation of the precise nature of this defect may provide the key to understanding the apparent contradiction of increased steroidogenesis in the face of abnormal and arrested follicle growth.

REFERENCES

1 Adams J, Polson DW, Abdulwahid N et al. Multifollicular ovaries: clinical and endocrine features and response to pulsatile gonadotrophin releasing hormone. *Lancet* (1985) **ii**: 1375–8.

2 Mason HD, Willis DS, Beard RW, Winston RML, Margara R, Franks S. Estradiol production by granulosa cells of normal and polycystic ovaries (PCO): relationship to menstrual cycle history and to concentrations of gonadotrophins and sex steroids in follicular fluid. *J Clin Endocrinol Metab* (1994) **791**: 1355–60.

3 Hughesden PE. Morphology and morphogenesis of the Stein–Leventhal ovary and of so-called

'Hyperthecosis'. Review. *Obstet Gynaecol Surv* (1982) **37**: 59–77.

4 McNatty KP. Hormonal correlates of follicular development in the human ovary. *Aust J Biol Sci* (1981) **34**: 249–68.

5 Tilly JL. Apoptosis and ovarian function. *Rev Reprod* (1996) **1**: 162–72.

6 Joseph-Horne R, Mason HD, Batty SC et al. Luteal phase progesterone excretion in ovulatory women with polycystic ovaries. *J Endocrinol* (1998) **156**(suppl.): P263.

7 Polson DW, Adams J, Wadsworth J, Franks S. Polycystic ovaries – a common finding in normal women. *Lancet* (1988) **i**: 870–2.

8 Short RV, London DR. Defective biosynthesis of ovarian steroids in the Stein–Leventhal syndrome. *Br Med J* (1961) **i**: 1724–7.

9 Axelrod LR, Goldzeiher JW. The polycystic ovary III. Steroid biosynthesis in normal and polycystic ovarian tissue. *Clin Endocrinol* (1962) **22**: 431–40.

10 Goldzeiher JW, Axelrod LR. Polycystic ovarian disease. *Fertil Steril* (1981) **35**: 371–94.

11 McNatty KP, More-Smith D, Makris A, Osathanondh R, Ryan KJ. The microenvironment of the human follicle: interrelationships among the steroid levels in antral fluid, the population of granulosa cells and the status of the oocyte in vivo and in vitro. *J Clin Endocrinol Metab* (1979) **49**: 851–60.

12 McNatty KP, Baird DT. Relationship between follicle-stimulating hormone, androstenedione and oestradiol in human follicular fluid. *J Endocrinol* (1978) **76**: 527.

13 Pache T, Hop WCJ, de Jong FH et al. 17β Oestradiol, androstenedione and inhibin levels in fluid from individual follicles of normal and polycystic ovaries, and in ovaries from androgen treated female to male transsexuals. *Clin Endocrinol (Oxf)* (1992) **36**: 565–71.

14 Agarwal SK, Judd HL, Magoffin DA. A mechanism for the suppression of estrogen production in the polycystic ovary syndrome. *J Clin Endocrinol Metab* (1996) **81**: 3686–91.

15 Hillier SG, van den Boogard AM, Reichert LE, van Hall EV. Alterations in granulosa cell aromatase activity accompanying preovulatory follicular development in the rat ovary with evidence that 5α-reduced C19 steroids inhibit the aromatase reaction in vitro. *J Endocrinol* (1980) **84**: 409–19.

16 Jakimiuk AJ, Weitsman SR, Magoffin DA. 5α-reductase activity in women with polycystic ovary syndrome. *J Clin Endocrinol Metab* (1999) **84**: 2414–18.

17 Takayama K, Fukaya T, Sasano H et al. Immunohistochemical study of steroidogenesis and cell proliferation in polycystic ovarian syndrome. *Hum Reprod* (1996) **11**: 1387–92.

18 Almahbobi G, Anderiesz C, Hutchinson P, McFarlane JR, Wood C, Trounson AO. Functional integrity of granulosa cells from polycystic ovaries. *Clin Endocrinol* (1996) **44**: 571–80.

19 Stein IF, Leventhal ML. Amenorrhoea associated with bilateral polycystic ovaries. *Am J Obstet Gynecol* (1935) **29**: 181–91.

20 Conway GS, Honour JW, Jacobs HS. Heterogeneity of the polycystic ovary syndrome; clinical, endocrine and ultrasound features in 556 patients. *Clin Endocrinol* (1989) **30**: 459–70.

21 Franks S. Review. Polycystic ovary syndrome: a changing perspective. *Clin Endocrinol* (1989) **31**: 87–120.

22 Kirschner MA, Bardin W. Androgen production and metabolism in normal and virilised women. *Metabolism* (1972) **21**: 667–88.

23 Vermeulin A. The androgens. In: Gray CH, James VHT, eds, *Hormones in Blood* 3 (Academic Press: London, 1979) 355–416.

24 McKenna TJ, Cunningham SK. Testing for adrenal abnormalities in polycystic ovary syndrome. In: Filicori M, Flamigni C, eds, *The Ovary: Regulation, Dysfunction and Treatment* (Elsevier: Amsterdam, 1996) 295–301.

25 Chang RJ, Laufer LR, Meldrum DR et al. Steroid secretion in polycystic ovarian disease after ovarian suppression by a long-acting gonadotrophin-releasing agonist. *J Clin Endocrinol Metab* (1983) **56**: 897–903.

26 Erickson GF, Magoffin DA, Dyer CA, Hofeditz C. The ovarian androgen producing cells; a review of structure/function relationships. *Endocr Rev* (1985) **6**: 371–99.

27 Polson DW, Reed MJ, Franks S, Scanlon MJ, James VHT. (1988) Serum 11-hydroxyandrostenedione as an indicator of the source of excess androgen production in women with polycystic ovaries. *J Clin Endocrinol Metab* **66**: 946–50.

28 Yen SCC. The polycystic ovary syndrome. *Clin Endocrinol* (1980) **12**: 177–207.

29 Garzo VG, Dorrington JH. Aromatase activity in human granulosa cells during follicular development and the modulation by follicle stimulating hormone and by insulin. *Am J Obstet Gynecol* (1984) **148**: 657–62.

30 Poretsky L, Kalin MF. The gonadotropic function of insulin. *Endocr Rev* (1987) **8**: 132–45.

31 Gilling-Smith C, Willis DS, Beard RW et al. Hypersecretion of androstenedione by isolated thecal cells from polycystic ovaries. *J Clin Endocrinol Metab* (1994) **79**: 1158–65.

32 Rosenfield RL, Barnes RB, Cara JF, Lucky AW. Dysregulation of cytochrome P450c 17α as the cause of polycystic ovarian syndrome. *Fertil Steril* (1990) **53**: 785–91.

33 White DM, Leigh A, Wilson C, Franks S. Gonadotrophin and gonadal steroid response to a single dose of a long-acting agonist of gonadotrophin-releasing hormone in ovulatory and anovulatory women with polycystic ovary syndrome. *Clin Endocrinol* (1995) **42**: 475–81.

34 Nelson VL, Legro RS, Strauss JF, McAllister JM. Augmented androgen production is a stable steroidogenic phenotype of propagated theca cells from polycystic ovaries. *Molec Endocrinol* (1999) **13**: 946–57.

35 Gharani N, Waterworth DM, Batty S et al. Association of the steroid synthesis gene CYP11a with polycystic ovary syndrome and hyperandrogenism. *Hum Molec Genet* (1997) **6**: 397–402.

36 Gharani N, Waterworth DM, Williamson R, Franks S. 5' polymorphism of the CYP17 gene is not associated with serum testosterone levels in women with polycystic ovaries [letter]. *J Clin Endocrinol Metab* (1996) **81**: 4174.

37 Watson H, Willis D, Mason HD, Wright C, Franks S. Comparison of the effects of insulin and insulin-like growth factor binding protein-1 (IGF) on ovarian stromal cell growth. *J Endocrinol* (1997) **152**(suppl.): P240.

38 Erickson GF, Hsueh AJW, Quigley ME, Rebar RW, Yen SS. Functional studies of aromatase activity in human granulosa cells from normal and polycystic ovaries. *J Clin Endocrinol Metab* (1979) **49**: 514–18.

39 McNatty KP, Moore-Smith D, Makris A et al. The intraovarian sites of androgen and estrogen formation in women with normal and hyperandrogenic ovaries as judged by in vitro experiments. *J Clin Endocrinol Metab* (1980) **50**: 755–63.

40 Franks S, Mason HD. Polycystic ovary syndrome: interaction of follicle stimulating hormone and polypeptide growth factors in oestradiol production by human granulosa cells. *J Steroid Biochem Mol Biol* (1991) **40**: 1–3, 405–9.

41 Willis DS, Mason HD, Gilling-Smith C, Franks S. Modulation by insulin of follicle stimulating hormone and luteinising hormone actions in human granulosa cells of normal and polycystic ovaries. *J Clin Endocrinol Metab* (1996) **81**: 302–9.

42 Erickson GF, Magoffin DA, Gabriel Garzo V, Cheung AP, Chang RJ. Granulosa cells of normal and polycystic ovaries: are they normal or abnormal? *Hum Reprod* (1992) **7**: 293–9.

43 Erickson G, Yen SCC. New data on follicle cells in polycystic ovaries: a proposed mechanism for the genesis of cystic follicles. *Semin Reprod Endocrinol* (1984) **2**: 231–43.

44 Giudice LC, Morales AJ, Yen SS. Growth factors and polycystic ovarian syndrome. *Semin Reprod Endocrinol* (1996) **14**: 3 203–8.

45 Urbanek M, Legro RS, Driscoll DA et al. Thirty-seven candidate genes for polycystic ovary syndrome: strongest evidence for linkage is with follistatin. *Proc Natl Acad Sci USA* (1999) **96**(15): 8573–8.

46 de Kretser DM, Phillips DJ. Mechanisms of protein feedback on gonadotrophin secretion. *J Reprod Immunol* (1998) **39**: 1–12.

47 Peng C, Ohno T, Khorasheh S, Leung PC. Activin and follistatin as local regulators in the human ovary. *Biol Sign* (1996) **5**: 81–9.

48 Erickson GF, Chung DG, Sit A, DePaolo LV, Shimasaki S, Ling N. Follistatin concentrations in follicular fluid of normal and polycystic ovaries. *Hum Reprod* (1995) **10**: 2120–4.

49 Khoury RH, Wang QF, Crowley WF et al. Serum follistatin levels in women: evidence against an endocrine function of ovarian follistatin. *J Clin Endocrinol Metab* (1995) **80**: 1361–8.

50 Schneyer AL. Intrafollicular inhibin/activin/follistatin in maturing human follicles across the normal menstrual cycle: comparison to PCOS follicles. *Proceedings of the 81st Meeting of the Endocrine Society*, San Diego 1999, S45–2.

51 Roberts VJ, Barth S, el-Roeiy A, Yen SS. Expression of inhibin/activin system messenger ribonucleic acids and proteins in ovarian follicles from women with polycystic ovarian syndrome. *J Clin Endocrinol Metab* (1994) **79**: 1434–9.

52 Willis DS, Mason HD, Watson H, Brincat M, Galea R, Franks S. Premature response to LH of granulosa cells from anovulatory women with PCOS: Relevance to mechanism of anovulation. *J Clin Endocrinol Metab* (1998) **83**: 3984–91.

6

Mechanism of hyperandrogenism

Robert L Rosenfield

Recent research suggests that most hyperandrogenism arises from abnormal regulation (dysregulation) of ovarian and adrenal androgen secretion and that insulin excess may be involved.[1,2] This chapter reviews this evidence as it pertains to polycystic ovary syndrome (PCOS).

THE OVARIAN SECRETORY ABNORMALITY IN PCOS

Classic polycystic ovary syndrome is a form of functional ovarian hyperandrogenism (FOH) which is usually due to dysregulation of ovarian androgen secretion.

FOH in classic PCOS

It is proposed that polycystic ovary syndrome is a form of FOH.[3,4] The model shown in Figure 6.1 hypothesizes that FOH is initiated by any disorder that causes a large increase in intraovarian androgens. This leads to hyperandrogenemia, which is responsible for the pilosebaceous manifestations of the syndrome.

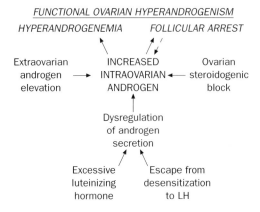

Figure 6.1 Model of the pathogenesis of functional ovarian hyperandrogenism. An increased intraovarian androgen concentration is central. It causes hyperandrogenemia, and the great local androgen excess promotes follicular maturation arrest which leads follicles to prematurely commit to follicular atresia. Increased intraovarian androgen concentration also may be caused by follicular atresia. Additional causes of increased intraovarian androgen levels include extraovarian virilizing disorders, ovarian steroidogenic blocks, and dysregulation of androgen secretion. The latter may result from LH excess or from augmentation of LH action by insulin, insulin-like growth factors (IGFs) and other peptides. Reproduced with permission from Rosenfield.[2]

It also causes follicular maturation arrest, which leads follicles to undergo atresia prior to the emergence of dominance, thus the anovulatory symptoms.

Several mechanisms may cause intraovarian androgen excess and hence secondary PCOS. *Arrest of follicular maturation* makes follicles androgenic by default because they lack aromatase. Consequently, follicular atresia contributes to increased intraovarian androgen concentration and potentially may initiate a vicious cycle which perpetuates ovarian androgen excess. Theoretically, processes leading to excessive follicular atresia could cause the syndrome, but have not been identified. *Frankly masculinizing extraovarian* states are known to bring about the morphology of PCOS, thecal hyperplasia and ovarian hyperandrogenism. This occurs most often in poorly controlled, virilizing congenital adrenal hyperplasia. *Steroidogenic blocks* also cause the PCOS picture. Disorders such as 3β-hydroxysteroid dehydrogenase (3β), 17β-oxidoreductase or aromatase deficiency hinder the formation of estrogen and lead to a predominance of androgen over estrogen within the ovary.

However, the vast majority of PCOS cases arise without an obvious cause (primary PCOS) and have an ovarian secretory abnormality, revealed by a test of coordinated ovarian function.[4] When women are given a single dose of a potent gonadotropin releasing hormone (GnRH) agonist such as nafarelin, a premature surge of luteinizing hormone (LH) and follicle-stimulating hormone (FSH) takes place which is of preovulatory magnitude and normally efficiently stimulates estrogen secretion (Figure 6.2, Table 6.1).[5,6]

Patients with classic PCOS (hyperandrogenism with LH and/or ultrasonographic abnormality) have a characteristic ovarian secretory response to gonadotropin stimulation which differs from that expected from any known enzyme block. Plasma 17-hydroxyprogesterone levels rise excessively in the vast majority of patients with classic PCOS (Figure 6.2). The intermediates from this point in the biosynthetic path onwards hyperrespond: androstenedione particularly, testos-

terone less so yet significantly, estrone and estradiol marginally. There is a slightly excessive rise in 3β-hydroxy intermediates. Similar 17-hydroxyprogesterone hyperresponsiveness to challenge with the LH analogue human chorionic gonadotropin has been reported.[7]

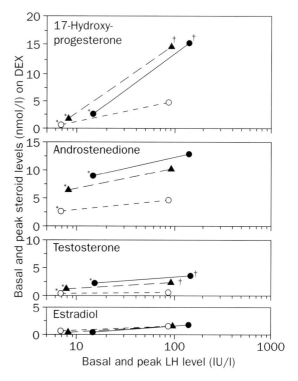

Figure 6.2 Gonadotropin releasing hormone agonist (nafarelin) tests after dexamethasone (DEX) pretreatment in women with FOH (classic PCOS, solid circles; nonclassic PCOS, triangles) and normal women (open circles). Baseline and peak blood levels of LH are plotted against these respective parameters for steroids. Baseline 17-hydroxyprogesterone, androstenedione, and testosterone levels differ among groups independently of LH according to analysis of covariance (*, $P < 0.05$). The apparent slopes of the LH–17-hydroxyprogesterone and LH–testosterone dose–response curves (Δsteroid/ΔLH) are significantly greater in both types of FOH than normal (†, $P < 0.05$). Modified with permission from Rosenfield et al.[6]

Table 6.1 Estradiol precursor steroids and steroid ratios during dexamethasone-suppressed nafarelin tests (mean ± SEM). Modified with permission from Rosenfield et al[6]

Group	Progesterone		17-Hydroxypregnenolone		DHA		Baseline ratios				Ratio of rises	
	Basal (nmol/l)	Rise (Δ) (nmol/l)	Basal (nmol/l)	Rise (Δ) (nmol/l)	Basal (nmol/l)	Rise (Δ) (nmol/l)	E_2/T	AD/DHA	17PROG/ PROG	T/AD	$\Delta E_2/\Delta T$	$\Delta AD/\Delta 17PROG$
Normal (n = 18)	0.23 ± 0.04	1.52 ± 0.40	0.36[a,c] ± 0.03	0.79[a,b] ± 0.09	2.38[c] ± 0.17	0.70 ± 0.20	1.32[a,b] ± 0.42	1.18[e,f] ± 0.10	4.05[a] ± 0.84	0.15[a] ± 0.02	5.84[a,b] ± 1.37	0.50[a,b] ± 0.05
FOH, LH high (n = 19)	0.45 ± 0.08	3.00 ± 0.42	0.81[c] ± 0.08	1.65[a] ± 0.23	3.97[c] ± 0.31	1.34 ± 0.31	0.15[a] ± 0.02	2.31[e] ± 0.18	13.3[e] ± 4.35	0.28[a] ± 0.03	2.14[b] ± 0.53	0.30[a] ± 0.04
FOH, LH normal (n = 18)	0.50 ± 0.14	2.74 ± 0.53	0.61[a] ± 0.06	1.69[b] ± 0.35	3.07 ± 0.30	1.83 ± 0.80	0.17[b] ± 0.03	2.41[f] ± 0.21	6.15 ± 0.84	0.24 ± 0.02	3.85[a] ± 1.98	0.29[b] ± 0.07
ANOVA	NS	<0.01	<0.001	<0.001	<0.01	NS	<0.002	<0.001	<0.05	<0.005	<0.003	<0.05

Significant differences exist among values designated by same superscript for a given parameter: [a,b]$P < 0.05$; [c,d]$P < 0.01$; [e,f]$P < 0.001$.
Abbreviations: AD, androstenedione; DHA, dehydroepiandrosterone; E_2, estradiol; FOH, functional ovarian hyperandrogenism; LH, luteinizing hormone; NS, not significant; PROG, progesterone; 17PROG, 17-hydroxyPROG; T, testosterone.

Dysregulation (abnormal regulation) of androgen secretion appears to account for this abnormality. This is particularly prominent at the level of 17-hydroxylase and 17,20-lyase activities, which are to a great extent two distinct activities of a single enzyme, cytochrome P450c17.

FOH in nonclassic PCOS

Classically PCOS patients with polycystic ovaries have gonadotropin abnormalities: LH is elevated or there is early LH hyperresponsiveness (at 0.5–1.0 hr) and FSH is low or hyporesponsive to GnRH agonist stimulation. However, this is not always the case. Furthermore, the ovarian dysfunction occurs independently of the gonadotropin abnormality.[6–9]

Functional ovarian hyperandrogenism due to a PCOS-like type of ovarian dysfunction is equally likely to occur with or without the classic ultrasonic or gonadotropic criteria for the diagnosis of PCOS. In a prospective study of hyperandrogenic women, the response of 17-hydroxyprogesterone to nafarelin correlated well with the free testosterone level after dexamethasone suppression of adrenal fraction ($r = 0.75$), with 85% concordance between the two tests.[4] This indicates that the GnRH agonist test and the dexamethasone androgen suppression test reflect related aspects of ovarian function. These two tests are nearly twice as sensitive for the diagnosis of FOH as gonadotropin or ultrasound criteria for PCOS. Approximately two-thirds of women with FOH identified by these tests have chronic hyperandrogenemia with oligomenorrhea. Thus, nonclassic PCOS resembles classic PCOS clinically as well as biochemically.

Therefore, the model (Figure 6.1) proposes that PCOS may arise from either LH excess or from escape from desensitization (downregulation) to LH stimulation. The latter may, as discussed below, be related to excessive production of insulin or intraovarian growth factors, such as insulin-like growth factor (IGF).

The ovarian secretory abnormality in PCOS/FOH as escape from downregulation

To elucidate the basis of ovarian dysregulation, an analysis was made of apparent LH–steroid dose–response relationships during nafarelin tests performed with concurrent dexamethasone administration to suppress coincidental adrenal steroid secretion.[6] The pattern of steroid secretion was similarly abnormal in classic and nonclassic PCOS, that is, whether or not serum LH levels were high (Figure 6.2).

Baseline 17-hydroxyprogesterone, androstenedione and testosterone levels differed among the groups. Abnormalities in these steroid concentrations were most severe in the high LH group, but were independent of LH levels. Baseline plasma estradiol concentration was slightly elevated in the classic PCOS group (268 pmol/l versus 235 pmol/l, $P < 0.05$), which appeared to be a function of their elevated serum LH levels.

Following nafarelin administration, the responses of estradiol in FOH patients fell along the normal LH–steroid dose–response slope, but those of estradiol precursors did not. The apparent slope of the LH–steroid dose–response relationship was markedly abnormal for 17-hydroxyprogesterone, above but parallel to normal for androstenedione, and slightly increased for testosterone in both types of PCOS. Table 6.1 shows that there were also increased levels or responses of all the other steroids studied beyond pregnenolone, but for each they were inconsistent (e.g. dehydroepiandrosterone), only marginally significant (e.g. progesterone), or modest (e.g. 17-hydroxypregnenolone).

Analysis of product/precursor ratios of plasma steroid levels (Table 6.1) was compatible with increased 17-hydroxylase activity (17PROG/PROG), 3β activity (AD/DHA), 17β-hydroxysteroid dehydrogenase activity (T/AD), and decreased aromatase activity ($\Delta E_2/\Delta T$). Although the $\Delta AD/\Delta 17PROG$ ratio was low, and thus compatible with inefficient 17,20-lyase activity, this appeared to be due to relative inefficiency rather than an absolute deficiency, since androstenedione levels were

elevated at baseline (and the high androstenedione levels are not due to a block in conversion to testosterone, the levels of which are
likewise increased in FOH).

These results were interpreted as indicating
that PCOS/FOH patients have generalized
overactivity of thecal steroidogenesis.
Steroidogenesis appears to be overactive
through the 17-hydroxylase step, leading to
excessive formation of 17-hydroxyproges-
terone. Apparent 17,20-lyase activity seems
excessive, too, but this step appears to be inefficient, which adds to the disproportionate
accumulation of 17-hydroxyprogesterone.
Testosterone formation seems to be increased,
in part because of its increased formation from
androstenedione (via 17β-hydroxysteroid dehydrogenase) and from dehydroepiandrosterone
(via 3β activity) and in part due to decreased
aromatase activity. The decrease in aromatase
activity appears to be compensatory (by negative feedback inhibition of FSH by estradiol) so
as to maintain a normal dose–response relationship between blood levels of LH and estradiol
and prevent frank hyperestrogenism. This
steroidogenic abnormality appears to be the
result of escape from normal downregulation of
precursor secretion by thecal cells, rather than
the result of overstimulation by LH, because the
steroid responses do not fall along the normal
LH–steroid dose–response curve.

Normal thecal cells are very sensitive to the
downregulating effect of LH levels (homologous desensitization) within the physiologic
range (Figure 6.3).[10,11] Maximal stimulation of
17-hydroxyprogesterone and androstenedione
in culture occurs at LH concentrations approxi-
mating the upper portion of the normal range
for serum LH levels, and a further increase in
LH dosage leads to no further rise. This resembles the situation in Leydig cells where overstimulation by LH, in a time- and dose-related
manner, initially causes downregulation of LH
receptors and cholesterol side-chain cleavage
activity, later causes downregulation of 17,20-
lyase, and finally causes downregulation of 17-
hydroxylase activities.[4] In the course of this
process, the ratio of 17-hydroxyprogesterone to
androgen production increases as LH rises into

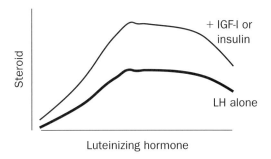

Figure 6.3 Effect of insulin or IGF on LH–steroid
dose–response curves in thecal cells. Luteinizing
hormone in the physiologic range stimulates thecal
steroid secretion. Doses above the physiologic range
– which in humans occurs at about 50 IU/l[11] –
completely desensitizes the ability of thecal cells to
respond to further increases in LH. The addition of
insulin or IGF-I to LH causes escape from this
downregulation and markedly augments steroid
production in response to LH. Reproduced with
permission from Rosenfield.[2]

the upper portion of the stimulatory range. It is
possible that the characteristic, disproportionate
17-hydroxyprogesterone response to ovarian
stimulation in PCOS/FOH is due to incipient
downregulation of 17,20-lyase at LH levels
stimulatory to 17-hydroxylation. Alternatively,
17-hydroxyprogesterone may simply accumulate in a 'metabolic cul-de-sac' because it is
inefficiently converted to androstenedione
by P450c17, which forms androstenedione
predominantly via dehydroepiandrosterone
(Figure 6.4).[4]

Thecal cells from PCOS patients in culture
have LH–steroid dose–response curves which
are displaced upwards and leftwards.[11]
Individual thecal cells secrete more steroid than
normal both at baseline and upon stimulation
with a low dose of LH. Thus, the abnormal
LH–steroid dose–response relationships both in
vivo and in vitro indicate that there is more to
the hyperandrogenism of PCOS than LH
excess.

The abnormality of the dose–response curves

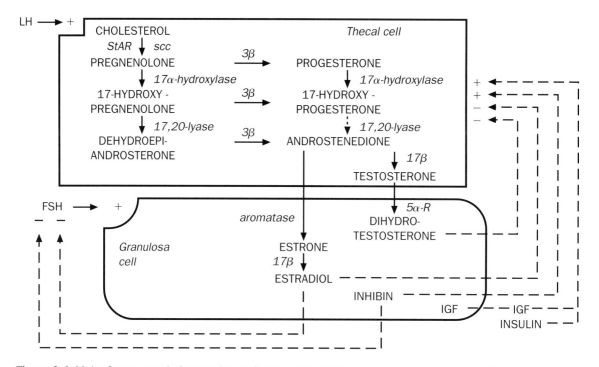

Figure 6.4 Major factors regulating ovarian androgen and estrogen secretion depicted according to the two-cell, two-gonadotropin model. Luteinizing hormone stimulates androgen formation within theca-interstitial-stromal (thecal) cells via the steroidogenic pathway common to the gonads and adrenal glands. Follicle-stimulating hormone regulates estradiol biosynthesis from androgen by granulosa cells. Long-loop negative feedback of estradiol and inhibin on gonadotropin secretion does not suppress LH at physiologic levels of estradiol. Androgen formation in response to LH appears to be modulated by intraovarian feedback at multiple levels, prominently including 17-hydroxylase and 17,20-lyase, both of which are to a great extent activities of cytochrome P450c17, and side-chain cleavage (SCC). Androgen, via dihydrotestosterone, and estradiol inhibit (minus signs) and inhibin, insulin, and insulin-like growth factors (IGF) stimulate (plus signs) enzyme activities. Other peptides probably also modulate the steroidogenic response to LH. 3β, 3β-hydroxysteroid dehydrogenase; 17β, 17β-hydroxysteroid dehydrogenase; 5α-R, 5α-reductase. Modified from Ehrmann et al,[4] with permission. StAR = steroidogenic acute regulatory protein.

in PCOS resembles the situation when normal cells are treated with insulin or IGF (see Figure 6.3). Insulin or IGF causes escape from homologous desensitization to LH. Insulin was initially reported to stimulate stromal androgen production in PCOS patients who had acanthosis nigricans, by Barbieri et al.[12] Insulin and IGF-I normally synergize with LH and augment the production of ovarian androgens in response to LH by interfering with LH-induced desensitization.[10] It is now known that IGFs and their binding proteins are produced within the ovary, as are a variety of other growth factors that modulate the steroidogenic responses to LH (see Figure 6.4).[4] The ovaries in PCOS behave as if responsive to a regulatory role of insulin or IGFs in a state of resistance to the glucose-metabolic effects of insulin. It has recently been shown that insulin itself is indeed active through its own receptor in polycystic ovaries.[13] Furthermore, reduction of insulin levels by a variety of mechanisms ameliorates the androgen excess.[14,15]

Serine phosphorylation was recently reported by Miller and colleagues to selectively increase the 17,20-lyase activity of P450c17 in forming dehydroepiandrosterone.[16] Serine phosphorylation also is known to decrease the activity of the insulin receptor. Therefore, it has been hypothesized that a single genetic defect that enhances serine phosphorylation could account for both the hyperandrogenism and the insulin resistance of PCOS. Recently, up-regulation of multiple steroidogenic enzymes has been found to be a stable characteristic of PCOS theca cells propagated in culture.[17]

Escape from downregulation – an abnormality of regulation of androgen and estrogen secretion

Androgens are a necessary evil in the ovary. Although androgens are obligate intermediates in estradiol biosynthesis, they arrest the process of follicular maturation. Therefore, androgen synthesis must be kept to the minimum necessary to optimize follicular development and prevent hyperestrogenism. This means that the synthesis of ovarian androgens needs to be coordinated with that of estrogen or some other follicular product.

There is not an efficient long-loop feedback mechanism (via pituitary LH) for regulating ovarian androgen secretion. Rather, ovarian androgen formation appears to be coordinated with estrogen formation by intraovarian mechanisms: androgen excess seems normally to be prevented primarily by downregulating the response to excessive LH stimulation (see Figure 6.4). A number of hormones and growth factors participate in the process by modulating steroidogenic responsiveness to LH. The activities of 17-hydroxylase and 17,20-lyase are major sites of this regulation. These activities are to a great extent separate functions of a single enzyme, cytochrome P450c17,[4,16] although androstenedione may be formed by other mechanisms not ordinarily considered.[18]

It appears likely that estrogen and androgen inhibit the response to LH by intraovarian negative feedback mechanisms. This inhibitory modulation of LH action seems to normally be counterbalanced by intraovarian growth factors which amplify P450c17 activities, including IGFs and inhibin, among others. Insulin is about as potent as IGFs in counteracting down-regulation.[19]

Consequently, the ovarian secretory abnormality of PCOS/FOH is postulated to be the result of the escape from the downregulatory response to LH stimulation which normally coordinates the ovarian synthesis of androgens with that of estrogens. The hyperinsulinemia of PCOS is a leading candidate as the cause of (or contributor to) the ovarian secretory abnormality in PCOS/FOH.

THE ADRENAL SECRETORY ABNORMALITY IN PCOS

Functional adrenal hyperandrogenism (FAH), glucocorticoid suppressible hyperandrogenemia with 17-ketosteroid hyperresponsiveness to adrenocorticotropic hormone (ACTH), is common in PCOS. It occurs in about 40% of FOH cases (Table 6.2). The vast majority of FAH is

Table 6.2 Relationship of adrenal to ovarian sources of androgen excess in hyperandrogenic women. Modified from Ehrmann et al,[24] with permission

	Adrenal androgens*	
	Abnormal (%)	Normal (%)
Ovarian androgens†		
Abnormal	30	40
Normal	20‡	10

* 17-ketosteroid hyperresponsiveness to ACTH.
† GnRH agonist or dexamethasone suppression test criteria.
‡ 1/40 with non-classic 21-hydroxylase deficiency.

idiopathic because less than 10% of adrenal hyperandrogenism can be incontrovertibly assigned to any well-established pathophysiologic entity, such as non-classical congenital adrenal hyperplasia (Table 6.3).[2] The cause of this primary FAH has fostered considerable debate.

Dysregulation of adrenal androgen secretion may be the mechanism that accounts for the

great majority of primary FAH. We have postulated that FAH results from abnormal regulation of 17-hydroxylase and 17,20-lyase activities, prominently involving cytochrome P450c17, in the adrenal glands (Figure 6.5), as in FOH ovaries. That is, excessive 17-ketosteroids are formed as by-products of ACTH stimulation of cortisol secretion. The evidence supporting this concept of dysregulation of adrenal steroidogenesis is as follows:

- Apparent overactivity of adrenal 17-hydroxylase/17,20-lyase is frequently associated with seeming overactivity of ovarian 17-hydroxylase/17,20-lyase. Hyperinsulinemia seems to potentiate both ACTH-stimulated 17-hydroxylase and 17,20-lyase activity, the former more prominently.[20] As in the ovary, insulin enhances the activities of these and other enzyme steps in the adrenal cortex.[21,22] These data are compatible with the concept that insulin excess causes adrenal dysregulation analogous to the ovarian dysregulation.
- The adrenal overproduction of 17-ketosteroids is associated with increased levels of the adrenarche marker dehydro-epiandrosterone sulfate in only a small minority of cases (approximately 20%), so the concept that this disorder is an exaggeration of adrenarche[23] seems unlikely.
- There is evidence of widespread but variable dysregulation of a number of aspects of corticosteroid secretion and metabolism, such as a tendency for cortisol to hyperrespond to ACTH and evidence of increased 11β-hydroxysteroid dehydrogenase activity.[4]

Most women with isolated FAH are eumenorrheic.[24] However, isolated FAH is the only secretory abnormality in about 20% of women with anovulatory hyperandrogenism. The mechanism by which adrenal androgen excess disturbs ovulation in this sizeable minority of cases is unclear. The plasma androgen levels do not seem sufficiently high to interfere directly with ovulation. Certainly the degree of elevation of plasma androgen levels is not sufficient to suppress gonadotropin levels; this requires frankly viriliz-

---

Table 6.3 Causes of female hyperandrogenism. From Rosenfield,[2] with permission

I   Functional gonadal hyperandrogenism
   A   Primary polycystic ovary syndrome/functional ovarian hyperandrogenism (ovarian dysregulation)
   B   Secondary polycystic ovary syndrome
      1   Extraovarian adrenal and pituitary disorders
      2   Ovarian steroidogenic blocks
      3   Syndromes of severe insulin resistance
   C   Hermaphroditism
   D   Chorionic gonadotropin-related
II   Functional adrenal hyperandrogenism
   A   Primary functional adrenal hyperandrogenism (adrenal dysregulation)*
   B   Congenital adrenal hyperplasia
   C   Cushing's disease
   D   Prolactin or growth hormone excess
   E   Abnormal cortisol action or metabolism
III   Peripheral androgen overproduction
   A   Obesity
   B   Idiopathic hyperandrogenism
IV   Tumoral hyperandrogenism

* Occasionally, this entity is the only abnormality in women with features of primary polycystic ovary syndrome.

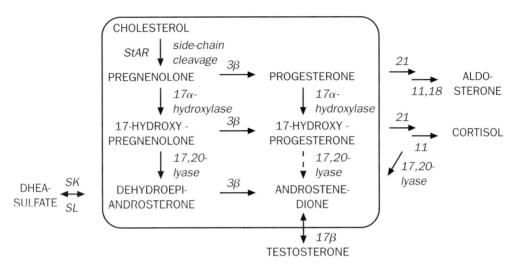

Figure 6.5 Major biosynthetic pathways in the adrenal cortex. The core pathway common to the adrenal and ovarian thecal cells is outlined. The 17-ketosteroids dehydroepiandrosterone and androstenedione are formed primarily by cytochrome P450c17, an enzyme with both 17-hydroxylase and 17,20-lyase activities. The steroidogenic enzymes are italicized. Abbreviations: 21, 21-hydroxylase; 11,18, 11β,18-hydroxylase; SK, sulfokinase; SL, sulfolyase; others as in Fig. 6.4. Modified from Rosenfield,[2] with permission.

ing amounts of androgen.[25] Perhaps heterogeneity in responsiveness to androgen accounts for the variable association of FAH with anovulation. Alternatively, one might speculate that the abnormal pulsatile release of plasma androgens subtly disturbs LH rhythmicity.[26]

Acknowledgments

These studies were supported in part by USPHS grant RR-00055. Jean Moore's expertise was essential in the preparation of the typescript.

REFERENCES

1 Rosenfield R. Ovarian secretory abnormalities in PCOS. In: Azzie R, Nestler J, Dewailly D, eds, *Androgen Excess Disorders in Women*, vol. 1 (Lippincott-Raven: Philadelphia, 1997) 303–13.

2 Rosenfield R. Current concepts of polycystic ovary syndrome. *Baillière's Clinical Obstetrics and Gynaecology* (1997) **11**: 307–33.

3 Barnes RB, Rosenfield RL. The polycystic ovary syndrome: pathogenesis and treatment. *Ann Int Med* (1989) **110**: 386–99.

4 Ehrmann DA, Barnes RB, Rosenfield RL. Polycystic ovary syndrome as a form of functional ovarian hyperandrogenism due to dysregulation of androgen secretion. *Endocr Rev* (1995) **16**: 322–53.

5 Barnes RB, Rosenfield RL, Burstein S, Ehrmann DA. Pituitary-ovarian responses to nafarelin testing in the polycystic ovary syndrome. *N Engl J Med* (1989) **320**: 559–65.

6 Rosenfield RL, Barnes RB, Ehrmann DA. Studies of the nature of 17-hydroxyprogesterone hyperresponsiveness to gonadotropin releasing hormone agonist challenge in functional ovarian hyperandrogenism. *J Clin Endocrinol Metab* (1994) **79**: 1686–92.

7 Ibañez L, Hall J, Potau N, Carrascoas A, Prat N, Taylor A. Ovarian 17-hydroxyprogesterone hyperresponsiveness to gonadotropin-releasing

hormone (GnRH) agonist challenge in women with polycystic ovary syndrome is not mediated by luteinizing hormone hypersecretion: evidence from GnRH agonist and human chorionic gonadotropin stimulation testing. *J Clin Endocrinol Metab* (1996) **81**: 4103–7.

8 Gilling-Smith C, Story H, Rogers V, Franks S. Evidence for a primary abnormality of thecal cell steroidogenesis in the polycystic ovary syndrome. *Clin Endocrinol* (1997) **47**: 93–9.

9 Arroyo A, Laughlin GA, Morales AJ, Yen SSC. Inappropriate gonadotropin secretion in polycystic ovary syndrome: influence of adiposity. *J Clin Endocrinol Metab* (1997) **82**: 3728–33.

10 Cara JF, Fan J, Azzarello J, Rosenfield RL. Insulin-like growth factor-I enhances luteinizing hormone binding to rat ovarian theca-interstitial cells. *J Clin Invest* (1990) **86**: 560–5.

11 Gilling-Smith C, Willis DS, Beard RW, Franks S. Hypersecretion of androstenedione by isolated theca cells from polycystic ovaries. *J Clin Endocrinol Metab* (1994) **79**: 1158–65.

12 Barbieri RL, Smith S, Ryan KJ. The role of hyperinsulinemia in the pathogenesis of ovarian hyperandrogenism. *Fertil Steril* (1988) **50**: 197–212.

13 Willis D, Franks S. Insulin action in human granulosa cells from normal and polycystic ovaries is mediated by the insulin receptor and not the type-I insulin-like growth factor receptor. *J Clin Endocrinol Metab* (1995) **80**: 3788–90.

14 Nestler J, Powers L, Matt D et al. A direct effect of hyperinsulinemia on serum sex-hormone binding globulin levels in obese women with the polycystic ovary syndrome. *J Clin Endocrinol Metab* (1991) **72**: 83–9.

15 Dunaif A, Scott D, Finegood D, Quintana B, Whitcomb R. The insulin-sensitizing agent troglitazone improves metabolic and reproductive abnormalities in the polycystic ovary syndrome. *J Clin Endocrinol Metab* (1996) **81**(9): 3299–306.

16 Zhang LH, Rodriguez H, Ohno S, Miller W. Serine phosphorylation of human P450c17 increases 17,20-lyase activity: implications for adrenarche and the polycystic ovary syndrome. *Proc Natl Acad Sci USA* (1995) **92**: 10 619–23.

17 Wickenheisser JK, Quinn PG, Nelson VL, Legro RS, Strauss III JF, McAllister JM. Differential activity of the cytochrome P450 17α-hydroxylase and steroidogenic acute regulatory protein gene promoters in normal and polycystic ovary syndrome theca cells. *J Clin Endocrinol Metab* (2000) **85**: 2304–11.

18 Lieberman S. Are estradiol-producing cells incompletely endowed? A chronicle of the emergence of certitude from conjecture. *Gynecol Obstet Invest* (1996) **41**: 147–72.

19 Cara JF, Rosenfield RL. Insulin-like growth factor-I and insulin potentiate luteinizing hormone-induced androgen synthesis by rat ovarian theca-interstitial cells. *Endocrinology* (1988) **123**: 733–9.

20 Moghetti P, Castello R, Negri C et al. Insulin infusion amplifies 17α-hydroxycorticosteroid intermediates response to ACTH in hyperandrogenic women: apparent relative impairment of 17,20-lyase activity. *J Clin Endocrinol Metab* (1996) **81**: 881–6.

21 Endoh A, Kristiansen S, Casson P, Buster J, Hornsby P. The zona reticularis is the site of biosynthesis of dehydroepiandrosterone and dehydroepiandrosterone sulfate in the adult human adrenal cortex resulting from its low expression of 3β-hydroxysteroid dehydrogenase. *J Clin Endocrinol Metab* (1996) **81**(10): 3558–65.

22 L'Allemand D, Penhoat A, Lebrethon MC et al. Insulin-like growth factors enhance steroidogenic enzyme and corticotropin receptor messenger ribonucleic acid levels and corticotropin steroidogenic responsiveness in cultured human adrenocortical cells. *J Clin Endocrinol Metab* (1996) **81**(11): 3892–7.

23 Lucky AW, Rosenfield RL, McGuire J, Rudy S, Helke J. Adrenal androgen hyperresponsiveness to ACTH in women with acne and/or hirsutism: adrenal enzyme defects and exaggerated adrenarche. *J Clin Endocrinol Metab* (1986) **62**: 840–8.

24 Ehrmann DA, Rosenfield RL, Barnes RB, Brigell DF, Sheikh Z. Detection of functional ovarian hyperandrogenism in women with androgen excess. *N Engl J Med* (1992) **327**: 157–62.

25 Rosenfield RL. Congenital adrenal hyperplasia and reproductive function in females. In: Flamigni C, Venturoli S, Givens J, eds, *Adolescence in Females* (Year Book: Chicago, 1985) 373–87.

26 Moll Jr G, Rosenfield RL, van Cauter E, Burstein S. Origin of episodic fluctuations of plasma testosterone in women: adrenal, ovarian, and TeBG contributions. In: Crowley WJ, Hofler J, eds, *The Episodic Secretion of Hormones* (John Wiley/Churchill Livingstone: New York, 1987) 403–14.

7

Hypersecretion of LH: effects and mechanisms

Adam Balen

Hypersecretion of luteinizing hormone (LH) occurs in approximately 40% of women who have polycystic ovaries.[1] The risk of infertility and miscarriage is raised in these patients.[1] Many reasons have been proposed for the aetiology of pituitary oversecretion of LH. These include increased pulse frequency of gonadotrophin releasing hormone (GnRH) secretion, altered pituitary sensitivity to GnRH, hyperinsulinaemic stimulation of the pituitary gland and perturbed ovarian-pituitary feedback of steroid hormones.[2] None of these hypotheses fully explains hypersecretion of LH and there is good evidence to suggest that hypersecretion of LH occurs secondary to a disturbance of non-steroidal ovarian-pituitary feedback.[2] A suggested hypothesis is that women with the polycystic ovary syndrome (PCOS) who hypersecrete LH have deficient production of an ovarian non-steroidal factor that normally inhibits LH secretion. Although this notion is attractive, the evidence to date remains inconclusive.

ADVERSE EFFECTS OF HYPERSECRETION OF LH

Inappropriate secretion of LH occurs either as tonic hypersecretion or as a 'premature' surge during ovulation induction regimens for assisted conception procedures such as in vitro fertilization (IVF). In a series of women undergoing IVF, a spontaneous, or premature, LH surge that occurred more than 12 hours before the administration of human chorionic gonadotrophin (hCG) resulted in a significant reduction in the rate of embryo cleavage.[3] Women with normal or polycystic ovaries may have a spontaneous LH surge during ovulation induction regimens, although the surge is often attenuated. Tonic hypersecretion of LH during the follicular phase of the cycle, however, only occurs in women with the PCOS.

Measurement of LH

It is important to discuss briefly the ways in which LH can be measured, as these may influence the findings of different groups. This complex heterogeneous hormone has variants that affect its amino acid sequence and oligosaccharide side chains. Since antibodies may react differently with these variants, potency estimates ('results') are critically dependent on the method used. Since the 1970s immunological methods of assay have become familiar to most clinicians and there are now more than forty commercially available kits. Broadly speaking the methods may be divided into radioimmunoassay (RIA) techniques, normally using polyclonal antisera to a highly purified human pituitary extract of LH, and two-site immunometric methods, often based on the use of monoclonal antibodies. Even when the same reference standard is used, RIAs generally give higher LH estimates than immunometric assays, particularly at low LH levels. The reason is unclear but may result from the restricted number of epitopes on the molecule that contribute to recognition by monoclonal antibodies. Recently in vitro bioassays for LH have also been applied, for example based on testosterone release by mouse Leydig cells. In general this type of bioassay gives numerical results similar to those produced by RIA.

Laboratory results of hormone assays are monitored in the UK by the National External Quality Assessment Scheme (NEQAS). Luteinizing hormone values obtained by RIA have been found to be on average 33% higher than those obtained by immunoradiometric assay (IRMA),[4] although this difference is now known to have been caused in part by miscalibration of a widely used IRMA. Conversely, measurements of serum follicle-stimulating hormone (FSH) by RIA were on average 17% lower than those obtained by IRMA. These differences have important implications for the interpretation of results, especially if the ratio of serum LH to FSH is used in the diagnosis of the PCOS.[5] The difference between the two types of assay is also illustrated by a study of women with PCOS who were given a gonadotrophin releasing hormone agonist to cause pituitary desensitization and suppression of serum LH levels prior to ovulation induction.[6] It was found that, in the same samples, LH levels were detectable when an RIA was used, but were below the limits of detection using an IRMA; it

was suggested that this was due to cross-reactivity of the RIA with free circulating alpha subunits of LH. It is therefore essential to interpret LH and FSH results against a properly determined reference range from the laboratory concerned.

Biological to immunological ratios (B:I ratios) have been used to try to circumvent these problems, although such ratios have their drawbacks and are still dependent upon the analytical systems that have been used to measure them. Exposure of the pituitary gland to different serum concentrations of steroids may affect the glycosylation and hence bioactivity of LH,[7] which in turn may influence ovarian steroid production. In contrast to this hypothesis, Fritz et al[8] found no differences between the excretion of bioactive or immunoactive LH at the time of the LH surge and observed that the surge characteristics were not influenced by physiological variations in steroid hormones.[8] Postmenopausal women have low serum concentrations of oestrogen and consequently secrete highly glycosylated LH which has a long half-life (and is found in hMG preparations).

Clinical consequences of hypersecretion of LH

It was first demonstrated in 1985 that oocytes obtained from women undergoing IVF who had a serum LH value greater than 1 standard deviation above the mean on the day of administration of hCG had a significantly reduced rate of fertilization and cleavage.[9] This relationship was confirmed in a series of 200 patients in whom elevated urinary LH excretion in the 2 days prior to hCG administration was associated with poor oocyte quality and embryo viability and reduced pregnancy rates (patients with an endogenous LH surge were excluded from the analysis).[10]

An important study of women undergoing 'natural cycle IVF' (that is, in unstimulated cycles) again found a reduction in fertilization rates in women who had elevated serum LH concentrations in either the early follicular

(45.5%) or midfollicular (50%) phase compared with an 87.5% fertilization rate in a control group who had normal serum LH concentrations.[11] In contrast to these findings, however, in a study of 596 women undergoing IVF, serum LH concentrations above either the 75th or 95th centile for more than 3 days had no significant effect on either fertilization or pregnancy rates.[12] Furthermore, another study found a closer relationship between an elevated serum progesterone concentration, but not elevated LH concentration, with respect to failure of fertilization during IVF.[13] The discrepancies between these studies may be a reflection of different study populations and are difficult to explain.

In patients with amenorrhoea undergoing treatment with pulsatile luteinizing hormone releasing hormone (LHRH) for induction of ovulation, follicular phase plasma LH concentrations were significantly higher in women with PCOS than in women with other diagnoses.[14] In an extension of this study it was found that the miscarriage rate was 33% in women with PCOS compared with 10.6% in those with hypogonadotrophic hypogonadism.[15] Furthermore, in women with PCOS there was a significantly reduced chance of conception and increased risk of miscarriage in those with an elevated follicular phase plasma LH concentration compared with those with PCOS and normal follicular phase LH levels.[15] The association of raised baseline and/or midfollicular phase plasma LH concentrations with a poor response to treatment was also demonstrated by Hamilton-Fairley et al in 100 women with PCOS who were treated with low-dose gonadotrophin therapy.[16] In this series patients with an elevated LH concentration also had a higher rate of miscarriage than the women with polycystic ovaries and normal LH levels.

In women attending a recurrent miscarriage clinic, Sagle et al reported that 82% had polycystic ovaries, as detected by ultrasound;[17] women attending that clinic were also found to have abnormalities of follicular phase LH secretion.[18] In a study of 538 patients undergoing IVF for conditions other than anovulatory infertility, polycystic ovaries were detected by ultrasound in 45.3% of those who miscarried compared with 31.4% of those with ongoing pregnancies ($P = 0.0038$).[19] A field study of 193 women planning to become pregnant showed that raised midfollicular phase serum LH concentrations were associated with both a lower conception rate (67%) and a much higher miscarriage rate (65%), compared with those in women with normal serum LH concentrations (88% and 12% respectively).[20]

In the three quoted studies of women undergoing IVF, late follicular phase LH secretion was assessed,[9,10,12] so it is difficult to make a clear distinction between tonic elevation of LH and the onset of the preovulatory LH surge, as in the study of Punnonen et al.[3] The studies of Homburg et al[15] and Regan et al,[20] however, determined pretreatment and midfollicular concentrations respectively, and so provide convincing evidence that tonic hypersecretion of LH is also detrimental to reproductive health.

Hypersecretion of LH and oocyte maturation

Luteinizing hormone leads to disruption of the processes that traverse the intercellular space between the cumulus granulosa cells and the oocyte, which results in a fall of cAMP levels within the oocyte – and hence a reduction in the 'oocyte maturation inhibitor' – and the resumption of meiosis.[21] Studies in pigs demonstrated that when ovulation was induced prematurely with hCG, there was an increase in the rate of polyspermic fertilization.[22] Moreover, delaying the insemination of rats was found to result in an increase in the number of abnormal pregnancies.[23] These findings are consistent with the notion that there is a species-specific interval between ovulation and fertilization and that if this interval is exceeded, physiologically aged oocytes are produced which may be subject to reproductive failure. An explanation of the adverse effect of hypersecretion of LH on human fertility may be that hypersecretion during the follicular phase results in an elevated concentration of intrafollicular LH which in turn results in premature oocyte maturation, with subsequent ovulation of a prematurely matured egg. Thus inappropriate release of LH may profoundly affect the timing of oocyte maturation such that the released egg is either unable to be fertilized,[15] or if fertilized miscarries.[20]

A number of alternative 'non-embryological' explanations of the association of hypersecretion of LH with reproductive disturbance have been offered. For example, it has been suggested that, rather than LH having its adverse effect upon the timing of oocyte maturation, it exerts its detrimental effect by causing over-secretion of ovarian androgens which then lead to suppressed granulosa cell function and follicular atresia. In the author's experience elevated androgen levels in women with the PCOS are associated with symptoms of hyperandrogenism (hirsutism, acne) rather than infertility, which is instead positively correlated with LH excess.[1] Furthermore, Shoham et al demonstrated that, in women treated with clomiphene citrate, high levels of LH during the follicular phase were associated with a reduced conception rate despite adequate follicular growth and corpus luteum function, as indicated by measurements of serum oestradiol concentrations in the follicular phase and of progesterone concentrations in the luteal phase.[24]

Another postulated explanation for the association of PCOS with miscarriage is an endometrial abnormality resulting from disordered prostaglandin synthesis.[25] However, a study of women treated by transfer of frozen embryos in natural cycles demonstrated no correlation between serum LH concentrations and the rates of conception and miscarriage.[26] The embryos in this study had been generated in IVF cycles in which pituitary desensitization had been used to achieve suppression of LH levels. Thus the elevated LH concentrations seen in the subsequent natural cycles of some of the women who received the frozen embryos could not have affected embryo quality and could only have exerted an effect by altering the endocrine or endometrial environments: in the event no effect on outcome was detected.

Obesity is a common finding in women with the PCOS and a moderate elevation of body mass index (BMI) to 25–27.5 kg/m^2 is associated with an increased rate of miscarriage, independent of LH levels.[27] While these factors may be important for a healthy pregnancy outcome they do not explain the reduced fertilization rates observed with oocytes removed from women with high serum LH concentrations. Thus we have concluded that it is abnormal oocyte maturation which is the main cause of reproductive failure in women who hypersecrete LH during the follicular phase of the ovulation cycle.

PROPOSED MECHANISMS OF HYPERSECRETION OF LH

The pituitary gonadotroph is central to reproductive function – its production and secretion of follicle-stimulating hormone and luteinizing hormone is directly stimulated by hypothalamic GnRH and is also influenced by integrated feedback mechanisms. Follicle-stimulating hormone provides the initial stimulus for follicular development and also promotes granulosa cell conversion of androgens to oestrogens by stimulating the aromatase enzymes. Luteinizing hormone, previously thought to be important mainly in the luteal phase by promoting progesterone secretion, also has a vital role in the follicular phase, inducing thecal androgen production (the substrate for oestrogen synthesis) and initiating oocyte maturation at mid-cycle.

Hypothalamic control of the gonadotroph

A single hypothalamic decapeptide, gonadotrophin releasing hormone, stimulates the release of both LH and FSH from the gonadotroph.[28] Pulsatile GnRH stimulation is required to maintain gonadotrophin secretion, whereas the continuous exposure of the pituitary to GnRH results in desensitization and a suppression of gonadotrophin secretion.[29] Changes in the pulsatility of GnRH are thought to alter the ratio of secretion of the two pituitary gonadotrophins throughout the menstrual cycle. When GnRH pulsatility is slow, FSH secretion predominates; when it is rapid, LH secretion predominates.[30] The action of GnRH is modulated at the level of the pituitary, thereby resulting in differential production and secretion of the two gonadotrophins. It both causes release of LH and FSH and has a self-potentiating effect on the gonadotroph.[31] The primary release of gonadotrophins and their secondary synthesis and storage have been termed the 'first pool' and 'second pool' of gonadotrophins respectively. Pituitary responsiveness to GnRH is increased by the self-priming action of GnRH, which is defined as the protein synthesis-dependent increase in GnRH-stimulated gonadotrophin secretion caused by previous exposure of the pituitary gland to GnRH.[32]

The sensitivity of the pituitary to GnRH varies during the menstrual cycle in synchrony with changes in circulating oestradiol concentrations.[33] In the early follicular phase, when oestradiol levels are low, pituitary sensitivity and gonadotrophin content are at a minimum; as oestradiol levels rise, consequent upon follicular development, both sensitivity and content increase – particularly the latter, as oestradiol has a stimulating effect on pituitary synthesis and storage and promotes the self-priming effect of GnRH on the pituitary.[33] At the time of the mid-cycle surge, sensitivity to GnRH is maximal, with the resultant release of large amounts of gonadotrophins. Oestradiol also potentiates GnRH responsiveness, increasing the number of GnRH receptors by directly stimulating the protein synthesis required for receptor formation.

The arcuate nucleus of the hypothalamus acts as a transducer for neuronal into endocrine signals, although the cellular nature of the GnRH 'pulse generator' is still unknown. Here the GnRH-secreting neurons act in a pulsatile manner, with varying frequencies throughout the normal ovulatory cycle, resulting in variable frequencies and amplitudes of gonadotrophin release. The control of the rhythmicity of the GnRH pulse generator is not fully understood. Although there does not appear to be feedback from within the pituitary itself,[34] gonadal steroids and other factors modulate GnRH action at the pituitary level, and possibly also at the level of the hypothalamus.

Some of the factors that influence GnRH activity include β-endorphin and opiate peptides, angiotensin II, serotonin, neuropeptide Y, neurotensin, somatostatin, corticotrophin releasing factor, dopamine, melatonin, noradrenaline, oxytocin and substance P. The interrelationship of these factors is unclear. Endogenous opioid tone is important in the regulation of LH and prolactin secretion. Opioids such as β-endorphin inhibit GnRH release from the human mediobasal hypothalamus. It has been postulated that withdrawal of endogenous opioid tone in the presence of sufficient quantities of oestradiol may contribute to the initiation of the LH surge. When opioid tone decreases, a chain of neurosecretory events is initiated, which, in the rat, activates neuropeptide-Y neurons which in turn, either alone or together with adrenergic transmitters, stimulate secretion of GnRH. The effects of opioids appear to be dependent upon the steroid hormone environment, in particular oestrogen, whose effect is augmented by progesterone:[35] thus the administration of an opioid antagonist, such as naloxone, during the early follicular phase has little effect on gonadotrophin levels, while greater effects are observed mid-cycle and the greatest effects are seen in the luteal phase.[36]

Circulating steroid levels also influence GnRH metabolism by altering the activity of proteolytic enzymes in the pituitary and peripheral circulation. For example, oestradiol has been shown to inhibit degradation of GnRH in rat and monkey pituitary glands and may thus enhance GnRH activity under conditions of high serum oestradiol concentrations.[37] Perhaps steroids also play such a role in women with the polycystic ovary syndrome.

Hypothalamic factors in the hypersecretion of LH

Tonic hypersecretion of LH in women with PCOS has been suggested as being caused, at least in part, by a combination of diminished opioid and dopaminergic tone.[38,39] There is also evidence that adrenergic activity is altered in women who hypersecrete LH.[40,41] Women with PCOS were found to be very sensitive to exogenous dopamine and it was proposed that these women had a deficiency in endogenous dopaminergic inhibition of GnRH secretion.[38] In normal women both dopamine receptor antagonists, such as metoclopramide, and opiate receptor antagonists, such as naloxone, elicit a rise in serum LH concentrations.[39] Conversely, administration of synthetic β-endorphin elicits a fall in serum LH concentration. In women with PCOS, the administration of metoclopramide, naloxone and β-endorphin did not alter LH secretory activity.[39] It was therefore proposed that an underlying hypothalamic defect might lead to hypersecretion of LH, through a reduction in endogenous dopaminergic and opioid control of GnRH secretion.[39]

Barnes and Lobo[42] performed naloxone infusion experiments in women with PCOS and weight-matched controls and found that LH responses were similar. Pretreatment using levodopa with carbidopa for one week resulted in an absence of naloxone-stimulated LH increase in normal women, but an exaggerated response of the rise in LH after naloxone in women with PCOS. It was suggested that central opioid tone is not decreased in PCOS and that dopaminergic tone and/or the interaction between the dopamine and opioid system might be altered in the PCOS. Further studies failed to demonstrate major alterations in brain dopaminergic activity in women with the PCOS,[43] although it is difficult to study the physiology of brain dopamine. Berga and Yen administered both progestogens and opioid antagonists to women with PCOS and found that there was an apparent link between an impairment of opioid and progesterone secretion in the genesis of hypersecretion of LH.[44] Yoshino et al studied women with PCOS and found abnormalities not only in dopamine metabolites but also in adrenergic metabolites.[41] It was also demonstrated that 4 weeks' treatment with naltrexone reduced pituitary sensitivity to GnRH in PCOS patients,[45] and so the question of the precise role of endogenous opioids in the control of LH secretion is unresolved.

The interactions of factors at the level of the hypothalamus are therefore complex and the factors that predominate in influencing LH secretion are unknown. Schoemaker reviewed the subject of neuroendocrine control in the PCOS and found a number of contrasting and sometimes contradictory theories.[46] He concluded that central disturbances in the PCOS (that is at the level of hypothalamus and pituitary) are secondary to 'one or more peripheral factors, which may be ovarian in origin'.

An area of further controversy is whether there is an increase in GnRH pulse frequency in women who hypersecrete LH. This is an important question: if steroids are the main ovarian product to influence LH secretion, they are able to cross the blood–brain barrier and so might be expected to effect GnRH pulsatility also; if, however, the primary defect is through perturbed secretion of an ovarian peptide, this would not be predicted to cross the blood–brain barrier to affect GnRH pulse frequency. While there is no disputing the increase in pulse amplitude, some studies have also described an increase in pulse frequency of LH.[47–49] Many groups, however, have failed to detect an increase in pulse frequency.[50–55] Some studies have also demonstrated an alteration of the circadian rhythm of LH secretion, with a persistence of high-amplitude LH pulses during the night.[53] The differing conclusions may result from different study populations; for this reason, differences in pulse frequency that have been detected may be too small to represent a central role for a primary disturbance of the hypothalamus in the hypersecretion of LH. Murdoch and coworkers, who extensively investigated the variability of LH measurements in women with the PCOS, found good reproducibility with repeated studies over a 1-year period.[55] They also assessed LH pulsatility by time-series analysis, which takes into consideration the complicated patterns of LH secretion which occur as superimposed pulses of differing frequency. No difference in pulse frequency was detected between 9 patients with PCOS and 12 normal women.[55]

Some women with hypogonadotrophic hypogonadism (HH) also have polycystic ovaries detected by pelvic ultrasound; when these women were treated with pulsatile GnRH to induce ovulation they had significantly higher serum LH concentrations than women with HH and normal ovaries.[56] Furthermore, the elevation in LH concentration was observed before serum oestradiol concentrations rose. Thus hypersecretion of LH occurred in these women when the hypothalamus was replaced by an artificial GnRH pulse generator (i.e. the GnRH pump), with a fixed GnRH pulse interval of 90 minutes (equivalent to the pulse interval in the early follicular phase). These results suggest that the cause of hypersecretion of LH involves a perturbation of ovarian-pituitary feedback, rather than a primary disturbance of hypothalamic pulse regulation. These findings are also consistent with the notion that there may be non-steroidal factors disturbing ovarian-pituitary feedback control of LH secretion.

The data collected in women with PCOS undergoing laparoscopic ovarian diathermy are also consistent with the hypothesis that it is altered ovarian-pituitary feedback that causes hypersecretion of LH. In these patients LH pulse amplitude decreased but no change in the (normal) pulse frequency was detected after the procedure.[57,58] Rossmanith et al found an attenuation of GnRH-stimulated LH secretion after laparoscopic ovarian diathermy,[58] a result consistent with abnormalities in the production of an ovarian factor that regulates LH secretion, rather than with the theory that the disorder starts at the level of either the hypothalamus or the pituitary.

Glycosylation of LH

Luteinizing hormone exists in multiple forms in both the pituitary gland and the peripheral circulation, primarily because of the considerable variations in the oligosaccharide side chains which may result in numerous LH 'glycoforms'.[59] The alpha and beta subunits of LH each have two N-linked glycosylation sites, and oligosaccharides form about 30% of the molecule. Individual glycoforms cannot be isolated and even the recently available recombinant gonadotrophins are likely to have a variety of glycoforms. The glycosylation isoforms that are more basic have a shorter half-life and a lower in vivo activity than the acidic isoforms – conversely, the basic isoforms have a higher biopotency, with higher receptor binding, steroidogenic and intracellular cAMP-stimulating abilities in vitro. These differences are not recognized by either immunoassays (as antibodies do not recognize oligosaccharides) or in vitro bioassays, which are not dependent on in vivo clearance mechanisms. Lectins bind to oligosaccharides and may have a future role in two-site lectin/antibody assays.

Luteinizing hormone is probably modified in the circulation, for example by proteolytic cleavage of part of the beta chain ('nicking').[60] Human chorionic gonadotrophin (hCG) differs from LH by having a single additional C-terminal peptide. There is evidence that hCG itself is secreted by the normal pituitary gland and may circulate at concentrations of about 1% that of LH.[59]

Exposure of the pituitary gland to different serum concentrations of steroids may affect glycosylation and hence bioactivity of LH, which in turn may influence ovarian steroid production. While animal studies have shown that gonadal steroids may act directly at the pituitary to control the biopotency of stored and secreted gonadotrophins, it is uncertain whether LH bioactivity is affected by the chronic alterations in steroid hormone secretion that are seen in women with the polycystic ovary syndrome. Some studies have shown that bioactive serum concentrations of LH are elevated in these patients.[61–64] Lobo et al suggested that the level of bioactive LH may be a more useful marker than the immunoactive LH concentration or the LH to FSH ratio,[61] although the degree of bioactivity did not correlate with dopaminergic activity or serum oestradiol concentrations.[62] Fauser et al found that bioactive LH levels correlated better with symptoms of PCOS (oligo/amenorrhoea) than did serum LH concentrations as measured by IRMA.[65] It has been suggested that women with PCOS may secrete LH isoforms with a high biological activity.[64,65] Further evidence for this was obtained by Ding and Huhtaniemi who performed isoelectric focusing on serum from women with normal and elevated concentrations of LH.[66] They found that those with high serum LH concentrations had the majority of LH isoforms distributed with an alkaline isoelectric point, and this correlated with a high biological activity.

Circulating serum concentrations of oestradiol, oestrone, androstenedione, testosterone or dehydroepiandrosterone sulfate (DHEA-S) were not found to correlate with either bioactive or immunoreactive LH levels.[65] Experiments in non-human primates have demonstrated that the administration of different doses of GnRH results in pituitary secretion of LH isoforms of varying bioactivity.[67] The pituitaries of women with the polycystic ovary syndrome might be sensitized to GnRH in such a way that higher-activity LH isoforms are secreted than in women with normal ovaries. Possibly a non-steroidal messenger from the ovary effects this phenomenon.

A genetic variant of LH (vLH) has been discovered with two missense point mutations in the LHβ gene (Trp[8]Arg and Ile[15]Thr), initially reported from Finland but now recognized as a common polymorphism with worldwide distribution and a mean population carrier frequency of 18.5% (28.9% in Finland, 16.8% in the UK, 14.1% in the USA and 11.2% in the Netherlands).[68] The biological activity of vLH is greater than wild-type LH in vitro, while its half-life in the circulation is shorter and the overall effect on bioactivity in vivo is unclear. The vLH carrier frequency appears to be similar in obese and non-obese controls but lower in obese subjects with PCOS. The authors suggested that obese women with vLH might be protected from developing symptomatic PCOS while those with wild-type LH might be more liable to develop the syndrome. Interestingly, in the four countries studied this relationship was true for all except subjects from the UK, who exhibited a higher frequency of vLH in obese PCOS than obese controls.

The possible role of insulin in the hypersecretion of LH

Insulin stimulates pituitary gonadotrophin secretion, at least in vitro.[69] It has therefore been proposed that the hyperinsulinaemia seen in many women with PCOS might have a causal relationship with hypersecretion of LH. Antilla et al studied obese and non-obese women with the polycystic ovary syndrome and found that the non-obese women had elevated serum concentrations of bioactive LH whereas obese women tended to have normal concentrations.[63] These differences could not be attributed to serum androgen concentrations. It was noted that bioactive (but not immunoactive) LH levels related to the serum insulin concentration, and Antilla proposed that the degree of hyperinsulinaemia in obese, insulin-resistant subjects had a direct effect on the glycosylation of LH.[63]

Women with PCOS often hypersecrete LH and this may result in increased thecal cell androgen secretion. A study of 556 women with polycystic ovaries demonstrated that the patients with the highest serum LH concentrations did not have the highest serum testosterone concentrations.[70] Indeed, it has been shown that lean women with PCOS and normal fasting serum insulin concentrations have higher serum LH concentrations than lean or obese women with polycystic ovaries and elevated fasting insulin levels.[71] Furthermore, it was found that lean and obese women with polycystic ovaries and elevated fasting insulin levels had higher serum testosterone concentrations than women with normal insulin levels, suggesting a stronger relationship between androgen secretion and circulating levels than with LH.[71]

Leptin

The adipose fat secretes the hormone leptin, a helical cytokine of the tumour necrosis factor group, which as well as affecting satiety, dietary intake and exercise appears to influence GnRH pulsatility. Within the hypothalamus leptin inhibits neuropeptide Y (NPY) synthesis and release,[72] and NPY is in turn an inhibitor of GnRH pulsatility. Hypersecretion of leptin in obese women with PCOS might therefore account for hypersecretion of LH in some of these individuals. It certainly appears that some women with PCOS have serum leptin concentrations that are higher than expected for their BMI and insulin sensitivity.[73] However, it has been reported that women with PCOS have a lower serum leptin concentration than expected for their BMI, which may be due to impaired action of insulin on the adipocyte caused by abnormalities in the insulin receptor.[74] Women with PCOS also accumulate more visceral fat, which secretes less leptin than subcutaneous fat. The leptin story is certainly a complex one and has yet to be fully elucidated.

Steroidal feedback on LH secretion

In their studies on the functional capacity of the human gonadotroph, with respect to its sensitivity to GnRH and its reserve storage of gonadotrophins, Lasley et al examined the effects of oestradiol and progesterone administration on GnRH-stimulated gonadotrophin secretion in normal women in the follicular phase of the cycle.[75] They found that oestradiol increased pituitary gonadotrophin secretion and this was augmented by the addition of progesterone – the effects being similar on FSH and LH secretion. The physiological significance of the amplification effect of progesterone on the oestrogen-primed pituitary is uncertain. Many studies have shown that various doses of exogenous oestrogen are able to induce an LH surge in monkeys and humans.[76,77] Both oestradiol and progesterone also inhibit pituitary gonadotrophin secretion and the differential effects may be dose and time dependent.[78] The main effect of progesterone has been proposed as being at the level of the hypothalamus,[79] although the finding of progesterone receptors on monkey gonadotrophs suggests a direct effect at the level of the pituitary also.[80] It is unlikely that progesterone plays a role in hypersecretion of LH as it is secreted in negligible quantities during the follicular phase of

women with both normal and high serum concentrations of LH.[14]

In a study of women with PCOS, Baird et al found that serum LH concentrations were lower after an ovulatory cycle than after a period of anovulation.[81] They also found that anovulatory women responded to exogenous GnRH by secreting larger pulses of LH than ovulatory women with PCOS, who did not differ in their response from women with normal ovaries. From these observations it was suggested that hypersecretion of LH was secondary to the increased secretion of ovarian steroids during periods of anovulation – in particular androgens which were then metabolized to oestrone in the peripheral fat. Ovulatory women with polycystic ovaries, however, have also been shown to have higher serum concentrations of LH than ovulatory women with normal ovaries,[82] and we too have observed elevated serum LH concentrations during ovulatory cycles of women with polycystic ovaries.[14] Women with polycystic ovaries treated with gonadotrophins to induce ovulation have also been shown to have an elevated serum concentration of LH at a time when they might be expected to have suppressed LH levels due to the ovarian secretion of LH-inhibitory factors.[83,84] These data support the notion that women with PCOS have a perturbation of ovarian-pituitary feedback control of LH secretion – even in the presence of exogenous gonadotrophins.

The precise role of oestrone in gonadotrophin secretion is not known. Plasma concentrations of oestrone are elevated in some women with PCOS and it has been postulated that oestrone may play a role in the hypersecretion of LH that is seen in these women.[85,86] The administration of exogenous oestrone to women with normal or polycystic ovaries over periods of 5–15 days did not, however, increase serum LH levels or the sensitivity of the pituitary to exogenously administered GnRH.[87]

Oestrogens have also been shown to be inhibitory to GnRH-mediated gonadotrophin secretion, usually in a biphasic pattern, with a subsequent stimulatory effect which may be secondary to a direct effect on the number of available GnRH receptors.[88–90] It appears that in pituitary cell cultures a 4-hour exposure to oestradiol decreases the rat pituitary response to GnRH, while a longer exposure of 24–48 hours is required before the response to GnRH is augmented.[89,90] The cellular mechanisms that result in this inhibitory effect are still to be elucidated. The concentration of oestradiol is critical, as high concentrations decrease the response, creating a bell-shaped dose–response curve.[90] When oestradiol was administered to both anovulatory and ovulatory hyperandrogenaemic women with PCOS there was no difference in the suppression of serum LH concentrations, which were also no different from those in normal control subjects.[91]

Androgens have been shown to inhibit gonadotrophin secretion by decreasing the number of GnRH receptors in a pituicyte culture,[92] and postreceptor events also appear to be affected by androgens. Studies in female-to-male transsexuals demonstrated that large doses of testosterone failed to block an oestradiol-induced LH surge.[93] It therefore appears that androgens do not play a significant role in the genesis of the LH surge, or, for that matter, in normal secretion of LH. The polycystic ovary often oversecretes androgens, which are metabolized to oestrogens. Exogenously administered androgens do not result in an elevation of either LH pulse amplitude or frequency, whether administered acutely or long-term. Indeed, supraphysiological levels of testosterone suppress LH secretion.[94]

Non-steroidal feedback on LH secretion

Since the isolation and characterization of inhibin it has become apparent that not only are there several members of the inhibin family of glycoprotein hormones, but there are also other non-steroidal gonadal signals that influence gonadotrophin secretion and help to fine-tune reproductive function. It has been established that ovarian inhibin exerts negative feedback on pituitary gonadotrophin production, preferentially affecting FSH.[95] More recently a feedback pathway that influences pituitary LH secretion

has been proposed, following in vivo and in vitro evidence that has suggested the presence of a putative inhibitory peptide, which has been named gonadotrophin surge inhibiting (or attenuating) factor (GnSIF or GnSAF).[96,97] The proposed actions of GnSIF and GnSAF are similar, although this will only be confirmed if and when it is purified. For the sake of clarity, the abbreviation GnSAF is used here when referring to published studies on this subject.[98,99]

Before the recognition of the complex endocrine and paracrine mechanisms that control ovulation, the hypothesized mechanism for the preovulatory gonadotrophin surge was, perhaps, improbably simple. The classic theory was that when a critical level of oestradiol was secreted by the ovary, this steroid hormone switched from a negative to a positive feedback effect both on hypothalamic pulsatility of GnRH and pituitary secretion of the gonadotrophins. In recent years, the use of superovulation regimens for assisted conception procedures has provided further insight into the mechanism of ovulation itself: in spite of supraphysiological levels of oestradiol in the early follicular phase of stimulated cycles, the preovulatory LH surge does not commence earlier in the cycle and when it does occur it is usually significantly attenuated. This phenomenon has led to the realization that there may be an additional factor (or factors) produced by the developing ovarian follicles that suppresses pituitary secretion of LH.

There has been debate as to whether the putative GnSAF could in fact be inhibin. Culler gave FSH to rats and found that the preovulatory gonadotrophin surge of FSH and LH was inhibited;[100] this effect was reversed by the administration of an anti-inhibin antibody, which suggested that inhibin was responsible for these observations. However, using Culler's anti-inhibin antibody it has been demonstrated that GnSAF bioactivity in human follicular fluid is retained after treatment with anti-inhibin.[101] It would seem reasonable to postulate that inhibin and other non-steroidal hormones have effects at different stages of the cycle and at different serum concentrations in the fine-tuning of pituitary secretion of the gonadotrophins.

The precise mechanism of action of the putative GnSAF will not be known until the hormone has been isolated. One theory is that its primary action is to reinstate the unprimed state of LH responsiveness of the pituitary gland to GnRH each time the gland has been exposed to GnRH.[102] Thus LH levels are kept low during the follicular phase preceding the surge. Increased stimulation by GnRH then overrules this suppressive action and converts the state of low (unprimed) pituitary responsiveness into a state of high (primed) responsiveness to GnRH – the self-priming effect of GnRH. Alternatively, it has been suggested that GnSAF attenuates both the readily releasable pool of LH (unprimed response) and the reserve pool of LH (primed response).[103] The site of action of GnSAF is probably within the gonadotroph itself, as receptor binding studies have indicated that GnSAF does not compete with GnRH for the GnRH receptor. There is now good evidence that both FSH and LH are secreted by the same cells.

Abnormalities of inhibin secretion have long been implicated in the pathogenesis of PCOS, with the notion that hypersecretion of inhibin-B by the ovary suppresses pituitary secretion of FSH to cause the relative imbalance in gonadotrophin concentrations observed in these patients.[104] A series of experiments have demonstrated significantly elevated serum levels of inhibin-B in women with PCOS, which has been postulated as being responsible both for the reversed FSH to LH ratio and the increased sensitivity of the polycystic ovary to exogenous FSH.[105]

Gonadotrophin biosynthesis and secretion are influenced by hypothalamic, paracrine and endocrine factors and there is considerable overlap between all three. The influence of nonsteroidal factors on pituitary and hypothalamic function is still being elucidated. Further work is required to examine both the pathophysiology of hypersecretion of LH and its effects at the level of the oocyte. The role of leptin is still uncertain, as is that of the members of the inhibin family – two continually unravelling subjects. The ultimate aim is to direct appropriate therapy in order to enhance the fertility and reduce the miscarriage rates of the 40% of women with the polycystic ovary syndrome who hypersecrete LH.

The effects of laparoscopic ovarian diathermy on ovarian-pituitary feedback

A prospective study compared unilateral with bilateral ovarian diathermy in order to observe which ovary responded by ovulating.[106] All of the patients had been unresponsive to treatment with clomiphene citrate in doses up to 100 mg per day for 5 days. Of the ten patients, six received bilateral diathermy and four had unilateral diathermy, three to the right and one to the left ovary. Ovarian diathermy was performed using the technique described by Armar et al.[107] Laparoscopy was performed under general anaesthesia. The pelvic organs were inspected and tubal patency confirmed by transcervical injection of methylene blue dye. About 300 ml of sodium chloride 0.9% solution was instilled into the pouch of Douglas via a suprapubic Verres needle. The ovary was lifted onto the anterior wall of the uterus, where it was cauterized at four points, with the diathermy setting on 4 (40 watts) for 4 seconds at each point. The ovary was cooled in the pool of saline both to minimize adhesion formation and to prevent heat trauma to adjacent viscera. The saline was left in the peritoneal cavity at the end of the procedure.

Five patients (50%) ovulated within 6 weeks of the procedure but the remaining five failed to ovulate by 12 weeks, although all subsequently ovulated in response to either clomiphene citrate or gonadotrophin therapy. Three of the four patients who received unilateral diathermy ovulated, all from the contralateral ovary in the first cycle and then alternately from each ovary.

There were no significant differences between the baseline hormone measurements of the responders and those of the non-responders. When the pre- and post-treatment values were compared, there were no differences in the serum FSH and testosterone concentrations in either the responders or the non-responders.

In the responders, however, there was a significant fall of the serum LH concentration after diathermy ($P = 0.045$, 95% CI 0.2 to 13.4), while in the non-responders there was no difference in the LH concentrations before and after treatment.

The therapeutic options for patients with anovulatory infertility who are resistant to anti-oestrogens (usually clomiphene citrate) are either parenteral gonadotrophin therapy or laparoscopic ovarian diathermy. The cumulative conception and live-birth rates have been published for 103 women with PCOS who did not ovulate with anti-oestrogen therapy.[108] While the cumulative conception and live-birth rates after 6 months were 62% and 54% respectively, and after 12 months 73% and 62% respectively, the rate of multiple pregnancy was 19% and there were three cases of moderate to severe ovarian hyperstimulation syndrome (although the rate of these complications fell after the introduction of real-time transvaginal ultrasound monitoring of follicular development). Ovarian diathermy is free of the risks of multiple pregnancy and ovarian hyperstimulation and does not require intensive ultrasound monitoring. Furthermore, it appears to be as effective as routine gonadotrophin therapy in the treatment of clomiphene-insensitive PCOS.[109]

The mechanism of ovulation induction by laparoscopic ovarian diathermy is uncertain. It appears, however, that minimal damage to an unresponsive ovary either restores an ovulatory cycle or increases the sensitivity of the ovary to exogenous stimulation. Furthermore, the finding of an attenuated response of LH secretion to stimulation with GnRH suggests an effect on ovarian-pituitary feedback and hence on pituitary sensitivity to GnRH. This study goes one step further by demonstrating that unilateral diathermy leads to bilateral ovarian activity, showing conclusively for the first time that ovarian diathermy achieves its effect by correcting a perturbation of ovarian-pituitary feedback. A suggested hypothesis is that the response of the ovary to injury leads to a local cascade of growth factors, and those such as IGF-I, which interact with FSH, result in stimulation of follicular growth and the production of the hormone gonadotrophin surge attenuating/inhibitory factor, which leads to a fall in serum LH concentrations.[110] Furthermore, minimal ovarian damage only is required to achieve this effect.

REFERENCES

1 Balen AH, Conway GS, Kaltsas G et al. Polycystic ovary syndrome: the spectrum of the disorder in 1741 patients. *Hum Reprod* (1995) **10**: 2107–11.

2 Balen AH, Tan SL, Jacobs HS. Hypersecretion of luteinising hormone – a significant cause of subfertility and miscarriage. *Br J Obstet Gynaecol* (1993) **100**: 1082–9.

3 Punnonen R, Ashorn R, Vilja P, Heinonen PK, Kujansuu E, Tuohimaa P. Spontaneous luteinizing hormone surge and cleavage of in vitro fertilized embryos. *Fertil Steril* (1988) **49**: 479–82.

4 Seth J, Hanning I, Jacobs HS, Jeffcoate SL. Measuring serum gonadotropins: a cautionary note. *Lancet* (1989) **i**: 671.

5 Robins S, Rodin DA, Deacon A, Wheeler MJ, Clayton RN. Which hormone tests for the diagnosis of polycystic ovary syndrome? *Br J Obstet Gynaecol* (1992) **99**: 232–8.

6 Buckler HM, Critchley HO, Cantrill JA, Shales SM, Anderson DC, Robertson WR. Efficacy of low dose purified FSH in ovulation induction following pituitary desensitisation in polycystic ovarian syndrome. *Clin Endocrinol* (1993) **38**: 209–17.

7 Warnt EL, Williams BE, Cowan BD, Lynch A, Lerner SP, Hodgen GD. Pulsatile pituitary gonadotropin secretion during maturation of the dominant follicle in monkeys: estrogen positive feedback enhances the biological activity of LH. *Endocrinology* (1981) **109**: 2270–2.

8 Fritz MA, McLachlan RI, Cohen NL, Dahl C, Bremner WJ, Soules MR. Onset and characteristics of the midcycle surge in bioactive and immunoactive luteinising hormone secretion in normal women: influence of physiological variations in periovulatory ovarian steroid hormone secretion. *J Clin Endocrinol Metab* (1992) **75**: 489–93.

9 Stanger JD, Yovich JL. Reduced in-vitro fertilisation of human oocyte from patients with raised basal luteinising hormone levels during the follicular phase. *Br J Obstet Gynaecol* (1985) **92**: 385–93.

10 Howles CM, Macnamee MC, Edwards RG, Goswamy R, Steptoe PC. Effect of high tonic levels of luteinising hormone on outcome of in-vitro fertilisation. *Lancet* (1986) **i**: 521–2.

11 Verma S, Monks N, Turner K, Hooper M, Kumar A, Lenton E. Influence of elevated LH during follicular phase on fertility as assessed in a natural IVF programme. Seventh Annual Meeting of the ESHRE and the 7th World Congress on IVF and Assisted Procreation (Paris, July 1991) 68.

12 Thomas A, Okamoto S, O'Shea F, Maclachlan V, Besanko M, Healy D. Do raised serum luteinizing hormone levels during stimulation for in vitro fertilisation predict outcome? *Br J Obstet Gynaecol* (1989) **96**: 1328–32.

13 Kagawa T, Yamano S, Nishida S, Murayama S, Aono T. Relationship among serum levels of luteinising hormone, estradiol and progesterone during follicle stimulation and results of in-vitro fertilisation and embryo transfer. *J Assist Reprod Genet* (1992) **9**: 106–12.

14 Abdulwahid NA, Adams J, Van der Spuy ZM, Jacobs HS. Gonadotrophin control of follicular development. *Clin Endocrinol* (1985) **23**: 613–26.

15 Homburg R, Armar NA, Eshel A, Adams J, Jacobs HS. Influence of serum luteinising hormone concentrations on ovulation, conception and early pregnancy loss in polycystic ovary syndrome. *Br Med J* (1988) **297**: 1024–6.

16 Hamilton-Fairley D, Kiddy D, Watson H, Paterson C, Franks S. Association of moderate obesity with a poor pregnancy outcome in women with polycystic ovary syndrome treated with low dose gonadotrophin. *Br J Obstet Gynaecol* (1992) **99**: 128–31.

17 Sagle M, Bishop K, Alexander FM et al. Recurrent early miscarriage and polycystic ovaries. *Br Med J* (1988) **297**: 1027–8.

18 Watson H, Hamilton-Fairley D, Kiddy D et al. Abnormalities of follicular phase luteinising hormone secretion in women with recurrent early miscarriage. *J Endocrinol* (1989) **123** (suppl.): abstr. 25.

19 Balen AH, Tan SL, MacDougall J, Jacobs HS. Miscarriage rates following in-vitro fertilisation are increased in women with polycystic ovaries and reduced by pituitary desensitisation with buserelin. *Hum Reprod* (1993) **8**: 959–64.

20 Regan L, Owen EJ, Jacobs HS. Hypersecretion of luteinising hormone, infertility and miscarriage. *Lancet* (1990) **336**: 1141–4.

21 Dekel N, Galiani D, Aberdam E. Regulation of rat oocyte maturation: involvement of protein kinases. In: Bavister BD, Cummins J, Roldan ERS, eds, *Fertilisation in Mammals* (Serono Symposia: Norwell, 1990) 17–24.

22 Hunter RHF, Cook B, Baker TG. Dissociation of response to injected gonadotrophin between Graffian follicle and oocyte in pigs. *Nature* (1976) **260**: 156–8.

23 Austin BR. The egg. In: Austin CR, Short RV, eds, *Reproduction in Mammals*. Part 1. *Germ Cells and Fertilisation*, 2nd edn (Cambridge University Press: Cambridge, 1982) 46–62.

24 Shoham Z, Borenstein R, Lunenfeld B, Pariente C. Hormonal profiles following clomiphene citrate therapy in conception and nonconception cycles. *Clin Endocrinol* (1990) **33**: 271–8.

25 Bonney RC, Franks S. The endocrinology of implantation and early pregnancy. *Baillière's Clinical Endocrinology and Metabolism* (1990) **4**: 207–31.

26 Polson DW, Chanda M, Bedi S, Troup S, Lieberman B. The effect of serum luteinising hormone concentrations on success rates of frozen embryo replacement into natural cycles. *Br Congr Obstet Gynaecol* (1992) abstr. 152.

27 Hamilton-Fairley D, Kiddy D, Watson H, Paterson C, Franks S. Association of moderate obesity with a poor pregnancy outcome in women with polycystic ovary syndrome treated with low dose gonadotrophin. *Br J Obstet Gynaecol* (1992) **99**: 128–31.

28 Schally AV, Arimura A, Kastin AJ et al. Gonadotropin-releasing hormone: one polypeptide regulates secretion of luteinizing and follicle stimulating hormones. *Science* (1971) **173**: 1036–7.

29 Belchetz PE, Plant TM, Nakai Y, Keogh EG, Knobil E. Hypophyseal responses to continuous intermittent delivery of hypothalamic GnRH. *Science* (1978) **202**: 631–3.

30 Dalkin AC, Haisenleder DJ, Ortolano GA, Ellis TR, Marshall JC. The frequency of GnRH stimulation differentially regulates gonadotropin subunit mRNA expression. *Endocrinology* (1989) **125**: 917–24.

31 Pickering AJMC, Fink G. Priming effect of luteinising hormone-releasing factor: in-vitro and in-vivo evidence consistent with its dependence upon protein and RNA synthesis. *J Clin Endocrinol Metab* **69**: 373–9.

32 Aiyer MS, Chiappa SA, Fink G. A priming effect of luteinizing releasing factor on the pituitary gland in the female rat. *J Endocrinol* (1974) **62**: 573–88.

33 Wang CF, Lasley BL, Lein A, Yen SSC. The functional changes of the pituitary gonadotrophs during the menstrual cycle. *J Clin Endocrinol Metab* (1976) **42**: 718–28.

34 Knobil E. Electrophysiological approaches to the hypothalamic GnRH pulse generator. In: Yen SSC, Vale WW, eds, *Neuroendocrine Regulation of Reproduction* (Serono Symposia: Norwell, 1990) 3–8.

35 Plosker SM, Marshall LA, Martin MC, Jaffe RB. Opioid, catecholamine and steroid interaction in prolactin and gonadotropin regulation. *Obst Gynec* (1990) **45**: 441–53.

36 Rosmanith WG, Wirth U, Sterzik K, Yen SS. The effects of prolonged opioidergic blockade on LH pulsatile secretion during the menstrual cycle. *J Endocrinol Invest* (1989) **12**: 245–52.

37 Danforth DR, Elkind-Hirsch K, Hodgen G. In-vivo and in-vitro modulation of GnRH metabolism by estradiol and progesterone. *Endocrinology* (1990) **127**: 319–24.

38 Quigley M, Rakoff J, Yen SSC. Increased luteinising hormone sensitivity to dopamine inhibition in the polycystic ovary syndrome. *J Clin Endocrinol Metab* (1981) **52**: 231.

39 Cumming DC, Reid RL, Quigley ME, Rebar RW, Yen SS. Evidence for decreased endogenous dopamine and opioid inhibitory influences on LH secretion in polycystic ovary syndrome. *Clin Endocrinol (Oxf)* (1984) **20**: 643–8.

40 Shoupe D, Lobo RA. Evidence for altered catecholamine metabolism in polycystic ovary syndrome. *Am J Obstet Gynecol* (1984) **150**: 566–70.

41 Yoshino K, Takahashi K, Shirai T, Nishigaki A, Araki Y, Kitao M. Changes in plasma catecholamines and pulsatile patterns of gonadotropins in subjects with a normal ovulatory cycle and with polycystic ovary syndrome. *Int J Fertil* **35**: 34–9.

42 Barnes R, Lobo R. Central opioid activity in the polycystic ovary syndrome with and without dopaminergic modulation. *J Clin Endocrinol Metab* (1985) **61**: 779.

43 Barnes RB, Mileikowsky GN, Cha KY, Spencer CA, Lobo RA. Effects of dopamine and metoclopramide in polycystic ovary syndrome. *J Clin Endocrinol Metab* (1986) **63**: 506–9.

44 Berga SL, Yen SSC. Opioidergic regulation of LH pulsatility in women with polycystic ovary syndrome. *Clin Endocrinol* (1989) **30**: 177–84.

45 Lanzone A, Apa R, Fulghesu AM, Cutillo G, Caruso A, Mancuso S. Long-term naltrexone treatment normalizes the pituitary response to gonadotrophin-releasing hormone in polycystic ovarian syndrome. *Fertil Steril* (1993) **59**: 734–7.

46 Schoemaker J. Neuroendocrine control in polycystic ovary-like syndrome. *Gynecol Endocrinol* (1991) **5**: 277–88.

47 Rebar R, Judd HL, Yen SCC, Rakoff J, Vandenberg G, Naftolin F. Characterization of the inappropriate gonadotropin secretion in polycystic ovary syndrome. *J Clin Invest* (1976) **57**: 1320–9.

48 Burger CW, Korsen T, Van Kessel H, Van Dop PA, Caron FJM, Schoemaker J. Pulsatile luteinizing hormone patterns in the follicular phase of the menstrual cycle, polycystic ovarian disease (PCOD) and non PCOD secondary amenorrhoea. *J Clin Endocrinol Metab* (1985) **61**: 1126–32.

49 Waldstreicher J, Santoro NF, Hall JE, Filicori M, Crowley W. Hyperfunction of the hypothalamic-pituitary axis in women with polycystic ovarian disease: indirect evidence for partial gonadotroph desensitization. *J Clin Endocrinol Metab* (1988) **66**: 165–72.

50 Baird DT, Corker CS, Davison DW, Hunter WM, Michie EA, Van Look PFA. Pituitary ovarian relationships in polycystic ovary syndrome. *J Clin Endocrinol Metab* (1977) **45**: 798–809.

51 Kazer RR, Kessel B, Yen SS. Circulating luteinizing hormone pulse frequency in women with polycystic ovary syndrome. *J Clin Endocrinol Metab* (1987) **65**: 233–6.

52 Sagel M, Kiddy M, Mason HD, Dobriansky D, Polson DW, Franks S. Evidence for normal hypothalamic regulation of LH in ovulatory women with the polycystic ovary syndrome. In: Rolland R, Heineman MJ et al, eds, *Neuroendocrinology of Reproduction* (Excerpta Medica: Amsterdam, 1987).

53 Venturoli S, Porcu E, Fabbri R et al. Episodic pulsatile secretion of FSH, LH, prolactin, oestradiol, oestrone and LH circadian variations in polycystic ovary syndrome. *Clin Endocrinol* (1988) **28**: 93–107.

54 Couzinet B, Thomas G, Thalabard JC, Brailly S, Schaison G. Effects of a pure antiandrogen on gonadotropin secretion in normal women and in polycystic ovarian disease. *Fertil Steril* (1989) **52**: 42–7.

55 Murdoch AP, Diggle PJ, White MC, Kendall-Taylor P, Dunlop W. LH in polycystic ovary syndrome: reproducibility and pulsatile secretion. *J Endocrinol* (1989) **121**: 185–91.

56 Schachter M, Balen AH, Patel A, Jacobs HS. Hypogonadotrophic patients with ultra-

sonographically diagnosed polycystic ovaries have aberrant gonadotropin secretion when treated with pulsatile gonadotrophin releasing hormone – a new insight into the pathophysiology of polycystic ovary syndrome. *Gynecol Endocrinol* (1996) **10**: 327–35.

57 Gadir AA, Khatim MS, Mowafi RS, Alnaser HMI, Alzaid HGN, Shaw RW. Hormonal changes in patients with polycystic ovarian disease after ovarian electrocautery or pituitary desensitization. *Clin Endocrinol* (1990) **32**: 749–54.

58 Rossmanith WG, Keckstein J, Spatzier K, Lauritzen C. The impact of ovarian laser surgery on the gonadotrophin secretion in women with PCOD. *Clin Endocrinol* (1991) **34**: 223–30.

59 Jeffcoate SL. Analytical and clinical significance of peptide hormone heterogeneity with particular reference to growth hormone and luteinising hormone in serum. *Clin Endocrinol* (1993) **38**: 113–21.

60 Iles RK, Lee CL, Howes I, Davies S, Edward R, Chard T. Immunoreactive β-core-like material in normal postmenopausal urine: human chorionic gonadotrophin or LH origin? Evidence for the existence of LH core. *J Endocrinol* (1992) **133**: 459–66.

61 Lobo RA, Kletzky OA, Campeau J, diZerega G. Elevated bioactive luteinising hormone in women with polycystic ovary syndrome. *Fertil Steril* (1983) **39**: 674–9.

62 Lobo RA, Shoupe D, Chang SP, Campeau J. The control of bioactive luteinising hormone secretion in women with polycystic ovary syndrome. *Am J Obstet Gynecol* (1984) **148**: 423–8.

63 Antilla L, Ding YQ, Ruutiainen K, Erkkola R, Irjala K, Huhtaniemi I. Clinical features and circulating gonadotropin, insulin and androgen interactions in women with polycystic ovarian disease. *Fertil Steril* (1991) **55**: 1057–61.

64 Fauser BCJM, Pache TD, Lamberts WJ, Hop WCJ, de Jong FH, Dahl KD. Serum bioactive and immunoreactive luteinising hormone and follicle stimulating hormone levels in women with cycle abnormalities, with or without polycystic ovary disease. *J Clin Endocrinol Metab* (1991) **73**: 811–17.

65 Fauser BCJM, Pache TD, Hop WCJ, de Jong FH, Dahl KD. The significance of a single serum LH measurement in women with cycle disturbances: discrepancies between immunoreactive and bioactive hormone estimates. *Clin Endocrinol* (1992) **37**: 445–52.

66 Ding YQ, Huhtaniemi I. Preponderance of basic isoforms of serum LH is associated with the high bio/immuno ratio of LH in healthy women and in women with polycystic ovarian disease. *Hum Reprod* (1991) **6**: 346–50.

67 Matteri RL, Djiershke DJ, Bridson WE, Rhutasel NS, Robinson JA. Regulation of the biopotency of primate LH by GnRH in-vitro and in-vivo. *Biol Reprod* (1990) **43**: 1045–9.

68 Tapanainen JS, Koivunen R, Fauser BCJM et al. A new contributing factor to polycystic ovary syndrome: the genetic variant of luteinizing hormone. *J Clin Endocrinol Metab* (1999) **84**: 1711–15.

69 Adashi EY, Hsueh AJW, Yen SSC. Insulin enhancement of luteinising hormone and follicle stimulating hormone release by cultured pituitary cells. *Endocrinology* (1981) **108**: 1441–9.

70 Conway GS, Honour JW, Jacobs HS. Heterogeneity of the polycystic ovary syndrome: clinical, endocrine and ultrasound features in 556 patients. *Clin Endocrinol* (1989) **30**: 459–70.

71 Conway GS, Clark PMS, Wong D. Hyperinsulinaemia in the polycystic ovary syndrome confirmed with a specific immunoradiometric assay for insulin. *Clin Endocrinol* (1993) **38**: 219–22.

72 Stephens TW, Basinski M, Bristow PK et al. The role of neuropeptide Y in the antiobesity action of the obese gene product. *Nature* (1995) **377**: 530–2.

73 Brzechffa PR, Jakimiuk AJ, Agarwal SK et al. Serum immunoreactive leptin concentrations in women with polycystic ovary syndrome. *J Clin Endocrinol Metab* (1996) **81**: 4166–9.

74 Jacobs HS, Conway GS. Leptin, polycystic ovaries and polycystic ovary syndrome. *Hum Reprod Update* (1999) **5**: 166–71.

75 Lasley BL, Wang CF, Yen SSC. The effects of estrogen and progesterone on the functional capacity of the gonadotrophs. *J Clin Endocrinol Metab* (1975) **41**: 820–6.

76 Karsch FJ, Weick RF, Butler WR et al. Induced LH surges in the rhesus monkey: strength-duration characteristics of the estrogen stimulus. *Endocrinology* (1973) **92**: 1740–7.

77 Liu JH, Yen SSC. Induction of midcycle gonadotropin surge by ovarian steroids: a critical evaluation. *J Clin Endocrinol Metab* (1983) **57**: 792–802.

78 Hsueh AJW, Erickson GF, Yen SSC. The sensitizing effect of estrogens and catechol estrogen on cultured pituitary cells to LHRH: its antagonism by progestins. *Endocrinology* (1979) **104**: 807–13.

79 Karsch FJ. Central actions of ovarian steroids in

the feedback regulation of pulsatile secretion of luteinising hormone. *Ann Rev Physiol* (1987) **49**: 365–82.

80 Sprangers SA, Brenner RM, Bethea CL. Estrogen and progesterone receptor immunocytochemistry in lactotropes versus gonadotropes of monkey pituitary cell cultures. *Endocrinology* (1989) **124**: 1462–70.

81 Baird DT, Corker CS, Davison DW, Hunter WM, Michie EA, Van Look PFA. Pituitary ovarian relationships in polycystic ovary syndrome. *J Clin Endocrinol Metab* (1977) **45**: 798–809.

82 Eden JA. The polycystic ovary syndrome. *Aust NZ J Obstet Gynaecol* (1989) **29**: 403–16.

83 McFaul PB, Traub AI, Thompson W. Premature luteinization and ovulation induction using human menopausal gonadotrophin or pure follicle stimulating hormone in patients with polycystic ovary syndrome. *Acta Eur Fertil* (1989) **20**: 157–61.

84 Mizunuma H, Andoh K, Yamada K, Takagi T, Kamijo T, Ibuki Y. Prediction and prevention of ovarian hyperstimulation by monitoring endogenous luteinising hormone release during purified follicle stimulating hormone therapy. *Fertil Steril* (1992) **58**: 46–50.

85 DeVane GM, Czekala NM, Judd HL, Yen SSC. Circulating gonadotropins, estrogens and androgens in polycystic ovarian disease. *Am J Obstet Gynecol* (1974) **38**: 476–81.

86 Rebar R, Judd HL, Yen SSC, Rakoff J, Vandenberg G, Naftolin F. Characterization of the inappropriate gonadotropin secretion in polycystic ovary syndrome. *J Clin Invest* (1976) **57**: 1320–9.

87 Chang RJ, Mandel FP, Lu JK, Judd HL. Enhanced disparity of gonadotropin secretion by estrone in women with polycystic ovarian disease. *J Clin Endocrinol Metab* (1982) **54**: 490–4.

88 Frawley LS, Neill JD. Biphasic effects of estrogen on GnRH-induced LH release in monolayer cultures of rat and monkey pituitary cells. *Endocrinol* (1984) **114**: 659–63.

89 Menon M, Peegel H, Katta V. Estradiol potentiation of gonadotrophin-releasing hormone responsiveness in the anterior pituitary is mediated by an increase in gonadotrophin-releasing hormone receptors. *Am J Obstet Gynecol* **151**: 534–40.

90 Emons G, Hoffmann HG, Brack C et al. Modulation of GnRH receptor concentration in cultured female pituitary cells by estradiol treatment. *J Steroid Biochem* (1988) **31**: 751–6.

91 Pemberton P, White DM, Franks S. The feedback effect of oestradiol on secretion of LH in ovulatory and anovulatory women with polycystic ovary syndrome. *J Endocrinol* **135** (suppl.): P97.

92 Giguere V, Lefebvre FA, Labrie F. Androgens decrease LHRH binding sites in rat anterior pituitary cells in culture. *Endocrinology* (1981) **108**: 350–2.

93 Goh HH, Ratnam SS. The gonadotrophin surge in humans: its mechanism and role in ovulatory function – a review. *Ann Acad Med* (1990) **19**: 524–9.

94 Spinder T, Spijkstra JJ, van den Tweel JG et al. The effects of long term testosterone administration on pulsatile luteinizing hormone secretion and on ovarian histology in eugonadal female to male transsexual subjects. *J Clin Endocrinol Metab* (1989) **69**: 151–7.

95 Burger HG, Igarashi M. Inhibin – definition and nomenclature. *J Clin Endocrinol Metab* (1988) **66**: 885–6.

96 Sopelak VM, Hodgen GD. Blockade of the estrogen-induced LH surge in monkeys: a non-steroidal, antigenic factor in porcine follicular fluid. *Fertil Steril* (1984) **41**: 108–13.

97 Messinis IE, Templeton A. Pituitary response to exogenous LHRH in superovulated women. *J Reprod Fert* (1989) **87**: 633–9.

98 Fowler PA, Templeton A. The nature and function of gonadotrophin surge attenuating factor/inhibiting factor (GnSAF/GnSIF). *Endocr Rev* (1996) **17**: 103–20.

99 Balen AH. Gonadotrophin surge attenuating factor – where are we now? *Clin Endocrinol* (1996) **44**: 177–80.

100 Culler MD. In-vivo evidence that inhibin is a gonado-trophin surge-inhibiting factor. *Endocrinology* (1992) **131**: 1556–8.

101 Balen AH, Er J, Rafferty B, Rose M. Evidence that gonadotrophin surge attenuating factor is not inhibin. *J Reprod Fert* (1995) **104**: 285–9.

102 Koppenaal DW, van Dieten JAMJ, Tijssen AMI, de Koning J. Induction of the gonadotrophin surge-inhibiting factor by FSH and its elimination: a sex difference in the efficacy of the priming effect of gonadotrophin-releasing hormone on the rat pituitary gland. *J Endocrinol* **138**: 191–201.

103 Fowler PA, Messinis IE, Cunningham P, Fraser M, Templeton AA. Effects of gonadotrophin surge-attenuating factor on the two pools of gonadotrophin-releasing hormone-induced LH secretion *in vitro*. *Hum Reprod* (1993) **8**: 822–8.

104 Lockwood GM, Muttukrishna S, Groome NP, Matthews DR, Ledger WL. Mid-follicular phase

pulses of inhibin B are absent in polycystic ovary syndrome and are initiated by successful laparoscopic ovarian diathermy: a possible mechanism for the emergence of the dominant follicle. *J Clin Endocrinol Metab* (1998) **83**: 1730–5.

105 Lockwood GM. The role of inhibin in PCOS. *Hum Fertil* (2000) **3**: 86–92.

106 Balen AH, Jacobs HS. A prospective study comparing unilateral and bilateral laparoscopic ovarian diathermy in women with the polycystic ovary syndrome. *Fertil Steril* (1994) **62**: 921–5.

107 Armar NA, McGarrigle HHG, Honour JW, Holownia P, Jacobs HS, Lachelin GCL. Laparoscopic ovarian diathermy in the management of anovulatory infertility in women with polycystic ovaries: endocrine changes and clinical outcome. *Fertil Steril* (1990) **53**: 45–9.

108 Balen AH, Braat DDM, West C, Patel A, Jacobs HS. Cumulative conception and live birth rates after the treatment of anovulatory infertility. An analysis of the safety and efficacy of ovulation induction in 200 patients. *Hum Reprod* (1994) **9**: 1563–70.

109 Gadir AA, Mowafi RS, Alnaser HMI, Alrashid AH, Shaw RW. Ovarian electrocautery versus hMG and pure FSH therapy in the treatment of patients with polycystic ovarian disease. *Clin Endocrinol* (1990) **33**: 585–92.

110 Balen AH, Jacobs HS. Gonadotrophin surge attenuating factor – a missing link in the control of LH secretion? *Clin Endocrinol* (1991) **35**: 399–402.

8

The role of the insulin-like growth factor system

Linda C Giudice

Polycystic ovary syndrome (PCOS) is a hetero-geneous syndrome characterized by persistent anovulation, oligomenorrhea or amenorrhea, and hyperandrogenism, in the absence of thy-roid, pituitary, and/or adrenal disease. At the level of the ovary, there are recruitment and growth of follicles to the small antral stage, with no selection of a dominant, preovulatory follicle. This leads to the accumulation of mul-tiple, small, antral follicles, which give the syn-drome its name.[1–3] There is also evidence of hyperfunctioning of the thecal compartment in addition to the relative hypofunctioning of the granulosa. While many women with PCOS have relatively high circulating levels of luteinizing hormone (LH) compared with folli-cle-stimulating hormone (FSH), this is not so in all women and does not account totally for the observed increase in thecal production of androgens or the relative quiescence and FSH resistance of the granulosa. This complex dis-order probably has its origins within, as well as outside, the hypothalamic–pituitary–ovarian axis. Clinical and basic research have high-lighted the roles, within the reproductive tract, of intraovarian autocrine and/or paracrine reg-ulators. Outside the reproductive axis, meta-bolic, neuroendocrine, and also endocrine regu-lators probably contribute to the pathogenesis of this disorder.[4–6] This chapter describes what is currently known about the ovarian insulin-like growth factor (IGF) system in normal folli-cle development and in PCOS. The focus is on insulin-like peptides, since the IGF family inte-grates endocrine and metabolic axes relevant to PCOS and the intraovarian IGF system may play a role in hyperandrogenemia and the arrest of follicular development observed in this disorder.[7–10]

INSULIN-LIKE GROWTH FACTOR SYSTEM

The IGF system comprises IGF peptides, IGF receptors, a family of high-affinity IGF binding proteins (IGFBPs), a family of IGFBP-related proteins, and a family of IGFBP proteases.[11–13] It is one of the most extensively studied systems in the ovary.[10] Both IGF-I and IGF-II are small, mitogenic and differentiative peptides that have insulin-like metabolic effects mediated upon binding to specific high-affinity mem-brane receptors. They also have antiapoptotic actions. Because of its known actions as a mediator of growth hormone IGF-I is also known as somatomedin C, and IGF-II has been classically viewed as a tumorigenic factor and a fetal growth factor. The IGF type I receptor is a typical growth factor receptor with signal transduction mediated via the tyrosine kinase pathway.[14] It is the primary receptor through which the IGFs exert their metabolic and growth-promoting actions in target cells. The type II IGF receptor is identical to the mannose 6-phosphate cation-independent receptor and is believed to play a role in IGF-II turnover. In addition, the type II receptor may mediate signals involved in angiogenesis[15] or other processes. The IGFs circulate bound primarily to IGFBP-3 as well as to other IGFBPs which prolong their half-lives and also facilitate transcapillary transport to tissues. In the circulation, IGFBP-1 regulates minute-to-minute availability of IGFs and is regulated (inhibited) by insulin.[16,17] Much attention has been focused on this IGFBP in the circulation of women with PCOS because of the hyperinsulinemia common in this syndrome.[6,10] Locally produced IGFBPs modulate (mostly inhibit) IGF actions at target cells.[11-13] The IGFBPs have affinities for the IGFs up to 2 orders of magnitude higher than that of the IGF receptors, and post-translational modifications, including phosphorylation, glycosylation, and proteolysis, increase IGF availability to their receptors. The IGFBPs may also have IGF-independent actions. A new group of these binding proteins has been identified that shares structural homology with other IGFBPs, although they have very low affinities for the IGFs, and thus have been termed 'IGFBP-related proteins' (IGFBP-rP).[13]

THE IGF SYSTEM IN NORMAL HUMAN OVARY

IGF and IGF receptor peptide and mRNA expression

In human ovary, IGF peptide expression is follicle stage-specific and is compartmentalized. The IGF-II messenger is expressed in theca and perifollicular vessels of all follicles.[18-20] In small antral follicles IGF-II mRNA and protein are expressed in granulosa and theca. In contrast, in atretic antral follicles, IGF-II is minimally expressed by thecal cells. It is abundantly expressed, however, in preovulatory follicle granulosa cells and granulosa-luteal cells harvested during oocyte retrieval after controlled ovarian hyperstimulation for in vitro fertilization.[18-22] Human preovulatory granulosa cells express IGF-II, but not IGF-I mRNAs, and whether IGF-I is expressed in human ovary at all is controversial.[18-20,23,24] While IGF-I demonstrates growth hormone dependence in some tissues, e.g. bone, it is unlikely that growth hormone effects on human ovary are mediated through IGF-I. This is true because human granulosa cells do not express IGF-I, although they do contain growth hormone receptors.[25] In contrast, while human thecal cells do express IGF-I, they do not have growth hormone receptors.[26] Gonadotropins regulate granulosa expression of IGF-II mRNAs as well as secretion of IGF-II peptide.[21,27] Also, FSH stimulates IGF-II mRNA in cultured human preantral follicles.[28] The IGF receptor mRNAs are expressed and specific binding sites have been demonstrated in granulosa and theca in human ovary.[18-20,24,29,30] Thus, gonadotropins appear to be the major regulators of members of the IGF family in the ovary.

IGF actions in ovary

The effects of primarily IGF-I have been investigated on human granulosa and theca in vitro, although the endogenous ligand in vivo is IGF-II. Actions of IGF on ovarian cellular constituents include mitogenic effects and augmentation of steroidogenesis, as well as inhibition of follicular apoptosis. Insulin-like growth factor stimulates DNA synthesis and basal estradiol (E_2) secretion in granulosa and granulosa-luteal cells.[31-36] It also synergizes with gonadotropins in augmenting E_2 and progesterone (P) production.[37-40] Insulin-like growth factor II stimulates basal progesterone and E_2 secretion in human granulosa[41,42] as well as granulosa proliferation in vitro.[43] In granulosa cells from unstimulated preovulatory follicles and gonadotropin-stimulated follicles, IGF-I alone, and synergistically with gonadotropins, stimulates cytochrome P450 aromatase activity and mRNA.[44] The IGFs also display actions in human thecal cells and oocytes. In cultured human thecae, IGF-I enhances DNA and androgen synthesis[45] and synergizes with LH in androstenedione production. Maturation of immature human oocytes in vitro can be augmented by IGF-I,[46] and IGF-I has also been shown to have antiapoptotic actions in ovarian follicles.[47] Follicular atresia is associated with apoptosis and regular cleavage of nuclear DNA by endonucleases.[48] In vitro this process is suppressed by IGF-I and gonadotropins and is enhanced by the presence of IGFBPs.[49]

IGFs in follicular fluid and serum

Constituents of follicular fluid (FF) derive from the circulation and from local, intraovarian production. In FF, IGF levels during gonadotropin-stimulated cycles are lower than in serum.[50–52] Levels of IGF-I are similar in FF from estrogen-dominant and androgen-dominant follicles, and are not correlated with follicular size,[53] suggesting that IGF-I in FF originates from the circulation by transudation. In contrast, FF IGF-II levels are higher in estrogen-dominant compared with androgen-dominant follicles and correlate positively with follicle size, cycle day and E_2, and inversely with androgen to estrogen (A : E) ratio.[53] Therefore, it is likely that FF IGF-II derives primarily by local production in the granulosa and perhaps theca, in addition to some contribution from the circulation. Circulating levels of IGF-I and IGF-II in normally cycling women are not menstrual cycle-dependent, underscoring the importance of the local intraovarian IGF system.[53] Circulating IGF-I is not a prerequisite for normal ovarian follicular development in humans, as evidenced by normal ovulation and fertility in patients with Laron dwarfism or growth hormone receptor deficiency (GHRD). Furthermore, in a GHRD woman whose serum growth hormone levels were markedly elevated, growth hor-

mone receptor deficient, and serum and FF levels of IGF-I barely detectable, normal follicular response to injectable gonadotropins, ovulation, and conception have been reported.[54–56] Serum IGF-II levels were about 25% of normal, but FF IGF-II was not measured. These clinical observations support the conclusion that circulating IGF-I is not essential for normal follicular development and that IGF-II is the major bioavailable IGF in human ovary.

IGF binding proteins: expression within the ovary

Of the six high-affinity IGFBPs that have been identified, five are expressed in human ovary.[19,20] Luteinizing granulosa cells synthesize IGFBP-1 and IGFBP-2 and secrete IGFBP-1, IGFBP-2, and IGFBP-3 in vitro.[57–62] The protein IGFBP-1 is expressed in granulosa of the dominant follicle as well as in the corpus lutuem;[63] IGFBP-2, -3, -4, and -5 are expressed in human thecal cells from small antral follicles and also dominant follicles. Proteins IGFBP-1, -2, and -3 are present in follicular fluid from gonadotropin-stimulated, luteinizing follicles,[64–67] whereas IGFBP-1, -2, -3, and -4 are detected in FF from cycling women.[62,66,67] The IGFBP profiles in FF from normally cycling women are dependent on the functional status of the follicle. Specifically, androgen-dominant follicles (with low estrogen to androgen ratios) have high levels of IGFBP-2 and IGFBP-4, compared with healthy estrogen-dominant follicles.[62,67,68] In addition, in situ hybridization studies reveal abundant IGFBP-2 mRNA expressed in granulosa of atretic follicles.[19] To date no reports on the four types of IGFBP-rP have appeared. However, IGFBP-rP-1 has extensive homology with follistatin,[69] and information should be forthcoming on this protein in the near future.

It is likely that IGFBPs act as modulators of IGF action in the ovary in vivo, based on their actions on ovarian cellular components in vitro: IGFBP-1 inhibits IGF-I-stimulated [^{3}H]thymidine incorporation,[31] and IGFBP-1 and IGFBP-3 inhibit IGF-I-stimulated E_2 and P production;[70]

IGFBP-4 inhibits IGF-II-stimulated granulosa steroidogenesis.[71–73] That IGFBP-2 and IGFBP-4 are involved in regulating follicular development is supported by the observation that these inhibitory IGFBPs are abundant in androgen-dominant follicles. It is possible that elevated levels of these inhibitory IGFBPs in androgen-dominant follicles in normally cycling women decrease intrafollicular levels of bioavailable IGFs, thereby contributing to follicular atresia in the ovary.

Regulation of ovarian IGFBPs

Since IGFBPs regulate IGF action, their own regulation assumes importance. Regulation is at the level of expression and in changing their affinities for their IGF ligands by partial proteolysis by IGFBP-specific proteases. Secretion of IGFBP by granulosa is regulated (mostly inhibited) by gonadotropins, insulin-like peptides, and activin-A.[10,61,70,74–76] Modulation of IGF action is further influenced by IGFBP proteases which affect the affinity of the IGFBPs for the IGFs. In human ovary, an IGFBP-4 protease is present in estrogen-dominant but not in androgen-dominant FF,[71] and IGFBP proteases have been found in media conditioned by human thecae.[77,78] The IGFBP-4 protease in human ovarian follicular fluid has recently been identified as pregnancy-associated plasma protein A (PAPP-A), a member of the metzincin superfamily of metalloproteinases.[79] Follicular fluid protease activity may be one of several mechanisms in E_2-dominant follicles to increase bioavailable IGF-II to synergize with gonadotropins for steroidogenesis and follicle growth.

A model for the role of the IGF system in normal human ovary

A model for proposed actions of the IGF system (IGF peptides, IGFBPs, and IGFBP proteases) in human granulosa and thecal steroidogenesis, follicle growth, and atresia, is presented in Figure 8.1. In growing, E_2-dominant follicles,

androgen from thecal cells is used as substrate for gonadotropin- and IGF-stimulated aromatase for the production of E_2. High levels of bioavailable IGF-II are effected within the follicle by a combination of decreased production of IGFBPs (mainly IGFBP-2) and increased degradation by IGFBP-specific proteases (mainly IGFBP-4). Granulosa-derived IGFBPs are in turn regulated by IGFs, insulin, LH, and activin-A. In contrast, in androgen-dominant follicles, the amount of bioavailable IGFs is markedly curtailed by high levels of inhibitory IGFBPs. What enables some androgen-dominant follicles to persist in the arrested state or to undergo atresia is currently unknown.

POLYCYSTIC OVARY SYNDROME

Polycystic ovary syndrome, the most common cause of anovulation in women, is a heterogeneous condition characterized by hyperandrogenism, persistent anovulation, oligomenorrhea or amenorrhea, hirsutism, elevated LH level and the accumulation of small cysts in the ovaries.[1–3] Many women with PCOS are obese, although there are also lean women with the syndrome, and insulin resistance and hyperinsulinism are common to both lean and obese women with PCOS.[6,80–83] Within the follicle, the initial stages of recruitment and growth to the small antral stage are not impaired in PCOS, although selection of a dominant preovulatory follicle does not occur, leading to accumulation of many small antral follicles in the ovary and persistent anovulation. Mechanisms underlying this disorder are not well understood, and in past years the pendulum has swung between invoking hypothalamic–pituitary dysfunction and intraovarian growth factor-mediated follicular dysfunction in attempting to explain the pathogenesis of this disorder. In addition, the spectrum of potential causes needs to be considered in the context of underlying insulin resistance and hyperinsulinemia. The potential contributions of insulin-like peptides in the pathogenesis of PCOS have been extensively reviewed[10] and are described briefly here.

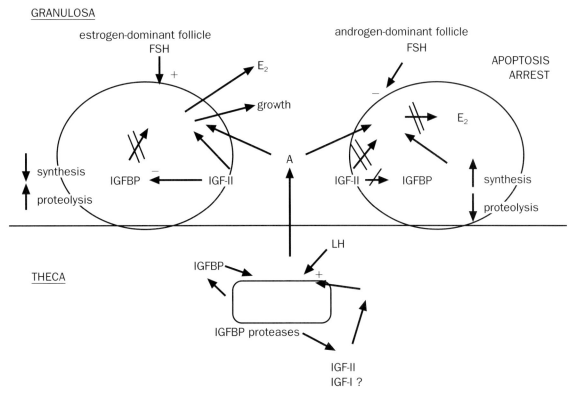

Figure 8.1 Model of gonadotropin, IGF, IGFBP, and IGFBP protease in human granulosa and theca (see text).

The intraovarian IGF system

In vitro IGFs stimulate granulosa proliferation and aromatase, processes that are characteristically absent in the PCOS follicle in vivo. The lack of stimulation of aromatase may be due to an abnormality in the aromatase gene in PCOS granulosa or to an abnormal protein product. It may also be due to inadequate levels of intrafollicular IGFs or FSH, or inhibition of IGF and/or FSH action within the PCOS follicle. In PCOS the follicles contain physiological levels of both FSH[84,85] and IGF-I,[86,87] and although PCOS granulosa cells produce little aromatase in vivo, they respond to FSH and/or IGF-I in vitro in a normal[88,89] or even elevated[90] fashion. Thus, the defect in PCOS is not an abnormality in the aromatase gene or enzyme or due to a lack of stimulating hormones *per se*. Nor is it due to decreased responsiveness of the granulosa to IGFs (or FSH) with regard to aromatase production. It has been postulated that locally active inhibitors of IGFs and/or FSH in FF of small antral PCOS follicles block stimulation of aromatase. The IGFBPs are likely candidates (see below).[9,10]

The IGFBP profiles in PCOS follicles are very similar to androgen-dominant, small antral (atretic) follicles obtained from regularly cycling women. There are high levels of IGFBP-2 and IGFBP-4,[62,68,91] in marked contrast to the near absence of these IGFBPs in estrogen-dominant follicles, detected by ligand binding techniques. In situ hybridization studies support these observations.[19] In addition, the IGFBP-4 protease is not detectable in the PCOS follicle,[92,93] like small, androgen-dominant follicles in normally cycling women and in marked contrast to healthy, estrogen-dominant follicles.[77] Localization of IGFBP-4 in antral follicles corresponds with insulin sensitivity,[94] with greater immunostaining observed in thecal cells compared with granulosa, in women with insulin resistance, and the reverse in ovaries of women without insulin resistance.

In estrogen-dominant follicles there is decreased IGFBP-2 production and increased IGFBP-4 degradation (effectively decreased inhibitory IGFBP levels), and elevated IGF-II levels, leading overall to increased IGF-II bioavailability. Androgen-dominant follicles that are atretic, arrested, or reside in ovaries of female-to-male transsexuals given high doses of androgens share several common features. Their IGFBP profiles are similar. Also, there is an absence of IGFBP-4 proteolysis in these follicles, and the FF levels of IGF-II (and IGF-I) are similar. These observations have led to the hypothesis that there is marked reduction of IGF bioavailability in androgen-dominant follicles.[77,91–93] The abundance of IGFBPs in androgen-dominant arrested follicles and in atretic follicles probably serves to inhibit IGF synergy with gonadotropins for aromatase induction and ovarian cellular mitosis. From available data in humans and in other species, it is likely that the IGF system (increased IGF-II, decreased IGFBP-2 and increased IGFBP-4 protease) is 'turned on' at the time of dominant follicle selection, augmenting the effects of FSH on the granulosa compartment (Fig. 8.2). It is currently unclear whether the changes in the IGF system participate in this transition or are a consequence of it. The IGFs inhibit ovarian follicle atresia, and the IGFBPs augment the atretic process. However, small androgen-dominant PCOS follicles that are rich in IGFBP and poor in bioavailable IGF are arrested in their development and are not atretic. The mechanisms (Figure 8.2) that underlie the transition from an androgen-dominant follicle to an atretic follicle, to an arrested PCOS follicle, or to an estrogen-dominant follicle are poorly understood, and

the participation of the IGF system in the choice of pathways is unclear and remains a challenge for future investigations.

In women the association between hyperinsulinism and hyperandrogenism is well established.[82,95,96] In vitro theca-interstitial cells obtained from women with hyperandrogenism release significantly more androgen per milligram of tissue than do those from non-hyperandrogenic women.[97] Since the insulin and type I IGF receptors are structurally similar[10] and insulin cross-reacts with the type I IGF receptor,[14] it has been suggested that excessive insulin action on the theca in insulin-resistant women with PCOS, resulting in hyperandrogenism, is via the type I IGF receptor in this compartment of the ovary (reviewed by Poretsky et al[10]). Levels of insulin needed to cross-react at the type I IGF receptor in thecae, however, would have to be several times higher than those observed clinically in PCOS women with insulin resistance and hyperinsulinemia. Several possibilities exist to explain the paradox of ovarian insulin sensitivity versus insulin resistance in most other tissues.[10] It is possible

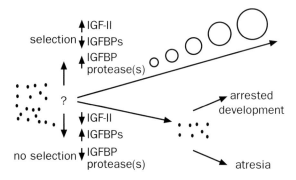

Figure 8.2 Changes in the IGF system in human ovary that correspond with follicle selection and no selection, and the enigma of what controls whether an androgen-dominant follicle will become atretic or will persist in an arrested state of development (as in PCOS).

that there is an altered or hybrid form of the insulin receptor in the ovary; alternatively, insulin receptors in the ovary may be differently regulated compared with those in other tissues.[10] Also postreceptor defects may explain the different effects of insulin on glucose metabolism and steroidogenesis.[83] With regard to the granulosa, why is there not excessive stimulation, since these cells are richly endowed with the type I IGF receptor, have abundant substrate for aromatase within the PCOS follicle, and bathe in physiologic FSH and IGF levels? Although an answer to this is not forthcoming currently, restriction of IGF bioavailability by high levels of intrafollicular inhibitory IGFBPs may contribute in part to this resistance to aromatase stimulation. Thus both elevated LH levels and hyperinsulinism – and perhaps IGFs – lead to hyperandrogenism observed in this disorder. In addition to direct action on the ovary, altered levels of sex hormone binding globulin can also contribute to increased bioavailable androgens in the circulation.

The circulating IGF system in PCOS

With regard to the IGF system and its potential role in the pathogenesis of hyperandrogenism in women with PCOS, elevated circulating levels of IGF-I may have effects similar to those proposed for hyperinsulinemia – i.e., synergism with LH in the thecal compartment. Most reports, however, demonstrate that serum IGF-I levels in PCOS women are in the normal range.[98,99] An alternative approach to elevate IGF bioactivity is through changes in IGFBPs. Since IGFs in serum are bound to a large extent to IGFBPs, and IGFBPs mostly have inhibitory effects on IGF actions, decreased IGFBP serum concentrations may lead to increased bioavailability of IGF within serum and thus in the ovary. Serum levels of the main circulating carrier of IGFs, IGFBP-3, are the same in normoovulatory women and women with PCOS.[5,53,91,100,101] Also, integrated 24-hour IGFBP-3 levels were observed in obese and lean women with PCOS, which also did not differ between obese and lean controls.[5] In a study

investigating the effect on IGFBP-3 of octreotide, which decreases insulin secretion in hyperinsulinemic women with PCOS,[102] octreotide increased serum IGFBP-3 levels by 42%, while decreasing serum IGF-I by 63%.[101] No change in IGFBP-3, but a small, yet significant, decrease in IGF-I were observed in controls. Octreotide's effect on insulin secretion does not explain the observed decrease in IGF-I since insulin does not modulate circulating IGFBP-3.[12] Also, the decrease in IGF-I does not explain IGFBP-3's increase in response to octreotide, since IGF-I does not regulate IGFBP-3. Thus, these observations suggest a central alteration in the growth hormone/IGF-I axis in PCOS.[4,5]

Since IGFBP-1 regulates minute-to-minute bioavailability of IGFs in the circulation and is regulated by insulin, its levels in the circulation of women with PCOS are particularly relevant and have been extensively investigated. Lower IGFBP-1 levels have been reported in PCOS patients than in controls, particularly in obese women with PCOS,[53,95,98,99,102–105] probably a consequence of hyperinsulinism. Fasting IGFBP-1 levels in sera are negatively correlated with insulin in all subjects, including women with PCOS.[16,17,99,106] Levels of IGFBP-1 in PCOS women decline during oral and intravenous glucose tolerance tests, mirroring the insulin response.[106,107] Weight loss increases IGFBP-1 levels,[108] although neither gonadotropin releasing hormone analog suppression of ovarian steroidogenesis nor ovarian electrocautery which normalizes ovulatory function has any effect on serum IGFBP-1 or insulin sensitivity in women with PCOS.[109–111] Thus, circulating IGFBP-1 levels reflect short-term fluctuations in circulating insulin,[112] and the degree of peripheral insulin resistance. Indeed, it has been proposed that IGFBP-1 levels in women with PCOS may be a useful clinical marker for insulin resistance.[110]

With lower levels of IGFBP-1 in women with PCOS and with hyperinsulinism, the amount of *free* IGF-I may be increased, with subsequent availability to synergize with LH, enhancing thecal androgen production and thus hyperandrogenemia. Total and free circulating levels of IGFs have been reported to be higher in PCOS than in normo-ovulatory women in one study[105] but not others.[95,99,113] Another study demonstrated that while free IGF-I levels were higher in women with PCOS, there was no correlation with circulating androgens.[53] However, in Laron dwarfism (growth hormone receptor deficiency), where circulating IGF-I levels are markedly suppressed,[56] IGF-I administration to affected women resulted in acne and other androgenic side effects.[114] These results suggest that IGF-I may indeed synergize with elevated LH on the thecal compartment for androgen production, an event not observed in this study probably because of its cross-sectional design.[53]

Higher levels of bioavailable IGFs (in serum or locally in the theca and stroma) may synergize with LH in stimulating thecal androgen production, resulting in hyperandrogenism, characteristic of this syndrome. Elevated levels of insulin may also contribute in this regard, probably acting through its own receptor. In the granulosa compartment, high levels of free IGFs may not synergize with FSH in stimulating aromatase activity, owing to high intrafollicular levels of IGFBPs in the androgen-dominant PCOS follicle.[91] Whether higher levels of free IGFs are present in the circulation or in the ovarian microenvironment (theca and stroma) of PCOS patients, compared with normo-ovulatory women, remains controversial and is worthy of further investigation. Studies have demonstrated that medium conditioned by thecal-interstitial cell explants contains an IGFBP-3 protease,[78] and so normal levels of circulating IGFBP-3, for example, probably do not reflect the state of IGF binding activity (and thus IGF bioavailability) within the follicular microenvironment.

CONCLUSION

The IGF system probably has a role in intra-ovarian regulation in PCOS. The profiles of IGFBPs, lack of IGFBP proteases, and levels of IGF-II in atretic follicles of normo-ovulatory women are similar to those observed in arrested follicles in the PCOS ovary. However, no evidence to date suggests that arrested follicles in the PCOS ovary are atretic. Therefore, a major question remains as to the role of the IGF system in the process of follicle selection and in follicle atresia (Fig. 8.2). A challenge to reproductive biology is to elucidate mechanisms underlying follicular selection. Whether the observed changes in the IGF system contribute to follicular selection or are a consequence of it remains unsettled. Furthermore, it is likely that other factors interact with the IGF system to prevent the arrested follicle from becoming atretic.

It is striking that hyperinsulinism is associated with PCOS, underscoring the endocrine aspect of this disorder. Emerging information on insulin-sensitizing agents and improvement of ovulation in insulin-resistant women using these agents and the role of insulin in follicle development are exciting areas of clinical reproductive endocrinology. Insulin sensitizers such as the biguanide metformin hold great promise in the therapy for PCOS. Agents that lower circulating insulin without affecting insulin sensitivity (e.g. diazoxide, octreotide) have adverse long-term effects on glucose tolerance that decrease their desirability as long-term therapy in women with PCOS.[10] Interestingly, metformin does not have a direct effect on ovarian steroidogenesis[114] or on the synthesis of IGFBP-1,[115] and its actions probably derive from its insulin-related effects.

Why is insulin so important for normal ovarian function? The answer to this and other questions will give insight into normal follicular development and atresia, and the pathogenesis of PCOS. A long-term goal is to design therapies to restore ovulation and decrease hyperandrogenemia in women at high risk for long-term hyperandrogenic and anovulatory-related health consequences.

REFERENCES

1 Yen SSC. The polycystic ovary syndrome. *Clin Endocrinol* (1980) **12**: 177–86.

2 Franks S. The polycystic ovary syndrome. *N Engl J Med* (1995) **333**: 853–61.

3 Futterweit W. Pathophysiology of polycystic ovarian syndrome. In: Redmond, GP, ed., *Androgenic Disorders* (Raven Press: New York, 1995) 77–166.

4 Kazer RR, Unterman TG, Glick RP. An abnormality of the growth hormone/insulin-like growth factor-I axis in women with polycystic ovary syndrome. *J Clin Endocrinol Metab* (1990) **71**: 958–62.

5 Morales AJ, Laughlin GA, Butzow T, Maheshwari H, Baumann G, Yen SSC. Insulin, somatotropic, and luteinizing hormone axes in lean and obese women with polycystic ovary syndrome: common and distinct features. *J Clin Endocrinol Metab* (1996) **81**: 2854–64.

6 Dunaiff A. Insulin resistance and the polycystic ovary syndrome: mechanism and implications for pathogenesis. *Endocr Rev* (1997) **18**: 774–800.

7 Giudice LC, Cataldo NA, van Dessel HJHM, Yap OWS, Chandrasekher YA. Growth factors in normal ovarian follicle development. *Semin Reprod Endocrinol* (1996) **14**: 179–96.

8 Giudice LC, Morales AJ, Yen SSC. Growth factors and polycystic ovary syndrome. *Semin Reprod Endocrinol* (1996) **14**: 203–8.

9 Cataldo NA. Insulin-like growth factor binding proteins: do they play a role in polycystic ovary syndrome? *Semin Reprod Endocrinol* (1997) **15**: 123–36.

10 Poretsky L, Cataldo NA, Rosenwaks Z, Giudice LC. The Insulin-related ovarian regulatory system in health and disease. *Endocr Rev* (1999) **20**: 535–82.

11 Jones JI, Clemmons D. Insulin-like growth factors and their binding proteins: biological actions. *Endocr Rev* (1995) **16**: 3–34.

12 Rajaram S, Baylink DJ, Mohan S. Insulin-like growth factor binding proteins in serum and other biological fluids: regulation and functions. *Endocr Rev* (1997) **18**: 801–31.

13 Hwa V, Oh Y, Rosenfeld RG. The insulin-like growth factor binding protein superfamily. *Endocr Rev* (1999) **20**: 761–87.

14 Nissley P, Lopaczynski W. Insulin-like growth factor receptors. *Growth Fact* (1991) **5**: 29–36.

15 Volpert O, Jackson D, Bouck N, Linzer DI. The insulin-like growth factor II/mannose-6-phosphate/insulin-like growth factor II receptor is required for proliferin-induced angiogenesis. *Endocrinology* (1996) **137**: 3871–6.

16 Lee PDK, Jensen MD, Divertie GD, Heiling VJ, Katz HH, Conover CA. Insulin-like growth factor binding protein-1 response to insulin during suppression of endogenous insulin secretion. *Metabolism* (1993) **42**: 409–14.

17 Lee PDK, Giudice LC, Conover CA, Powell DR. Insulin-like growth factor binding protein-1: recent findings amd new directions. *Proc Soc Exp Biol Med* (1997) **116**: 319–57.

18 El-Roeiy A, Chen X, Roberts VJ, LeRoith D, Roberts CT, Yen SSC. Expression of insulin-like growth factor-I (IGF-I) and IGF-II and the IGF-I, IGF-II, and insulin receptor genes and localization of the gene products in the human ovary. *J Clin Endocrinol Metab* (1993) **77**: 1411–18.

19 El-Roeiy A, Chen X, Roberts VJ et al. Expression of the genes encoding the insulin-like growth factors, the IGF and insulin receptors, and IGF-binding proteins-1–6 and the localization of their gene products in normal and polycystic ovary syndrome ovaries. *J Clin Endocrinol Metab* (1994) **78**: 1488–96.

20 Zhou J, Bondy C. Anatomy of the human ovarian insulin-like growth factor system. *Biol Reprod* (1993) **48**: 467–70.

21 Voutilainen R, Miller WL. Coordinate trophic hormone regulation of mRNAs for insulin-like growth factor II and the cholesterol side-chain cleavage enzyme, P450ssc, in human steroidogenic tissues. *Proc Natl Acad Sci USA* (1987) **84**: 1590–5.

22 Voutilainen TR, Franks S, Mason HD, Marktikainen H. Expression of insulin-like growth factor (IGF), IGF-binding protein and IGF receptor messenger ribonucleic acids in normal and polycystic ovaries. *J Clin Endocrinol Metab* (1996) **81**: 1003–8.

23 Geisthovel F, Moretti-Rojas IM, Asch RH, Rojas FJ. Expression of insulin-like growth factor-II (IGF-II) messenger ribonucleic acid (mRNA), but not IGF-I mRNA in human preovulatory granulosa cells. *Hum Reprod* (1989) **4**: 899–903.

24 Hernandez ER, Hurwitz A, Vera A et al. Expression of the genes encoding the insulin-like growth factors and their receptors in the human ovary. *J Clin Endocrinol Metab* (1992) **74**: 419–25.

25 Carlsson B, Bergh C, Bentham J et al. Expression of functional growth hormone receptors in human granulosa cells. *Hum Reprod* (1992) **7**: 1205–9.

26 Katz E, Riciarelli E, Adashi EY. The potential relevance of growth hormone to female reproductive physiology and pathophysiology. *Fertil Steril* (1993) **59**: 8–34.

27 Ramasharma K, Li CH. Human pituitary and

placental hormones control human insulin-like growth factor II secretion in human granulosa cells. *Proc Natl Acad Sci USA* (1987) **84**: 2643–8.

28 Yuan W, Giudice LC. Insulin-like growth factor-II mediates the steroidogenic and growth promoting actions of follicle stimulating hormone on human ovarian pre-antral follicles in vitro. *J Clin Endocrinol Metab* (1999) **84**: 1479–82.

29 Gates GS, Bayer S, Seibel M, Poretsky L, Flier JS, Moses AC. Characterization of insulin-like growth factor binding to human granulosa cells obtained during *in vitro* fertilization. *J Recept Res* (1987) **7**: 885–9.

30 Balboni GC, Vannelli GB, Barni T, Orlando C, Serio M. Transferrin and somatomedin C receptors in human ovarian follicles. *Fertil Steril* (1987) **48**: 706–10.

31 Olsson JH, Carlsson B, Hillensjo T. Effect of insulin-like growth factor-I on deoxyribonucleic acid synthesis in cultured human granulosa cells. *Fertil Steril* (1990) **54**: 1052–7.

32 Angervo M, Koistinen R, Suikkari AM, Seppala M. Insulin-like growth factor binding protein-1 inhibits the DNA amplification induced by insulin-like growth factor I in human granulosa-luteal cells. *Hum Reprod* (1991) **6**: 770–3.

33 Yong EL, Baird DT, Yates R, Reichert LE, Hillier SG. Hormonal regulation of the growth and steroidogenic function of human granulosa cells. *J Clin Endocrinol Metab* (1992) **74**: 842–50.

34 Wood AM, Lambert A, Hooper MAK, Mitchell GG, Robertson WR. Exogenous steroids and the control of estradiol secretion by human granulosa-lutein cells by follicle stimulating hormone and insulin-like growth factor-I. *Hum Reprod* (1994) **9**: 19–25.

35 Erickson GF, Garzo VG, Magoffin DA. Insulin-like growth factor-I regulates aromatase activity in human granulosa and granulosa-luteal cells. *J Clin Endocrinol* (1989) **69**: 716–20.

36 Erickson GF, Magoffin DA, Cragun RJ, Chang RJ. The effects of insulin and insulin-like growth factors-I and-II on estradiol production by granulosa cells of polycystic ovaries. *J Clin Endocrinol Metab* (1990) **70**: 894–902.

37 Bergh C, Olsson JH, Hillensjo T. Effect of insulin-like growth factor-I on steroidogenesis in cultured human granulosa cells. *Acta Endocrinol (Copenh)* (1991) **125**: 177–81.

38 Christman GM, Randolph JG, Peegel H, Menon KM. Differential responsiveness of luteinized human granulosa cells to gonadotropins and insulin-like growth factor-I for induction of aro-

matase activity. *Fertil Steril* (1991) **55**: 1099–105.

39 Mason HD, Margara R, Winstron RML, Beard RW, Reed MJ, Franks S. Inhibition of oestradiol production by epidermal growth factor in human granulosa cells of normal and polycystic ovaries. *Clin Endocrinol* (1990) **33**: 511–17.

40 Erickson GF, Garzo VG, Magoffin DA. Progesterone production by human granulosa cells cultured in serum free medium: effects of gonadotrophins and insulin-like growth factor-I (IGF-I). *Hum Reprod* (1991) **6**: 1074–81.

41 Kamada S, Kubota T, Taguchi M, Wen-Rong H, Sakamoto S, Aso T. Effects of insulin-like growth factor-II on proliferation and differentiation of ovarian granulosa cells. *Horm Res* (1992) **37**: 141–5.

42 Kubota T, Kamada S, Ohara M et al. Insulin-like growth factor-II in follicular fluid of the patients with in vitro fertilization and embryo transfer. *Fertil Steril* (1993) **59**: 844–9.

43 Di Blasio AM, Vigano P, Ferrari A. Insulin-like growth factor-II stimulates human granulosa-luteal cell proliferation in vitro. *Fertil Steril* (1994) **61**: 483–7.

44 Steinkampf MP, Mendelson CR, Simpson ER. Effects of epidermal growth factor and insulin-like growth factor I on the levels of mRNA encoding aromatase cytochrome P-450 of human ovarian granulosa cells. *Mol Cell Endocrinol* (1988) **59**: 93–8.

45 Hillier SG, Yong EL, Illingworth PJ, Baird DT, Schwall RH, Mason AJ. Effect of recombinant activin on androgen synthesis in cultured human thecal cells. *J Clin Endocrinol Metab* (1991) **72**: 1206–11.

46 Gomez E, Tarin JJ, Pellicer MD. Oocyte maturation in humans: the role of gonadotropins and growth factors. *Fertil Steril* (1993) **60**: 40–6.

47 Hsueh AJW, Billig H, Tsafriri A. Ovarian follicle atresia: a hormonally controlled apoptotic process. *Endocr Rev* (1994) **15**: 707–24.

48 Tilly JL, Kowalski KI, Schomberg DW, Hsueh AJW. Apoptosis in atretic ovarian follicles is associated with selective decreases in messenger ribonucleic acid transcripts for gonadotropin receptors and cytochrome P450 aromatase. *Endocrinology* (1992) **131**: 1670–5.

49 Chun SY, Billig H, Tilly JL, Furuta I, Tsafriri A, Hsueh AJW. Gonadotropin suppression of apoptosis in cultured preovulatory follicles: mediatory role of endogenous insulin-like growth factor-I. *Endocrinology* (1994) **135**: 1845–53.

50 Geisthovel F, Moretti-Rojas IM, Rojas FJ, Asch RH. Immunoreactive insulin-like growth factor I in human follicular fluid. *Hum Reprod* (1989) **4**: 35–40.

51 Rabinovici J, Dandekar P, Angle M, Rosenthal S, Martin M. Insulin-like growth factor I levels in follicular fluid from human preovulatory follicles: correlation with serum IGF-I levels. *Fertil Steril* (1990) **54**: 428–33.

52 Giudice LC, Farrell EM, Pham H, Rosenfeld RG. Identification of insulin-like growth factor binding protein-3 (IGFBP-3) and IGFBP-2 in human follicular fluid. *J Clin Endocrinol Metab* (1990) **71**: 1330–8.

53 Van Dessel HJHM, Lee PDK, Faessen GH, Chandrasekher YA, Fauser BCHM, Giudice LC. Elevated serum levels of free insulin-like growth factor (IGF)-I in polycystic ovary syndrome. *J Clin Endocrinol Metab* (1999) **84**: 3030–5.

54 Lunenfeld B, Menashe Y, Dor Y, Pariente C, Insler V. The effect of growth hormone, growth factors, and their binding globulins on ovarian responsiveness. *Contracept Fertil Sex* (1991) **19**: 133–6.

55 Menashe Y, Sack J, Mashiach S. Spontaneous pregnancies in two women with Laron-type dwarfism: are growth hormone and circulating insulin-like growth factor mandatory for induction of ovulation? *Hum Reprod* (1991) **6**: 670–1.

56 Dor J, Ben-Shlomo I, Lunenfeld B et al. Insulin-like growth factor-I (IGF-I) may not be essential for ovarian follicular development: evidence from IGF-I deficiency. *J Clin Endocrinol Metab* (1992) **74**: 539–42.

57 Suikkari AM, Jalkanen J, Koistinen R et al. Human granulosa cells synthesize low molecular weight insulin-like growth factor-binding protein. *Endocrinology* (1989) **124**: 1088–92.

58 Jalkanen J, Suikkari AM, Koistinen R et al. Regulation of insulin-like growth factor binding protein-1 production in human granulosa-luteal cells. *J Clin Endocrinol Metab* (1989) **69**: 1174–80.

59 Hamori M, Blum WF, Torok A et al. Immunoreactive insulin-like growth factor binding protein-3 in the culture of human luteinized granulosa cells. *Acta Endocrinol (Copenh)* (1991) **124**: 685–90.

60 Giudice LC, Milki AM, Milkowski DA, El-Danasouri I. Human granulosa contain messenger ribonucleic acids (mRNAs) encoding insulin-like growth factor binding proteins (IGFBPs) and in culture secrete IGFBPs. *Fertil Steril* (1991) **56**: 475–80.

61 Cataldo NA, Woodruff TK, Giudice LC. Regulation of insulin-like growth factor binding protein production by human luteinizing granulosa cells cultured in defined medium. *J Clin Endocrinol Metab* (1993) **76**: 207–15.

62 San Roman GA, Magoffin DA. Insulin-like growth factor binding proteins in healthy and atretic follicles during natural menstrual cycles. *J Clin Endocrinol Metab* (1993) **76**: 625–32.

63 Seppala M, Wahlstrom T, Koskimes AI et al. Human preovulatory follicular fluid, luteinized cells of hyperstimulated preovulatory follicles, and corpus luteum contain placental protein 12. *J Clin Endocrinol Metab* (1984) **58**: 505–10.

64 Hartsthorne GM, Bell SC, Waites GT. Binding proteins for insulin-like growth factors in the human ovary: identification, follicular fluid levels and immunohistological localization of the 29–32 kd type 1 binding protein, IGF-bp1. *Hum Reprod* (1990) **5**: 649–60.

65 Hamori M, Blum WF, Torok A et al. Insulin-like growth factors and their binding proteins in human follicular fluid. *Hum Reprod* (1991) **6**: 313–18.

66 Holly JMP, Eden JA, Alaghband-Zadeh J et al. Insulin-like growth factor binding proteins in follicular fluid from normal dominant and cohort follicles, polycystic and multicystic ovaries. *Clin Endocrinol (Oxf)* (1990) **33**: 53–7.

67 Cataldo NA, Giudice LC. Insulin-like growth factor binding protein profiles in human ovarian follicular fluid correlate with follicular functional status. *J Clin Endocrinol Metab* (1992) **74**: 821–9.

68 Schuller AGP, Lindenbergh-Kortleve DJ, Pache TD, Zwarthoff EC, Fauser BCJM, Drop SLS. Insulin-like growth factor binding protein-2, 28 kDa and 24 kDa IGF-BP levels are decreased in fluid of dominant follicles, obtained from normal and polycystic ovaries. *Regul Pept* (1993) **48**: 157–63.

69 Kato MV, Sato H, Tsukada T, Ikawa Y, Aizawa S, Nagayoshi M. A follistatin-like gene, mac-25, may act as a growth suppressor of osteosarcoma cells. *Oncogene* (1996) **12**: 1361–4.

70 Mason H, Margara R, Winston RML, Seppälä M, Koistinen R, Franks S. Insulin-like growth factor-1 (IGF-1) inhibits production of IGF-binding protein-1 while stimulating estradiol secretion in granulosa cells from normal and polycystic human ovaries. *J Clin Endocrinol Metab* (1993) **76**: 1275–9.

71 Chandrasekher YA, Van Dessel HJHM, Fauser BCJM, Giudice LC. Estrogen- but not androgen-

dominant human ovarian follicular fluid contains an IGFBP-4 protease. *J Clin Endocrinol Metab* (1995) **80**: 2734–9.

72 Mason HD, Cwyfan-Hughes S, Holly JMP, Franks S. Potent inhibition of human ovarian steroidogenesis by insulin-like growth factor binding protein-4 (IGFBP-4). *J Clin Endocrinol Metab* (1998) **83**: 284–7.

73 Iwashita M, Kudo Y, Takeda Y. Effect of follicle stimulating hormone and insulin-like growth factors on proteolysis of insulin-like growth factor binding protein-4 in human granulosa cells. *Mol Hum Reprod* (1998) **4**: 401–5.

74 Mason H, Willis D, Seppala M, Franks S. Insulin inhibits insulin-like growth factor binding protein-1 (IGFBP-1) production by granulosa, theca, and stroma from human ovaries. *J Endocrinol* (1993) **137**: 179–85.

75 Cataldo NA, Fujimoto VY, Jaffe RB. Interferon-g and activin A promote insulin-like growth factor-binding protein-2 and -4 accumulation by human luteinizing granulosa cells and interferon-g promotes their apoptosis. *J Clin Endocrinol Metab* (1998) **83**: 179–86.

76 Poretsky L, Chandrasekher YA, Bai C, Liu HC, Rosenwaks HC, Giudice LC. Insulin receptor mediates inhibitory effect of insulin, but not of insulin-like growth factor (IGF)-I, on IGF binding protein-1 (IGFBP-1) production in human granulosa cells. *J Clin Endocrinol Metab* (1996) **81**: 493–6.

77 Chandrasekher YA, Clark CR, Faessen GH, Giudice LC. Insulin-like growth factor binding protein profile in theca explant cultures from normal human ovaries. *Proceedings of the Endocrine Society 77th Annual Meeting*, Washington, DC, 1995, 166.

78 Mason HD, Cwyfan-Hughes SC, Heinrich G, Franks S, Holly JMP. Insulin-like growth factor-I (IGF-I), IGF-II, IGF binding protein (IGFBP), and IGFBP proteases are produced by theca and stroma of normal and PCOS human ovaries. *J Clin Endocrinol Metab* (1996) **81**: 276–84.

79 Conover CA, Oxvig C, Overgaard MT, Christiansen M, Giudice LC. Evidence that the insulin-like growth factor binding protein-4 protease in human ovarian follicular fluid is pregnancy associated plasma protein-A. *J Clin Endocrinol Metab* (1999) **84**: 4742–5.

80 Burghen GA, Givens JR, Kitabchi AE. Correlation of hyperandrogenism with hyperinsulinism in polycystic ovarian disease. *J Clin Endocrinol Metab* (1980) **50**: 113–21.

81 Chang RJ, Nakamura RM, Judd HL, Kaplan SA. Insulin-resistance in non-obese patients with polycystic ovarian disease. *J Clin Endocrinol Metab* (1983) **57**: 356–62.

82 Dunaif A, Segal KR, Futterweit W, Dobrjansky A. Profound peripheral insulin resistance, independent of obesity, in polycystic ovary syndrome. *Diabetes* (1989) **38**: 1165–74.

83 Dunaif A, Segal KR, Shelley D, Green G, Dobrjansky A, Licholai T. Evidence for distinctive and intrinsic defects in insulin action in polycystic ovary syndrome. *Diabetes* (1992) **41**: 1257–65.

84 Fauser BCJM, Pache TD, Lamberts SW, Hop WC, De Jong FH, Dahl KD. Serum bioactive and immunoreactive luteinizing hormone and follicle-stimulating hormone levels in women with cycle abnormalities, with or without polycystic ovarian disease. *J Clin Endocrinol Metab* (1991) **73**: 811–17.

85 Erickson GF, Magoffin DA, Garzo VG, Cheung AP, Chang RJ. Granulosa cells of polycystic ovaries: are they normal or abnormal? *Hum Reprod* (1992) **7**: 293–9.

86 Eden JA, Jones J, Carter GD, Alagnband-Zadeh J. A comparison of follicular fluid levels of insulin-like growth factor-I in normal dominant and cohort follicles, polycystic and multicystic ovaries. *Clin Endocrinol* (1988) **29**: 327–36.

87 Eden JA, Jones J, Carter GD, Alaghband-Zadeh J. Follicular fluid concentrations of insulin-like growth factor 1, epidermal growth factor, transforming growth factor-alpha and sex-steroids in volume matched normal and polycystic human follicles. *Clin Endocrinol* (1990) **32**: 395–405.

88 Erickson GF, Hsueh AJW, Quigley ME, Rebar RW, Yen SSC. Functional studies of aromatase activity in human granulosa cells from normal and polycystic ovaries. *J Clin Endocrinol Metab* (1979) **49**: 514–19.

89 Mason HD, Margara R, Winstron RML, Beard RW, Reed MJ, Franks S. Inhibition of oestradiol production by epidermal growth factor in human granulosa cells of normal and polycystic ovaries. *Clin Endocrinol* (1990) **33**: 511–17.

90 Mason HD, Willis DS, Holly JMP, Franks JMP. Insulin preincubation enhances insulin-like growth factor-II (IGF-II) action on steroidogenesis in human granulosa cells. *J Clin Endocrinol Metab* (1994) **78**: 1265–7.

91 Cataldo NA, Giudice LC. Follicular fluid insulin-like growth factor binding protein profiles in polycystic ovary syndrome. *J Clin Endocrinol*

Metab (1992) **74**: 695–7.

92 Yap OWS, van Dessel HJHM, Chandrasekher YA, Fauser BCJM, Giudice LC. Similar insulin-like growth factor binding protein profiles in androgen-dominant follicular fluid from normal, polycystic ovary syndrome, and androgen-treated female-to-male transsexual human ovaries. Society for the Study of Reproduction, Sacramento, CA, July 1995.

93 Yap OWS, van Dessel HJHM, Chandrasekher YA, Fauser BCJM, Giudice LC. Insulin-like growth factors (IGFs) and IGF binding protein proteases in follicles from normally cycling women and androgen-treated female-to-male transsexuals. *Fertil Steril* (1997) **68**: 252–8.

94 Peng X, Maruo T, Samoto T, Mochizuki M. Comparison of immunocytologic localization of insulin-like growth factor binding protein-4 in normal and polycystic ovary syndrome human ovaries. *Endocrine J* (1996) **43**: 269–78.

95 Conway GS, Jacobs HS, Holly JMP, Wass JAH. Effects of luteinizing hormone, insulin, insulin-like growth factor-1 and insulin-like growth factor small binding protein 1 in the polycystic ovary syndrome. *Clin Endocrinol* (1990) **33**: 593–603.

96 Poretsky L, Peiper B. Insulin resistance, hypersecretion of LH, and a dual-defect hypothesis for the pathogenesis of polycystic ovary syndrome. *Obst Gynec* (1994) **84**: 613–21.

97 Barbieri RL, Makris S, Randall RW, Daniels G, Kistner RW, Ryan KJ. Insulin stimulates androgen accumulation in incubations of ovarian stroma obtained from women with hyperandrogenism. *J Clin Endocrinol Metab* (1986) **62**: 904–10.

98 Lanzone A, Fulghesu AM, Pappalardo S et al. Growth hormone and somatomedin-C secretion in patients with polycystic ovarian disease. Their relationships with hyperinsulinism and hyperandrogenism. *Gynecol Obstet Invest* (1990) **11**: 143–56.

99 Homburg R, Pariente C, Lunenfeld B, Jacobs HS. The role of insulin-like growth factor-1 (IGF-1) and IGF binding protein-1 (IGFBP-1) in the pathogenesis of polycystic ovary syndrome. *Hum Reprod* (1992) **7**: 1379–83.

100 El-Roeiy A, Baxter RC, Chen X, Laughlin G, Yen SSC. The role of growth hormone, insulin growth factors (IGF-I and IGF-II) and their binding proteins (IGFBP-3 and IGFBP-1) in PCO syndrome. Society for Gynecologic Investigation, San Antonio, TX, March 1991, abstract no. 517.

101 Morris RS, Carmina E, Vijod MA, Stanczyk FZ, Lobo RA. Alterations in the sensitivity of serum insulin-like growth factor I and insulin-like growth factor binding protein-4 to octreotide in polycystic ovary syndrome. *Fertil Steril* (1995) **63**: 742–6.

102 Fulghesu A, Lanzone A, Andreani CL, Pierro E, Caruso A, Mancuso S. Effectiveness of a somatostatin analogue in lowering luteinizing hormone and insulin-stimulated secretion in hyperinsulinemic women with polycystic ovary disease. *Fertil Steril* (1995) **64**: 703–8.

103 Pekonen F, Laatikainen T, Buyalos R, Rutanen EM. Decreased 34K insulin-like growth factor binding protein in polycystic ovarian disease. *Fertil Steril* (1989) **51**: 972–5.

104 Suikkari AM, Ruutiainen K, Erkkola R, Seppala M. Low levels of low molecular weight insulin-like growth factor-binding protein in patients with polycystic ovarian disease. *Hum Reprod* (1989) **4**: 136–9.

105 Iwashita M, Mimuro T, Watanabe M et al. Plasma levels of insulin-like growth factor-1 and its binding protein in polycystic ovary syndrome. *Horm Res* (1990) **33**(suppl. 2): 21–6.

106 Buyalos RP, Pekonen F, Halme JK, Judd HL, Rutanen EM. The relationship between circulating androgens, obesity, and hyperinsulinemia on serum insulin-like growth factor binding protein-1 in the polycystic ovarian syndrome. *Am J Obstet Gynecol* (1995) **172**: 932–9.

107 Hamilton-Fairley D, Kiddy D, Anyaoku V, Koistinen R, Seppala M, Franks S. Response of sex hormone binding globulin and insulin-like growth factor binding protein-1 to an oral glucose tolerance test in obese women with polycystic ovary syndrome. *Clin Endocrinol (Oxf)* (1993) **39**: 363–7.

108 Kiddy DS, Hamilton-Fairley D, Seppala M et al. Diet-induced changes in sex hormone binding globulin and free testosterone in women with normal or polycystic ovaries: correlation with serum insulin and insulin-like growth factor-1. *Clin Endocrinol* (1989) **31**: 757–63.

109 Greenblatt E, Casper RF. Endocrine changes after laparoscopic ovarian cautery in polycystic ovarian syndrome. *Am J Obstet Gynecol* (1987) **156**: 279–85.

110 Tiitinen AE, Tenhunen A, Seppala M. Ovarian electrocauterization causes LH-regulated but not insulin-regulated endocrine changes. *Clin Endocrinol* (1993) **39**: 181–4.

111 Homburg R, Orvieto R, Bar-Hava I, Ben-Rafael

Z. Serum levels of insulin-like growth factor-I, IGF binding protein-1 and insulin and the response to human menopausal gonadotrophins in women with polycystic ovary syndrome. *Hum Reprod* (1996) **11**: 716–19.

112 Hamilton-Fairley D, White D, Griffiths M, Anyaoku V, Koistinen R, Seppala M, Franks S. Diurnal variation of sex hormone binding globulin and insulin-like growth factor binding protein-1 in women with polycystic ovary syndrome. *Clin Endocrinol (Oxf)* (1995) **43**: 159–65.

113 Suikkari AM, Tiitinen A, Stenman UU, Seppala M, Laatikainen T. Oral contraceptives increase insulin-like growth factor binding protein-1 concentration in women with polycystic ovarian disease. *Fertil Steril* (1991) **55**: 895–9.

114 Klinger B, Anin S, Silbergeld A, Eshet R, Laron Z. Development of hyperandrogenism during treatment with insulin-like growth factor-I (IGF-I) in female patients with Laron syndrome. *Clin Endocrinol* (1998) **48**: 81–7.

9

Insulin resistance and obesity

Dror Meirow

INTRODUCTION

Polycystic ovary syndrome (PCOS), which is an exceptionally common endocrinopathy in premenopausal women, is characterized by significant metabolic abnormalities. It is the most common cause of anovulatory infertility with clinical or biochemical evidence of hyperandrogenism. Since the early 1980s it has become clear that PCOS is associated with obesity, glucose intolerance and biochemical evidence of hyperinsulinism.[1]

The association between diabetes mellitus, glucose intolerance and hyperandrogenism was first described in 1921 by Archard and Thiers ('diabetes of the bearded women'). Since then many studies have focused on the correlation between glucose intolerance, type 2 diabetes mellitus (non-insulin-dependent), hyperinsulinemia and hyperandrogenic disorders. Obesity, especially upper-body obesity, correlates positively with hyperandrogenism and insulin resistance, and indeed obesity is common in PCOS. This chapter presents the place of hyperinsulinism and obesity in the pathogenesis of PCOS, and discusses the role of weight reduction and the use of insulin sensitizing agents in the treatment of patients with PCOS.

INSULIN RESISTANCE, GLUCOSE INTOLERANCE AND OBESITY IN HYPERANDROGENIC DISORDERS

Several syndromes reported between 1947 and 1976 link severe insulin resistance and hyperandrogenism. Severe cases of insulin resistance are congenital, and include leprechaunism, Robson–Mendenhall syndrome and lipoatrophy. In the adolescent and adult form of lipoatrophy, severe hyperandrogenism is a major feature of the syndrome. In 1976 Kahn et al reported on adolescent girls with hyperandrogenism (true virilization), insulin resistance and acanthosis nigricans – Kahn type A syndrome.[2] These patients had mutations of the insulin receptor gene or other genetic defects in insulin action. Another rare syndrome combining severe insulin resistance and hyperandrogenism was identified in adult women with insulin receptor autoantibodies, and is known as Kahn type B syndrome. The association between those features is called the HAIR-AN syndrome (HA, hyperandrogenism; IR, insulin resistance; AN, acanthosis nigricans). However, these extreme forms of insulin resistance and hyperandrogenism are rare and account for only a minor section of the female population who suffer from insulin resistance and hyperandrogenism.

The most common hyperandrogenic disorder in women is PCOS. It was first identified in 1980,[1] and several studies subsequently confirmed that women with PCOS were hyperinsulinemic, suggesting the presence of insulin resistance. Dunaif et al have shown that insulin resistance exists in at least 50% of PCOS patients independent of obesity.[3]

The exact incidence of obesity in PCOS has not been determined and there are probably ethnic variations. However, most investigations have found that at least 50% of women with PCOS are obese. It has been estimated that 20% of these obese patients have glucose intolerance or type 2 diabetes mellitus by the age of 40 years.[4]

When less strict criteria were used, the prevalence of glucose intolerance in obese women with PCOS was recorded as being as high as 40%, the majority of women being in the third or fourth decade of life.[5,6] Whether the prevalence of glucose intolerance in these patients is 20% or 40%, this incidence is significantly higher than the reported population rate which is 5–10%.[7]

Insulin resistance is recognized as a major risk factor for the development of type 2 diabetes mellitus. One retrospective case–control study from Scandinavia has reported a prevalence of type 2 diabetes mellitus in patients with PCOS of 15%, compared with 2.3% in control subjects.[8] The opposite is also true. Conn et al found that 82% of women with type 2 diabetes mellitus had polycystic ovaries on ultrasound scan, and of these women, 52% had clinical evidence of cutaneous hyperandrogenism and/or menstrual disturbance.[9] The authors concluded that there is a higher prevalence of polycystic ovaries in women with type 2 diabetes mellitus compared with the general population. However, not all type 2 diabetes mellitus patients with hyperinsulinaemia develop PCOS, suggesting that hyperinsulinaemia alone is not sufficient cause for the expression of the syndrome. In addition, an increased incidence of glucose intolerance or

gestational diabetes mellitus was found in a group of pregnant women with PCOS who did not have diabetes or glucose intolerance before pregnancy.[10]

Hyperandrogenism is the second defining characteristic of PCOS. Clinically, it is usually manifested as hirsutism and acne. Depending on the androgen measured and the technique employed, between 50% and 90% of women with PCOS have elevated serum androgen levels. The biological effect of the most potent androgen, testosterone, is determined by the amount of sex hormone binding globulin (SHBG), since only the unbound fraction is active. Levels of SHBG are controlled by sex hormones and by insulin.[11]

Obesity is a well-known feature in PCOS and affects about 50% of patients. Obesity influences the clinical and biochemical features of PCOS patients in several ways: menstrual disturbances are more common in obese patients than in non-obese ones. A higher percentage of obese women with PCOS complain of hirsutism. Biochemical evaluation shows that obese patients had significantly lower serum levels of SHBG and higher levels of free testosterone.[12–14]

The author's group has investigated the clinical symptoms and hormone levels of patients with PCOS in Israel, and the connection with a hyperinsulinemic state. The occurrence of insulin resistance was determined by measuring insulin and glucose levels following a standard 75 g oral glucose load. All patients were evaluated by anthropometric measurements and endocrine profile. Following the oral glucose challenge test, insulin resistance was found in approximately half of the patients. The insulin-resistant group of patients were found to be significantly more obese, with a higher body mass index (BMI) ($P < 0.0001$), a higher percentage of body fat and upper-body obesity type (high waist/hip ratio, $P < 0.005$) and were more hirsute ($P < 0.002$) than patients who did not show insulin resistance (Figs 9.1, 9.2).[15] Hormonal profile evaluation showed that the insulin-resistant group had significantly higher testosterone levels ($P < 0.027$) with significantly lower levels of SHBG ($P < 0.02$). Thus, the

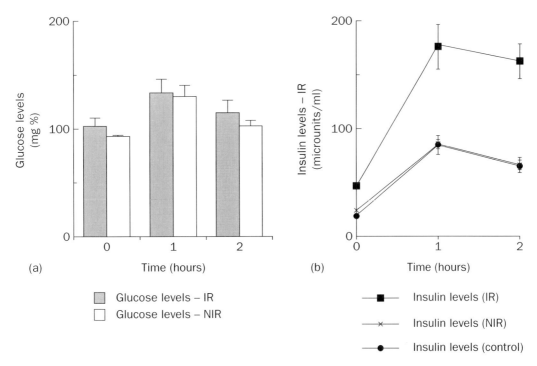

Figure 9.1 Mean (SEM) glucose (a) and insulin (b) levels at time zero and every hour for 2 hours following administration of 75 g glucose orally in group of patients with PCOS from Israel. In all patients glucose levels were within normal limits, hence none of the patients was diabetic. Fasting insulin levels and insulin levels in response to glucose administration were found to be significantly higher in one group of PCOS patients than in the other and in healthy, normally ovulating female subjects, thus defining two distinct subgroups: insulin-resistant (IR) and non-insulin-resistant (NIR). From Meirow et al,[15] with permission.

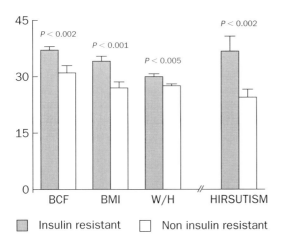

Figure 9.2 Body composition fat (BCF) assessed by means of Futrex 5000, fat distribution assessed by the waist-to-hip ratio (W/H), body mass index (BMI), the ratio between weight and body surface measured as weight/height^2, and hirsutism score (according to the Ferriman–Gallwey scoring) in insulin-resistant (IR) versus non-insulin-resistant (NIR) PCOS patients. The IR patients (grey bars) were significantly more obese and more hirsute compared with NIR patients, (white bars). From Meirow et al,[15] with permission.

BCF – Body composition fat
BMI – Body mass index
W/H – Waist to hip ratio

T/SHBG index was substantially higher when compared with the non-insulin-resistant subjects (22 versus. 5; $P < 0.0009$). An impaired luteinizing hormone/follicle-stimulating hormone (LH/FSH) ratio was only found in the non-insulin-resistant group of patients, while a normal ratio was found in the insulin-resistant group (2.94 vs. 1.34), ($P < 0.0001$).[15] Several other studies have stressed that a high BMI and insulin resistance are not associated with an increase in LH levels or LH/FSH ratio.[16–19]

HYPERINSULINISM AND HYPERANDROGENISM: CAUSE AND EFFECT

Even though the concomitant elevation of androgens and insulin is well established, the cause and effect relation between them should be appraised.

The effects of high levels of androgens on insulin levels

Androgens may cause insulin resistance and therefore hyperinsulinemia. Androgen administration can induce a moderate degree of insulin resistance, though much less severe than the insulin resistance seen in patients with PCOS.[20] Glucose clamp studies in oophorectomized female rats have shown that testosterone administration results in a marked decrease in insulin sensitivity.[21] In addition, modest changes in insulin sensitivity were found during antiandrogen therapy in non-obese PCOS patients without insulin resistance.[22]

Several studies have argued against the possibility that insulin resistance in patients with PCOS is caused by hyperandrogenism. Complete ovarian suppression with gonadotropin releasing hormone analog (GnRH-a) for up to 6 months in PCOS patients resulted in a sharp reduction of androgen levels with no change in insulin resistance. Administration of antiandrogens did not significantly alter insulin sensitivity in patients with PCOS.[23,24] Furthermore, men have high androgen levels

but have the same population rate of insulin resistance as women.

The effects of high insulin levels on androgens

Several observations and studies support the concept that high insulin levels can induce a hyperandrogenic state. Different diseases cause insulin resistance and hyperinsulinemia and all result in hyperandrogenism when they occur in premenopausal women. This includes genetic defects of the insulin receptor, or postreceptor defects, autoantibodies to insulin receptor (Kahn type B syndrome) or hypersecretion of insulin.[25]

Studies in vivo using a euglycemic, hyperinsulinemic clamp technique, carried out on normal men and women, obese women and hyperandrogenic women, have shown that in all groups, high levels of insulin were associated with an elevation of plasma androgens.[26,27] Conversely, a decrease in insulin levels following treatment with oral hypoglycemic agents in PCOS has been shown to result in a decrease in androgen levels. Nestler et al treated obese PCOS patients with diazoxide, measuring insulin levels both before and 28 days after diazoxide administration.[28] After treatment, there was a significant decrease in both basal and dynamic insulin levels followed by a decline in androgen levels: total testosterone was reduced by 17% and free testosterone was reduced by 28%. Studies in vitro have confirmed that insulin can stimulate ovarian androgen production (as well as estrogen and progesterone production).[29,30] Insulin administration stimulates androgen accumulation in incubations of ovarian stroma cells obtained from women with hyperandrogenism.[31]

In addition to directly increasing the production of androgens, insulin also plays a role in other important aspects of the regulation of the metabolism of androgens. Insulin has been shown to inhibit the production of SHBG in vitro by human hepatoma cells.[32] Furthermore, in PCOS patients treated with GnRH-a, suppression of insulin production by oral hypoglycemic agent results in a significant increase of serum SHBG with no change in androgen levels, indicating the direct effect of insulin on SHBG production.[11,33]

Studies examining the direct effects of insulin on pituitary–gonadotropin release in PCOS patients have yielded conflicting results. Insulin stimulates both basal and GnRH-induced LH and FSH release in isolated rat pituitary cells.[34] Also, decreased LH levels were observed after long-term administration of oral hypoglycemic agents.[35,36] In contrast, in short-term hyper-glycemic, euglycemic clamp studies performed in PCOS and normal women, insulin infusion did not alter LH or FSH plasma levels.[37] It seems that insulin can modify gonadotropin secretion and thus contribute also by this path-way to the changes in androgen production in humans.

In conclusion, hyperandrogenism can only be a contributing factor in the insulin resistance seen in women with PCOS, not the primary cause, and therefore does not explain the insulin resistance in this population. On the contrary, insulin can directly stimulate andro-gen production, modulate secretion and deter-mine free serum androgen level by manipulation of SHBG production.

THE MECHANISM OF HYPERINSULINEMIA IN PCOS

Hyperinsulinemia can result from any one of – or a combination of – the following reasons: increased insulin production by beta cells, insulin resistance in target cells, or impaired hepatic insulin clearance. Which is the cause of hyperinsulinemia in PCOS?

Beta cell function

In PCOS patients exaggerated beta cell reactiv-ity and insulin production were reported following glucose stimulation.[38] Abnormalities in insulin secretion have been reported in stud-ies of women with PCOS, with and without a family history of type 2 diabetes mellitus. Fasting hyperinsulinemia is present in obese women with PCOS and is, in part, secondary to increased basal insulin secretion.[39] Increased beta cell reactivity is also more pronounced in obese patients. Aging causes beta cell failure, leading to glucose intolerance which may result in type 2 diabetes mellitus, and this may explain the high incidence of diabetes in the older population of PCOS patients. The dispro-portionate beta cell effect is dependent on the insulin gene and its regulatory site. The VNTR (variable number tandem repeats) minisatellite which lies 5' to the insulin gene on chromo-some 11p15.5 is directly involved in the regula-tion of insulin secretion and has been associated with hyperinsulinemia and susceptibility to type 2 diabetes mellitus. At this locus, there is bimodal distribution of the 14–15 base pairs repeats, a short sequence of I alleles with about 40 repeats and a long sequence of III alleles with an average of 157 repeats which correlate with hyperinsulinemia and an insulin-resistant state. Studies have demonstrated that class III alleles are associated with PCOS in different populations and most strongly with anovula-tory PCOS patients.[40,41] It is proposed that class III alleles of the VNTR predispose a person to the sort of alterations in insulin secretion found in PCOS, which in turn cause hyperinsulinemia and insulin resistance.

Insulin clearance in PCOS

Decreased insulin clearance is present in hyper-insulinemic PCOS patients. This may be directly related to hyperinsulinemia which decreases the number of hepatic receptors for insulin, or secondary to hyperandrogenicity which also decreases hepatic insulin clearance.[42]

Target cell insulin resistance

Insulin resistance can exist when cellular response does not occur following exposure to insulin. The causes for such abnormal cellular response to insulin are impaired insulin recep-tor binding due to receptor defect (type A syn-drome) or autoantibodies to insulin receptor (type B syndrome); or a defect in insulin signaling which is mediated through a tyrosine kinase receptor causing activation of a number of phosphorylation–dephosphorylation steps.

A family with a severe form of insulin resistance resulting from a receptor defect is currently being treated at the author's clinic. Four out of five sisters in this family suffer from severe insulin resistance associated with acanthosis nigricans and hyperandrogenism. All four are obese, with severe hirsutism and irregular menstruation but without virilization. Endocrine studies show extremely high insulin levels (fasting insulin 360–760 pmol/l and post-glucose load of 75 g insulin levels above 1000 pmol/l) and high androgen levels with low SHBG. On ultrasonography all sisters showed the presence of classic polycystic ovaries. Molecular scanning techniques identified deletion of exon 3 of the insulin receptor gene. The resulting protein product is deformed, lacking 95% of its amino acids, including most of its extracellular, transmembrane and intracellular domains.[43] Patients with severe insulin resistance syndromes due to insulin receptor mutations or autoantibodies can also be virilized at a young age, or may present like this family with PCOS and acanthosis nigricans.[2]

However, insulin receptor mutations were not demonstrated in most patients with PCOS. Studies in lymphocytes, adipocytes and peripheral muscle cells have demonstrated that approximately 50% of PCOS patients have a postreceptor insulin signaling defect. In these women, the insulin receptor constantly undergoes serine phosphorylation, which in turn decreases its tyrosine kinase activity.[5,44] The biochemical effect of serine phosphorylation has been shown to terminate insulin signaling.[45] The result of continuous phosphorylation of the receptor is slightly increased basal insulin activity but with decreased response to insulin administration. It has been assumed that serine phosphorylation of the insulin receptor is important in the pathogenesis of hyperglycemia-induced insulin resistance.[46] However, the mechanism for the serine phosphorylation defect in PCOS has not been elucidated.[13] Figure 9.3 summarizes the different mechanisms of insulin resistance in PCOS patients.

INSULIN EFFECT ON THE POLYCYSTIC OVARY: HOW CAN A RESISTANT ORGAN HYPERRESPOND?

Insulin receptors are present in the stroma of the ovary and studies in vitro have demonstrated that insulin can directly stimulate steroidogenesis.[29] Decreased ability of insulin to control glucose metabolism is a hallmark of insulin resistance. Paradoxically, however, in PCOS the resistance of insulin action does not extend to ovarian steroidogenesis. A few hypotheses have been proposed to explain the ability of the polycystic ovary to hyperrespond to high insulin levels in the presence of an insulin-resistant state. There can be tissue-specific responses to insulin action, and differences among adipocytes, fibroblasts and ovarian stroma cells may exist. Also, a selective defect in peripheral and ovarian sensitivity to insulin has been demonstrated in some patients with PCOS who had severe metabolic insulin resistance (in terms of glucose metabolism) but maintained mitogenic insulin signaling pathways sensitivity.[47] The most convincing hypothesis suggests that the actions of insulin on steroidogenesis may be mediated by insulin-like growth factor (IGF) receptors that are present in ovarian tissues. Insulin has been shown to bind to type 1 IGF receptors at high concentrations and can mimic IGF-I actions.[48,49] It is likely that under physiological conditions, IGF-I rather than insulin stimulates steroidogenesis. However, in the presence of hyperinsulinemia, insulin may directly act on IGF receptors. Also, the affinity of the IGF-I receptor for insulin varies by tissue; thus data on receptor affinity cannot be extrapolated from one tissue to another. There are also 'atypical' IGF-I receptors that bind IGF-I and insulin with similar affinity. Dimmers of the insulin and IGF-I receptor can assemble together to form a hybrid.[25,50] All these have been proposed as a mechanism for insulin-mediated hyperandrogenism.

Hyperinsulinemia can result in upregulation

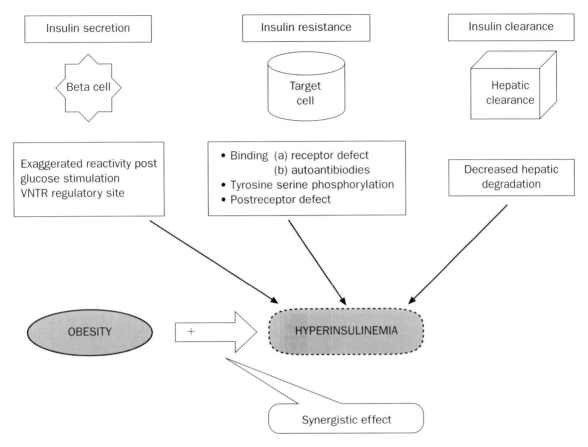

Figure 9.3 The different pathways that can cause hyperinsulinemia in women with PCOS. Obesity has a synergistic effect, thus increasing hyperinsulinemia and insulin resistance. Changes in the VNTR regulatory site are strongly associated with PCOS. A postreceptor insulin signaling defect is found in approximately 50% of patients with PCOS. In these women the insulin receptor is constantly serine phosphorylated, which in turn decreases its tyrosine kinase activity.

of ovarian IGF-I binding sites, and this may provide yet another mechanism by which insulin can amplify growth factor action.[51] Insulin-like growth factor binding proteins (IGFBPs) are major regulators of IGF action: they can specifically bind IGF-I and modulate its cellular actions by altering its bioavailability. Insulin decreases hepatic production of IGFBP-1 and may thus make IGF-I more biologically available.[52]

An intrinsic ovarian hypothesis has been suggested to explain the etiology of PCOS. Studies on PCOS patients have found dysregulation of the P450c17 enzyme function in the ovaries which performs both 17-hydroxylation and 17,20-lyase functions.[53] It has recently been proposed that hyperinsulinemia with insulin resistance and increased ovarian cytochrome P450c17 activity, two features of the syndrome, are pathogenetically linked. Serine phosphorylation of this enzyme selectively induces increase of the 17,20-lyase activity, thus producing more androgens.[54] As previously described, approximately 50% of patients with PCOS have a defect in serine phosphorylation of the insulin receptor, making this hypothesis tempting. Lowering insulin levels (following administration of metformin) leads to a reduction in stimulated ovarian cytochrome P450c17 activity in women with PCOS.[55]

High insulin levels associated with PCOS may also contribute to the increased plasma levels of adrenal androgens. La Marca et al have shown that with the administration of metformin to women with PCOS a decrease in the adrenal steroid response was recorded following an ACTH stimulation test.[56]

Most of the reported actions of insulin on steroidogenesis in vitro are enhanced by the addition of gonadotropins and are clinically observed only in PCOS patients. In normal women no significant changes in androgen pro-duction are present following manipulation in insulin levels.[30,35,57]

A summary of the possible insulin action in the polycystic ovary is presented in Figure 9.4.

OBESITY

The association between obesity, hyperandro-genism and hyperinsulinemia is well recog-nized. Obesity, however, is not a prerequisite for insulin resistance. Hyperinsulinemia in non-obese hyperandrogenic patients, with or with-out acanthosis nigricans, has been described.[3]

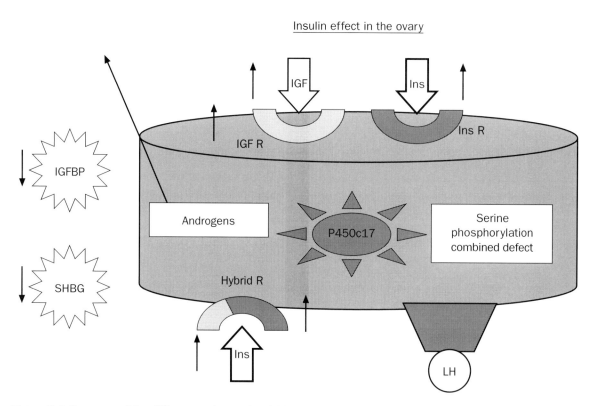

Figure 9.4 Summary of the different pathways by which hyperinsulinemia increases free androgen levels in the serum. High levels of insulin (Ins) activate insulin receptors (Ins R) in the theca cell, increase production of insulin-like growth factor (IGF), increase the number of IGF receptors (IGF R) and decrease hepatic production of IGF binding proteins (IGFBP). Insulin can also easily activate hybrid insulin and IGF receptors (Hybrid R). Thus, in the presence of luteinizing hormone (LH), insulin increases androgen production by the theca cells. There can also be a combined defect in the P450c17 system that causes both increased androgen production and insulin resistance. Freee androgen levels are even higher due to decreased production and serum levels of sex hormone binding globulin (SHBG).

Among obese subjects, the most unfavorable endocrine profiles have been demonstrated in those with upper-body obesity. Obese PCOS patients without insulin resistance usually have gynecoid obesity.[15]

An increased waist-to-hip ratio is associated with increased androgenicity (decreased SHBG level and increased percentage of free testosterone), increased basal and post-glucose-load blood insulin levels, and diminished insulin sensitivity in vivo.[58] Independent of obesity, increased waist-to-hip ratio predicts development of diabetes.[59]

Mechanisms of obesity-induced insulin resistance are not well understood, but appear to involve a decrease in the number of insulin receptors in target tissues and an inhibition of postreceptor events.[60] This form of insulin resistance appears to be reversible. It therefore appears that obesity is an additional, but not essential, risk factor predisposing to insulin resistance.[61]

TREATMENT

Diet and weight loss

Weight loss in women with PCOS can cause spontaneous resumption of menses and can lower circulating androgen levels.[62,63] These changes have been reported with a weight loss as small as 5% of the initial weight. As little as 7% reduction in body weight can restore fertility in obese women with PCOS.[62,64,65] Weight loss decreases circulating insulin levels,[62] and exercise has additional beneficial effects in lowering insulin levels in women with type 2 diabetes.[66,67] The decrease in unbound testosterone levels after weight loss may largely be mediated through increases in SHBG, which is negatively regulated by insulin levels.[62,64] It must be concluded that weight loss is an effective method of treatment of anovulatory infertile PCOS patients.

Antidiabetic drugs

Agents that lower insulin levels by improving insulin sensitivity may provide a new therapeutic option for patients with PCOS. Studies assessing the effects of attenuation of hyperinsulinemia and insulin resistance obtained by insulin sensitizing agents in women with PCOS have suggested potential scope for these drugs in treating the whole spectrum of reproductive, endocrine and metabolic abnormalities.

The initial experience with antidiabetic drugs in PCOS has shown promise; drugs that improve insulin action have consistently been found to improve reproductive abnormalities in women with PCOS. Short-term use of agents that lower insulin secretion, such as diazoxide, has shown beneficial effects.[35,68]

The insulin-sensitizing agent metformin works primarily by suppressing hepatic gluconeogenesis, which is accompanied by a reduction in circulating insulin levels. When used in PCOS it can decrease androgen levels and at times results in resumption of menses.[35,69,70] Randomized studies on metformin have shown improvement in insulin action and lowered serum androgen levels in women with POCS.[35,71] However, other studies have not consistently shown improvement in PCOS women; some showed that the beneficial effects of metformin were accompanied by weight loss, and it was difficult to separate out the effects of weight loss on improved insulin action from those of the medication.[70,71] Moghetti et al evaluated the effect of long-term administration (6 months) of metformin 500 mg three times a day to obese patients with PCOS (BMI $30.0 \pm 1.1 \, \text{kg/m}^2$) who maintained their usual eating habits.[72] Following this treatment, striking amelioration of menstrual abnormalities was noticed in about 50% of subjects. Women given metformin showed reduced plasma insulin levels and increased insulin sensitivity ($P < 0.05$). Concurrently, ovarian hyperandrogenism was attenuated, as indicated by significant reductions in serum free testosterone following stimulation test ($P < 0.05$). No changes were found in the placebo group. In 10 subjects whose menses proved regular after treatment, about 80% of cycles became ovulatory. This was despite the fact that only relatively minor changes in body mass index occurred both in the metformin group and in the placebo group. In conclusion, metformin treatment reduced hyperinsulinemia and hyperandrogenemia in women with PCOS, independently of changes in body weight. In a large number of subjects these changes were associated with striking, sustained improvements in menstrual abnormalities and resumption of ovulation.

The effect of metformin on spontaneous and clomiphene-induced ovulation was evaluated in 61 obese PCOS patients.[73] Metformin 500 mg three times a day or placebo was given for 35 days, and women who did not ovulate were treated with clomiphene citrate. In the metformin group about 40% of patients had spontaneous ovulation and as many as 90% ovulated following metformin and clomiphene citrate treatment. In the placebo-treated group only 1 out of 26 patients ovulated and following administration of clomiphene citrate a total of only 2 out of 26 patients had ovulation. This is, of course, a relatively small study.

Troglitazone is an agent that directly reduces insulin resistance and circulating insulin levels. Troglitazone administration to women with PCOS resulted in an improvement in insulin sensitivity and reduced circulating androgen levels.[36,74] Results of the study suggest a dose–response relationship, with an improved response at a daily dose of 400 mg compared with 200 mg. The effect of troglitazone on ovulatory performance was evaluated in women with insulin-resistant PCOS.[75] Administration of clomiphene citrate resulted in ovulation in 35% (15 out of 43) of women; with troglitazone administration 42% (11 out of 26) ovulated, and with co-administration of troglitazone and clomiphene citrate as many as 73% (8 out of 11) of women ovulated.

It should be remembered that both drugs have side effects that require careful monitoring such as abdominal discomfort, nausea, diarrhea, anorexia (with metformin) and elevated liver function tests, and in extremely rare cases troglitazone has caused hepatic necrosis. Although both medications are listed as cat-

egory B, with no known human teratogenic effects, there is a lack of substantial experience in women of reproductive age. The long-term efficacy (beyond 6 months) of these medications also needs to be established, as well as their usefulness in treating peripheral hyperandrogenism, such as acne or hirsutism. As yet, there is no study of adequate power or design to recommend this as a standard therapy in PCOS women, and pregnancy rates following administration of these medications were not monitored.

Patients with PCOS do not belong to a homogenic population with ethnic variations, and presumably underlying genetic differences. In insulin resistance may explain the fact that metformin appears effective in certain populations, such as Venezuelan or Finnish women, but not so in American or Turkish populations. Patients may or may not be insulin-resistant. Non-obese women with PCOS who are not absolutely insulin-resistant or hyperinsulinemic will not respond; they may not tolerate all antidiabetic agents, and may require special consideration. It is hoped that the molecular mechanism of insulin resistance in PCOS will be discovered and lead to the development of an appropriate pharmacological treatment. It may be beneficial to offer patients with PCOS a simple glucose tolerance test measuring both glucose and insulin levels (as described above) which will allow judicious selection of patients for insulin- sensitizing treatments.

REFERENCES

1 Burghen GA, Givens JR, Kitabachi AE. Correlation of hyperandrogenism with hyperinsulinism in polycystic ovarian disease. *J Clin Endocrinol Metab* (1980) **50**: 113–16.

2 Kahn CR, Flier JS, Bar RS et al. The syndromes of insulin resistance and acanthosis nigricans. *N Engl J Med* (1976) **294**: 739–45.

3 Dunaif A, Futterweit W, Segal KR, Dobrjansky A. Profound peripheral insulin resistance, independent of obesity, in the polycystic ovary syndrome. *Diabetes* (1989) **38**: 1165–74.

4 Dunaif A. Hyperandrogenic anovulation (PCOS): a unique disorder of insulin action associated

with an increased risk of non-insulin-dependent diabetes mellitus. *Am J Med* (1995) **98**: 33S.

5 Dunaif A, Segal KR, Shelley DR, Green G, Dobrjansky A, Licholai T. Evidence for distinctive and intrinsic defects in insulin action in polycystic ovary syndrome. *Diabetes* (1992) **41**: 1257–66.

6 Dunaif A, Sorbara L, Delson R, Green G. Ethnicity and polycystic ovary syndrome are associated with independent and additive decreases in insulin action in Caribbean Hispanic women. *Diabetes* (1993) **42**: 1462–68.

7 Harris MI, Hadden WC, Knowler WC, Bennett PH. Prevalence of diabetes and impaired glucose tolerance and plasma glucose levels in US population aged 20–74 yr. *Diabetes* (1987) **36**: 523–34.

8 Dahlgren E, Johansson S, Lindstedt F et al. Women with polycystic ovary syndrome wedge resected in 1956 to 1965: a long term follow-up focusing on natural history and circulating hormones. *Fertil Steril* (1992) **57**: 505–13.

9 Conn JJ, Jacobs HS, Conway GS. The prevalence of polycystic ovaries in women with type 2 diabetes mellitus. *Clin Endocrinol (Oxf)* (2000) **52**: 81–6.

10 Lanzone A, Caruso A, Di Simone N, De Carolis S, Fulghesu AM, Mancuso S. Polycystic ovary disease. A risk factor for gestational diabetes? *J Reprod Med* (1995) **40**: 312–16.

11 Nestler JE, Powers LP, Matt DW et al. A direct effect of hyperinsulinemia on serum sex hormone-binding globulin levels in obese women with polycystic ovary syndrome. *J Clin Endocrinol Metab* (1991) **72**: 83–9.

12 Kiddy DS, Sharp PS, White DM et al. Differences in clinical endocrine features between obese and non-obese subjects with polycystic ovary syndrome: an analysis of 263 consecutive cases. *Clin Endocrinol* (1990) **32**: 213–20.

13 Taylor AE. Polycystic ovary syndrome. *Endocr Metab Clin North Am* (1990) **27**: 877–902.

14 Franks S, Kiddy D, Sharp P et al. Obesity and polycystic ovary syndrome. *Ann N Y Acad Sci* (1991) **626**: 201–6.

15 Meirow D, Yossepowitch O, Rosler A et al. Insulin resistant and non-resistant polycystic ovary syndrome represent two clinical and endocrinological subgroups. *Hum Reprod* (1995) **10**: 1951–6.

16 Conway GS, Honour JW, Jacobs HS. Heterogeneity of the polycystic ovary syndrome: clinical, endocrine, and ultrasound features in 556 patients. *Clin Endocrinol* (1989) **30**: 459–70.

17 Dale PO, Tanbo T, Vaaler S et al. Body weight, hyperinsulinemia, and gonadotropin levels in the polycystic ovary syndrome: evidence of two distinct populations. *Fertil Steril* (1992) **58**: 487–91.

18 Lobo RA, Kletzky OA, Campeau JD. Elevated bioactive luteinizing hormone in women with the polycystic ovary syndrome. *Fertil Steril* (1983) **39**: 674–8.

19 Pasquali R, Casimirri F, Venturoli S. Insulin resistance in patients with polycystic ovaries: its relationship to body weight and androgen levels. *Acta Endocrinol (Copenh)* (1983) **104**: 110–16.

20 Billar RB, Risharadson D, Schwartz R, Posner B, Little B. Effect of chronically elevated androgen or estrogen on the glucose tolerance test and insulin response in female rhesus monkeys. *Am J Obstet Gynecol* (1987) **157**: 1297–302.

21 Holmang A, Larsson BM, Brzezinska Z, Bjorntorp P. Effects of short-term testosterone exposure on insulin sensitivity of muscles in female rats. *Am J Physiol* (1992) **25**: E851–5.

22 Moghetti P, Tosi F, Castello R et al. The insulin resistance in women with hyperandrogenism is partially reversed by antiandrogen treatment: evidence that androgens impair insulin action in women. *J Clin Endocrinol Metab* (1996) **81**: 952–60.

23 Dunaif A, Green G, Futterweit W et al. Suppression of hyperandrogenism does not improve peripheral or hepatic insulin resistance in the PCOS. *J Clin Endocrinol Metabol* (1990) **70**: 699–704.

24 Geffner ME, Kaplan SA, Bersch N, Golde DW, Landaw EM, Chang RJ. Persistence of insulin resistance in polycystic ovarian disease after inhibition of ovarian steroid secretion. *Fertil Steril* (1986) **45**: 327–33.

25 Dunaif A. Insulin resistance and the polycystic ovary syndrome: mechanism and implications for pathogenesis. *Endocr Rev* (1997) **18**: 774–800.

26 Stuart CA, Prince MJ, Peters EJ, Meyer WJ. Hyperinsulinemia and hyperandrogenemia: in vivo androgen response to insulin infusion. *Obstet Gynecol* (1987) **69**: 921–5.

27 Stuart CA, Nagamani M. Insulin infusion acutely augments ovarian androgen production in normal women. *Fertil Steril* (1990) **54**: 788–92.

28 Nestler JE, Barlascini CO, Matt DW et al. Suppression of serum insulin by diazoxide reduces serum testosterone levels in obese women with polycystic ovary syndrome. *J Clin Endocrinol Metab* (1989) **68**: 1027–32.

29 Nestler JE, Strauss JF. Insulin as an effector of human ovarian and adrenal steroid metabolism. *Endocr Metab Clin North Am* (1991) **20**: 807–23.

30 Dunaif A. Insulin resistance and ovarian hyperandrogenism. *Endocrinologist* (1992) **2**: 248–60.

31 Barbieri RL, Makris A, Randall RW et al. Insulin stimulates androgen accumulation in incubations of ovarian stroma obtained from women with hyperandrogenism. *J Clin Endocrinol Metab* (1986) **62**: 904–10.

32 Plymate SR, Matej LA, Jones RE, Freidl KE. Inhibition of sex hormone-binding globulin production in the human hepatoma (Hep G2) cell line by insulin and prolactin. *J Clin Endocrinol Metab* (1988) **67**: 460–4.

33 Nestler JE. Sex hormone binding globulin. A marker for hyperinsulinemia and/or insulin resistance? *J Clin Endocrinol Metab* (1993) **76**: 273–4.

34 Adashi EY, Hseueh AJW, Yen SSC. Insulin enhancement of luteinizing hormone and follicle-stimulating hormone release by cultured pituitary cells. *Endocrinology* (1981) **108**: 1441–9.

35 Nestler JE, Jakubowicz DJ. Decreases in ovarian cytochorme P450c17a activity and serum free testosterone after reduction of insulin secretion in polycystic ovary syndrome. *N Engl J Med* (1996) **335**: 617–23.

36 Dunaif A, Scott D, Finegood D, Quintana B, Whitcomb R. The insulin sensitizing agent troglitazone: a novel therapy for the polycystic ovary syndrome. *J Clin Endocrinol Metab* (1996) **81**: 3299–306.

37 Dunaif A, Graf M. Insulin administration alters gonadal steroid metabolism independent of changes in gonadotropin secretion in insulin-resistant women with the polycystic ovary syndrome. *J Clin Invest* (1989) **83**: 23–9.

38 Ehrmann D, Sturis J, Byrne MM, Karrison T, Rosenfield RL, Polonsky KS. Insulin secretory defects in polycystic ovary syndrome. Relationship to insulin sensitivity and family history of non-insulin-dependent diabetes mellitus. *J Clin Invest* (1995) **96**: 520–7.

39 O'Meara NM, Blackman JD, Ehrmann DA et al. Defects in β-cell function in functional ovarian hyperandrogenism. *J Clin Endocrinol Metab* (1993) **76**: 1241–7.

40 Franks S, Gharani N, Waterworth DM et al. The genetic basis of polycystic ovary syndrome. *Hum Reprod* (1997) **12**: 2641–8.

41 Waterworth DM, Bennett ST, Gharani N et al. Linkage and association of insulin gene VNTR regulatory polymorphism with polycystic ovary syndrome. *Lancet* (1997) **349**: 986–90.

42 Peiris AN, Mueller RA, Struve MF, Smith GA, Kissebah AH. Relationship of androgenic activity to splanchnic insulin metabolism and peripheral glucose utilization in premenopausal women. *J Clin Endocrinol Metab* (1987) **64**: 162–9.

43 Wertheimer E, Litvin Y, Ebstein RP et al. Deletion of Exon 3 of the insulin receptor gene in a kindred with a familial form of insulin resistance. *J Clin Endocrinol Metab* (1994) **78**: 1153–8.

44 Dunaif A, Xia J, Book C, Schenker E, Tang Z. Excessive insulin receptor serine phosphorylation in cultured fibroblasts and in skeletal muscle: a potential mechanism for insulin resistance in the polycystic ovary syndrome. *J Clin Invest* (1995) **96**: 801–10.

45 Theroux SJ, Latour DA, Stanley K, Raden DL, Davis RJ. Signal transduction by the epidermal growth factor receptor is attenuated by a COOH-terminal domain serine phosphorylation site. *J Biol Chem* (1992) **267**: 16620–6.

46 Kruszynska YT, Olefsky JM. Cellular and molecular mechanisms of non-insulin dependent diabetes mellitus. *J Invest Med* (1996) **44**: 413–28.

47 Book CB, Dunaif A. Selective insulin resistance in the polycystic ovary syndrome. *J Clin Endocrinol Metab* (1999) **84**: 3110–16.

48 Rechler MM, Nissley SP. Insulin-like growth factor (IGF)/somatomedin receptor subtypes: structure, function, and relationships to insulin receptors and IGF carrier proteins. *Horm Res* (1986) **24**: 152–9.

49 Froesch ER, Zapf J. Insulin-like growth factors and insulin: comparative aspects. *Diabetologia* (1985) **28**: 485–93.

50 Moxham CP, Jacobs S. Insulin/IGF-I receptor hybrids: a mechanism for increasing receptor diversity. *J Cell Biochem* (1992) **48**: 136–40.

51 Poretsky L, Glover B, Laumas V, Kalin M, Dunaif A. The effects of experimental hyperinsulinemia on steroid secretion, ovarian insulin binding, and ovarian insulin-like growth-factor I binding in the rat. *Endocrinology* (1988) **122**: 581–5.

52 Leroith D, Werner H, Beitner-Johnson D, Roberts CT. Molecular and cellular aspects of the insulin-like growth factor I receptor. *Endocr Rev* (1995) **16**: 143–63.

53 Gilling-Smith C, Story H, Rogers V. Evidence for a primary abnormality of thecal cell steroidogenesis in the polycystic ovary syndrome. *Clin Endocrinol* (1997) **47**: 93–9.

54 Zhang LH, Rodriguez H, Ohno S. Serine phosphorylation of human P450c17 increases 17,20-lyase activity: implications for adrenarche and the polycystic ovary syndrome. *Proc Natl Acad Sci USA* (1995) **92**: 10619–23.

55 La Marca A, Egbe TO, Morgante G et al. Metformin treatment reduces ovarian cytochrome P-450c17alpha response to human chorionic gonadotrophin in women with insulin resistance-related polycystic ovary syndrome. *Reprod 2000* (2000) **15**: 21–3.

56 La Marca A, Morgante G, Paglia T, Ciotta L, Cianci A, De Leo V. Effects of metformin on adrenal steroidogenesis in women with polycystic ovary syndrome. *Fertil Steril* (1999) **72**: 985–9.

57 Nestler JE, Singh R, Matt DW, Clore JN, Blackard WG. Suppression of serum insulin level by diazoxide does not alter serum testosterone or sex hormone-binding globulin levels in healthy, non-obese women. *Am J Obstet Gynecol* (1990) **163**: 1243–6.

58 Evans DJ, Hoffman RG, Kalkoff RK, Kissebah AH. Relationship of androgenic activity to body fat topography, fat cell morphology, and metabolic aberrations in premenopausal women. *J Clin Endocrinol Metab* (1983) **57**: 304–10.

59 Ohlson LO, Larsson B, Svardsudd K. The influence of body fat distribution on the incidence of diabetes mellitus. *Diabetes* (1985) **34**: 1055–8.

60 Flier JS, Eastman RC, Minaker KL, Matteson D, Rowe JW. Acanthosis nigricans in obese women with hyperandrogenism. Characterization of an insulin-resistant state distinct from the type A and B syndromes. *Diabetes* (1985) **34**(2): 101–7.

61 Kissebah AH, Vydelingum N, Murray R. Relation of body fat distribution to metabolic complications of obesity. *J Clin Endocrinol Metab* (1982) **54**: 254–60.

62 Kiddy DS, Hamilton-Fairley D, Bush A, Short F, Anyaoku V, Reed MJ. Improvement in endocrine and ovarian function during dietary treatment of obese women with polycystic ovary syndrome. *Clin Endocrinol* (1992) **36**: 105–11.

63 Guzick DS, Wing R, Smith D, Berga SL, Winters SJ. Endocrine consequences of weight loss in obese, hyperandrogenic, anovulatory women. *Fertil Steril* (1994) **61**: 598–604.

64 Franks, S, Kiddy D, Sharp P et al. Obesity and polycystic ovary syndrome. *Ann NY Acad Sci* (1991) **626**: 201–6.

65 Holte J, Bergh T, Berne C, Wide L, Lithell H. Restored insulin sensitivity by persistently increased early insulin secretion after weight loss in obese women with polycystic ovary syndrome. *J Clin Endocrinol Metab* (1995) **80**: 2586–93.

66 Braun B, Zimmerman MB, Kretchmer N. Effects of exercise intensity on insulin sensitivity in women with non-insulin-dependent diabetes mellitus. *J Appl Physiol* (1995) **78**: 300–6.

67 Jaatinen TA, Anttila L, Erkkola R et al. Hormonal responses to physical exercise in patients with polycystic ovary syndrome. *Fertil Steril* (1993) **60**: 262–7.

68 Prelevic GM, Wurzburger MI, Balint-Peric L, Nesic JS. Inhibitory effect of sandostatin on secretion of luteinising hormone and ovarian steroids in polycystic ovary syndrome. *Lancet* (1990) **336**(8720): 900–3.

69 Velazquez EM, Mendoza S, Hamer T, Sosa F, Glueck CJ. Metformin therapy in polycystic ovary syndrome reduces hyperinsulinemia, insulin resistance, hyperandrogenemia, and systolic blood pressure, while facilitating normal menses and pregnancy. *Metabolism* (1994) **43**: 647–54.

70 Velazquez E, Acosta A, Mendoza SG. Menstrual cyclicity after metformin therapy in polycystic ovary syndrome. *Obstet Gynecol* (1997) **90**: 392–5.

71 Crave JC, Fimbel S, Lejeune H, Cugnardey N, Dechaud H, Pugeat M. Effects of diet and metformin administration on sex hormone-binding globulin, androgens, and insulin in hirsute and obese women. *J Clin Endocrinol Metab* (1995) **80**: 2057–62.

72 Moghetti P, Castello R, Negri C et al. Metformin effects on clinical features, endocrine and metabolic profiles, and insulin sensitivity in polycystic ovary syndrome: a randomized, double-blind, placebo-controlled 6-month trial, followed by open, long-term clinical evaluation. *J Clin Endocrinol Metab* (2000) **85**: 139–46.

73 Nestler JE, Jakubowicz DJ, Evans WS, Pasquali R. Effects of metformin on spontaneous and clomiphene-induced ovulation in the polycystic ovary syndrome. *N Engl J Med* (1998) **338**(26): 1876–80.

74 Ehrmann DA, Schneider DJ, Sobel BE, Cavaghan MK. Troglitazone improves defects in insulin action, insulin secretion, ovarian steroidogenesis, and fibrinolysis in women with polycystic ovary syndrome. *J Clin Endocrinol Metab* (1997) **82**: 2108–16.

75 Hasegawa I, Murakawa H, Suzuki M, Yamamoto Y, Kurabayashi T, Tanaka K. Effect of troglitazone on endocrine and ovulatory performance in women with insulin resistance-related polycystic ovary syndrome. *Fertil Steril* (1999) **71**(2): 323–7.

10

Symptomatic treatment of acne and hirsutism

Gordana M Prelevic

Hirsutism is present in over 70% of women with polycystic ovary syndrome (PCOS). In a proportion of these women it is accompanied by other skin disorders such as alopecia, seborrhoea and acne, all of which are the results of increased androgen production and/or increased skin sensitivity to androgens.

The individual drugs used in the treatment of hirsutism affect different aspects of androgen metabolism (Table 10.1).

They may:

- decrease androgen production
- increase metabolic clearance rate of androgens
- inhibit androgen receptors
- inhibit or block enzymes involved in the peripheral production of testosterone or conversion of testosterone to dihydrotestosterone (DHT)
- increase the amount of sex hormone binding globulin (SHBG).[1]

Suppression of androgen excess alone will not cure hirsutism; an antiandrogen is also required. The response to treatment varies from 20% to 95%, depending on the drug, the dosage used and the individual response,

Table 10.1 Treatment of hirsutism in polycystic ovary syndrome

Medical management	Other therapies
Combined oral contraceptive pill	Weight reduction
Antiandrogens	Cosmetic procedures
Cyproterone acetate	Antibiotics and topical therapies
Spironolactone	Psychological intervention
Flutamide	
Finasteride	
GnRH agonists (plus add-back therapy)	

and overall is far from being completely successful.

The growth cycle of hair is long, 6–24 months, and the conversion of vellus to terminal hair is irreversible. Once hair growth has been stimulated by excessive androgen levels, maintenance of the same growth rate requires much less androgen. Drug treatment is essentially directed toward arresting growth of new hair until the hair that is present enters the catagen stage and is eventually shed from the follicle. Patients must therefore be advised that a response to therapy may not be seen for 6–12 months, and that although it is possible to prevent further conversion of vellus to terminal hair, little change will be seen in the total number of terminal hairs. Some women may note a lighter hair colour, a slowing of the rate of regrowth and a decrease in the diameter of the hair shaft. As there are wide variations in response, treatment must be individualized and continued beyond the growth cycle of the relevant hairs before benefit can be assessed. The response to therapy varies greatly not only between individuals but also between different sites on the body, depending on the local rate of hair growth. Of all signs of hyperandrogenism, alopecia is the slowest to respond as scalp hair has a growth cycle of over 3 years.[2]

The patient should be clearly informed from the onset that treatment is effective only while the medication is in use. Most patients report worsening of hirsutism, acne and oily skin after stopping medication. Patients with a relatively short history of hirsutism tend to respond better to treatment than those with long-standing hyperandrogenaemia and severe hirsutism. It is also easier to prevent hair growth than to treat established hirsutism. Adolescent girls who are beginning to develop hirsutism therefore respond best to the medical therapy.[3]

Women who respond to treatment may notice changes in unwanted hair growth by the third month, but most do not until the sixth month. Beneficial effect will be obvious after 12 months, although the effectiveness of treatment increases to a maximum at approximately 2 years. Treatment may be withdrawn subsequently on a trial basis or maintained at the lowest dose.

Once therapy has started the patient's progress can be monitored on the basis of both clinical appearance and laboratory tests. The effectiveness of treatment is best assessed in terms of a reduction in the time a woman spends in mechanically removing the hair. Patients who exhibit progressive hirsutism or whose circulating androgens fail to decrease as expected on hormonal therapy should undergo further evaluation.[1]

When adequate suppression of serum androgens has been maintained for 6–12 months but a satisfactory reduction in new hair growth has not been achieved, other therapeutic options should be tried. The dose of the current medication can be increased, a new medication can be substituted, or a new medication can be added. Maximal doses are often only slightly, if at all, more effective than mid-range doses.[3] In theory, a combination of drugs that act at different sites may offer the best results. Adding an oral contraceptive has other benefits such as contraceptive protection, which is a necessary part of antiandrogen treatment, or cycle control.

COMBINED ORAL CONTRACEPTIVE PILLS

The drugs most widely used to suppress ovarian androgen production are combined oestrogen/progestogen oral contraceptive pills (OC),[4,5] and these should be the treatment of choice for mild hirsutism of PCOS. However, some of the progestogens (norethindrone, norgestrel, ethynodiol diacetate) in OC are 19-nor-testosterone derivatives and have androgenic properties. It is therefore of utmost importance to choose a combination that does not have androgenic activity and preferably has antiandrogenic effects, such as cyproterone acetate (CPA).

Ovarian androgen secretion is reduced as a result of suppression of gonadotrophins. The oestrogen component stimulates SHBG production, further lowering free androgen levels. In addition to suppression of gonadotrophins, OCs induce a decrease in adrenal androgen production.[6] This is of obvious therapeutic benefit since at least a third of patients with PCOS have additional adrenal hyperandrogenism. The magnitude of this decrease is 30–60% in terms of dehydroepiandrosterone sulfate (DHEA-S) levels. At least three cycles of an oral contraceptive regimen are required to reach an endocrine equilibrium as reflected in levels of luteinizing hormone, follicle-stimulating hormone, SHBG and sex steroids.[7]

Treatment with OC containing 2 mg of CPA (Dianette) has marked beneficial effects on acne, seborrhoea and hirsutism. The rate of clearing facial acne seems to be faster in women under 25 years old than in those who are older (42% and 30% respectively within the first 3 months of therapy).[8] While the effect on acne and seborrhoea is evident shortly after introducing treatment, eight to twelve cycles are needed for the effect on hirsutism to become clinically evident in most patients, and the longer treatment is continued the better are the results achieved.

The beneficial effect of Dianette on hirsutism is the result of general reduction of biologically active androgens in circulation and antiandrogen effects at the target organ. Individual variations in susceptibility to treatment are considerable. Mild facial hirsutism regresses completely in 25–34% of cases after nine to twelve cycles, but in patients with severe hirsutism, additional CPA is required to improve the effect of Dianette (see below).

In the author's series treatment with Dianette resulted in marked clinical improvement with significantly decreased hirsutism scores – 16.8% after the first year and 42.7% over 3 years (Figure 10.1), disappearance of acne and seborrhoea, normalization of hormonal profile (Figure 10.2) and a reduction of ovarian volume in hirsute women with PCOS (Table 10.2).[7] Beneficial effects were observed on fertility, as a proportion of these patients conceived soon after discontinuing Dianette. This clinical observation of potential beneficial effect on future fertility is most probably the result of the

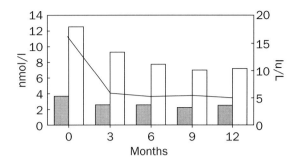

Figure 10.2 Mean serum LH (line), testosterone (shaded bars) and androstenedione (open bars) concentrations during treatment with cyproterone acetate and ethinyloestradiol (Dianette) in hirsute women with PCOS. From Prelevic et al.[7]

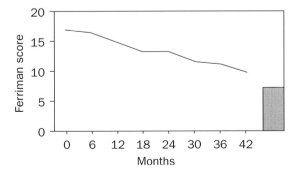

Figure 10.1 Changes in the mean hirsutism score (line) during treatment with cyproterone acetate and ethinyloestradiol (Dianette) and the mean difference (shaded bar) between pretreatment and end-of-study scores in hirsute women with PCOS. From Prelevic et al.[7]

Table 10.2 Beneficial effects of low-dose combined oestrogen–antiandrogen preparation (Dianette) in PCOS
On hormonal disturbances
Decrease in LH levels
Decrease in ovarian and adrenal androgen levels
Increase in SHBG concentrations
On clinical signs
Decrease in hirsutism score
Improvement in acne and seborrhoea
Good control of menstrual cycle
On ovarian size
Decrease in ovarian volume
On future fertility
Possible favourable profertility effect

improved hormonal milieu and ovarian suppression during treatment and is consistent with other studies which showed that normalization of luteinizing hormone (LH) and ovarian androgens in the early follicular phase has a beneficial effect on ovulatory performance.[9,10] Several clinicians share the opinion that normalizing the hormonal milieu (particularly the suppression of androgens with a low-dose oestrogen/antiandrogen pill) in adolescents with PCOS has beneficial effects on these patients' subsequent clinical presentation, not only in terms of their fertility potential but also in terms of hirsutism.

The side effects of Dianette are those of any OC: breast tenderness, headache, dizziness, nausea, nervousness and depression. Patients reported a decrease of libido in some studies. Fluctuations of body weight of more than 2 kg were recorded in 18.2% of patients after 36 cycles of treatment. Side effects of Dianette in our study were transient and experienced during the first six cycles of treatment. On a long-term basis cycle control was good, the drug is well tolerated and patient compliance is excellent.[7] Thromboembolic disease and hypertension are more likely to occur in women over 35 years old who are obese and who smoke. Insulin levels during an oral glucose tolerance test were significantly increased in women with PCOS on Dianette.[11] In some studies there was also an increase in levels of total cholesterol, high-density lipoprotein (HDL) and low-density lipoprotein (LDL) cholesterol in these women. Significantly increased levels of triglycerides and total lipids were observed in all studies.[11,12]

ANTIANDROGENS

Antiandrogens interfere with androgen action at the target organ. They vary in structure and mode of action and either block enzyme reactions (thereby limiting the formation of potent androgens) or specifically block the androgen receptor; some antiandrogens affect both enzyme reactions and androgen receptor. These drugs may have no hormonal activity or may

be converted to other steroid derivatives that have little or no androgenic potency. No antiandrogen has been shown to be superior in a well-designed clinical trial on hirsute women. In theory, however, cyproterone acetate should be the best for women with PCOS and elevated testosterone levels.[3]

A male fetus in utero is at risk of developing feminized external genitalia if his mother is having treatment with an antiandrogen. Concurrent use of adequate contraception is therefore an essential component of any treatment regimen using an antiandrogen. Additionally, most antiandrogens have side effects, some of which are potentially dangerous. Consideration of the risk-benefit ratio is therefore of utmost importance in choosing an antiandrogen drug, as the underlying condition, however distressing, is benign.[13] More recent comparative clinical studies, particularly with low-dose regimens, suggest that these agents are well tolerated.

Cyproterone acetate

Cyproterone acetate, a steroid derived from 17-hydroxyprogesterone, has been the most widely used antiandrogen in Europe since the 1970s. It has progestational and antigonadotrophic actions in addition to antiandrogen activity.[14] The clinical improvement observed with CPA is therefore due to both central antigonadotrophic activity and antiandrogen effect at the end organ. The antiandrogen effect results from inhibition of testosterone and DHT binding to their intracellular receptors; the reduction in concentrations of circulating androgens is the result of inhibition of ovarian androgen production through suppression of LH release. Cyproterone acetate also increases the metabolic clearance of androgens by hepatic enzyme induction as well as an indirect reduction in the androgen-dependent 5α-reductase enzyme activity.

Cyproterone acetate is lipophilic and has a prolonged progestogenic effect, so treatment has to be interrupted for relatively long periods to ensure withdrawal bleeding. Hence a 'reverse sequential' regimen is best prescribed, in which CPA (25–100 mg daily) is given orally on days 5–15 of the cycle and ethinyloestradiol (20–30 μg) is given on days 5–26 of the cycle.[14,15] Most commonly, CPA is used with the combined oral contraceptive pill instead of with ethinyloestradiol alone. This regimen is a highly effective treatment for severe hirsutism and provides excellent cycle control and contraception. Moderate doses of CPA (50 mg daily for 10 days) combined with an OC suppress LH and testosterone at least as much as a gonadotropin releasing hormone (GnRH) analogue.[3] This combination therapy reduces plasma testosterone and androstenedione levels, suppresses gonadotrophins and increases SHBG. This regimen is the treatment of choice for women with PCOS. Cyproterone acetate could also be used with transdermal oestrogens.[16] Monotherapy with CPA (for 10 days in each cycle or month) could be an option for women who do not tolerate oestrogens provided adequate contraception is used. However, it often induces amenorrhoea, particularly in obese women. With a higher dose of CPA (100 mg) a definite improvement, even in severe hirsutism, has been reported in 50% of patients at 6 months and in 70% at 1 year. When a satisfactory reduction in hirsutism has been achieved the dose of CPA may be reduced every 3–6 months, first to 50 mg daily and then to 25 mg daily for the first 10 days of the reverse sequential regimen. Alternatively, a regimen with 10 mg CPA during the first 15 days of the OC can be employed in cases of recurrence or of less severe hirsutism. When a satisfactory clinical reduction in hirsutism is observed it is justifiable to continue treatment with a lower-dose preparation containing 2 mg of CPA and 35 μg of ethinyloestradiol (Dianette) with no added CPA.

Because of the lipophilic nature of CPA it is important to stop therapy at least 3 months before attempting conception. In practice we recommend that women stop CPA and use a low-dose pill for another three cycles.

Side effects of CPA include weight gain, loss of libido, headache, nausea and fatigue, and mood changes,[17] and are more frequently associated with high-dose treatment. However, when ethinyloestradiol is added to CPA these complaints diminish in frequency and the major side effects are those of a combined oral contraceptive.[1] Metabolic changes, which may be subtle, occur with the reverse sequential regimen. There is a tendency toward hyperinsulinaemia and glucose intolerance in patients using CPA.[18]

Although hepatotoxicity of CPA is related to high-dose therapy in men with prostate carcinoma, the Committee on Safety of Medicines in the UK has reported five cases of hepatotoxicity in women taking the drug: four of these occurred in women on low-dose combined pills containing 2 mg of CPA.[19] The prevailing attitude of practising clinicians is that CPA in the doses used for the treatment of hirsutism can be considered relatively safe for long-term use. However, assessment of liver function is advisable before the start of treatment, at 2–3 months and thereafter every 6 months. Adrenal suppression with long-term administration of CPA observed in laboratory animals has not been a clinical problem in our experience.

Spironolactone

Spironolactone, an aldosterone antagonist, is also a potent antiandrogen which competitively binds to the androgen receptor within the hair follicle. It possesses antiandrogenic properties and exerts its peripheral antiandrogenic effects in the hair follicle by competing for androgenic receptors and displacing DHT at both nuclear and cytosol receptors as well as interfering with translocation of the receptor complex to the nucleus.[20] It acts by forming a biologically inactive spironolactone–receptor complex. Spironolactone exerts an additional effect on androgen metabolism by interfering with cytochrome P450 mono-oxygenases.[21] This interference results in defective steroidogenesis and a decrease in testosterone production from the ovary.

In clinical practice doses of spironolactone range from 50 mg to 200 mg daily, but most patients require at least 100 mg. This dosage has been associated with significant improvement in 70–75% of hirsute women after 6 months.[22] Comparative studies showed it to be as effective as CPA in the management of hirsutism.[23] The combination of spironolactone with Dianette may have a synergistic effect on hirsutism score.[24]

Serum levels of SHBG, DHEA-S and DHEA are unaltered by treatment with spironolactone, but testosterone levels will drop within a few days of treatment. The incidence of side effects reported with spironolactone therapy seems to be dose-related. Gastrointestinal side effects (abdominal discomfort, nausea, vomiting and diarrhoea) occur in 20% of patients at doses of 200 mg daily.[20] Similarly, menstrual irregularities and menorrhagia were reported in 27% of women treated with 200 mg of spironolactone. This problem could be overcome either by lowering the dose or adding a low-dose OC. The mechanism of abnormal bleeding is unclear but in women with PCOS and oligomenorrhoea, resumption of normal menses may occur. Hyperkalaemia is almost never seen in patients with normal renal function. Hypotension is rare except in older women. Monitoring is, however, imperative for electrolytes and blood pressure within the first 2 weeks at each dose level. Women taking higher doses should have electrolytes estimated at intervals because of the small risk of hyperkalaemia.

Spironolactone can increase fasting insulin concentrations.[25] It should be avoided in women using drugs such as angiotensin converting enzyme inhibitors or angiotensin II receptor blockers which are otherwise the first-choice therapy for hypertension in women with PCOS.

The Committee on Safety of Medicines in the UK advised against the use of spironolactone as first-line therapy, except in patients with hyperaldosteronism, because of animal studies that showed leukaemia developing in rats exposed to large amounts of spironolactone. No case of leukaemia has been seen in humans on this drug.

Flutamide

Flutamide is a non-steroidal compound which is a pure peripheral androgen antagonist. It is metabolized to hydroxyflutamide, an active metabolite which acts by competitive inhibition of cytoplasmic and nuclear binding of androgens to the receptor.[26] Some data, however, suggest that flutamide may also reduce the synthesis of androgens and/or increase their metabolism to inactive molecules. Flutamide induces a significant reduction in total and free testosterone, 5α-dihydrotestosterone, DHEA, DHEA-S and androstenedione levels.

Doses of 250 mg three times daily resulted in improvement of hirsutism after only 3 months' therapy.[27] In comparative studies it has been shown to be either better than[28] or similarly effective to[29] spironolactone. Flutamide seems to be the fastest of all antiandrogens in decreasing hair diameter.[30] Lower doses (250 mg or even 125 mg per day) may be equally effective.[30–32]

Side effects of flutamide include nausea, vomiting, deterioration in liver function tests, cholestatic jaundice and hepatic necrosis. Drug-induced hepatitis occurs in less than 0.5% of patients[33] but deaths from severe hepatic injury have been reported.[26] Assessment of liver function is mandatory before the start of treatment and after 6–8 weeks. In view of its high risk-benefit ratio the use of this compound has to be carefully considered. However, evidence of the effectiveness and almost complete absence of side effects with low dosages (125–250 mg per day) will probably encourage use of this drug. An additional benefit is a favorable effect on lipid profile in women with PCOS.[34]

Finasteride

Finasteride is a potent competitive 5α-reductase inhibitor which does not bind to the androgen receptor.[35] It therefore blocks the conversion of testosterone to the more potent DHT. Although finasteride is more effective against 5α-iso-enzyme type 2 (present in genital skin and the prostate) than the type 1 isoenzyme (present in non-genital skin and scalp), the specificity of the two enzymes seems to be incomplete,[36] explaining its effectiveness in hirsute women.

Finasteride induces a decrease in DHEA-S and 5α-dihydrotestosterone and an increase in testosterone level.[30,37] Comparative randomized trials showed that finasteride (5 mg daily) has a clinical effect on hirsutism similar to that of spironolactone and flutamide.[30,31,38] It appears to be the drug with the slowest onset of action but is highly effective. Animal data suggest that it might be particularly useful in women with androgenic alopecia.[39] The drug is well tolerated and no side effects have been noted in humans.[3,40]

GnRH AGONISTS

Gonadotrophin releasing hormone agonists such as nafarelin, leuprorelin or buserelin decrease ovarian steroid production by suppressing LH and FSH secretion. This treatment is highly effective in women with PCOS or ovarian hyperthecosis and is particularly indicated in those with concurrent severe premenstrual syndrome.[41] Over a period of 6 months' therapy hair growth was reduced in the majority of patients and skin oiliness was eliminated in all.[42]

Suppression of ovarian steroid production was associated with postmenopausal symptomatology, such as hot flushes and vaginal dryness. Decreased levels of oestradiol increase the risk of bone loss and coronary heart disease with prolonged administration. This can successfully be overcome by combining GnRH agonist treatment with oestrogen add-back therapy – either an oral contraceptive[43] or low-dose hormone replacement therapy.[44,45] Such regimens enhance the effects of GnRH analogue treatment while preventing most of the side effects of GnRH analogue given alone. In addition to profound ovarian androgen suppression, this combination also increases SHBG concentration. The combined regimen may allow the more prolonged treatment necessary for hirsutism. An added benefit for women with PCOS could be improved insulin sensitivity.[46]

KETOCONAZOLE

Ketoconazole, an imidazole derivative, inhibits ergosterol synthesis in fungi. In larger doses it also interferes with glandular cytochrome P450-linked steroidogenesis. Its principal inhibitory role involves inhibition of the 17,20-desmolase and 11 β-hydroxylase steps in steroidogenesis,[47] which explains why androgens are suppressed more than cortisol, although both adrenal gland and ovary are affected.

Ketoconazole has been used in the treatment of Cushing's syndrome and prostatic cancer. Because of its significant ovarian suppressive effects its use has also been suggested for ovarian androgen suppression in hirsutism.[48] Improvement has been noted with 400 mg per day in PCOS as well as with 1000 mg per day in stromal hyperthecosis.[49] In women with PCOS low-dose ketoconazole attenuated serum androgen levels, and inhibited ovarian steroidogenesis in vitro.[50]

There is concern regarding the side effects of this drug, which include nausea, vomiting, pruritus and alterations in hepatic functions. Some 10% of patients may have transient hepatic dysfunction, and although true hepatotoxicity is rare ($<1\%$) long-term use of this drug in patients with PCOS is not recommended.

OTHER TREATMENTS

Metformin

Metformin (500 mg three times a day) is increasingly used in the treatment of PCOS. It significantly reduces hyperinsulinaemia and hyperandrogenism independent of changes in body weight. However, in spite of significant reductions in serum androgens, improvement in menstrual irregularities and resumption of ovulation, hirsutism scores did not improve over 18 months of therapy.[51]

Weight reduction

One third of women with PCOS are overweight and it is recognized that obesity worsens hirsutism, although the relationship is complex.[52,53] Failure to respond to antiandrogen therapy is much more common in the obese than in slim patients[13] and weight reduction often has beneficial effect on menstrual abnormalities and hirsutism.[54,55]

Short-term (4 weeks) very low-energy diets in women with PCOS resulted in a reduction in serum free testosterone, insulin and insulin-like growth factor I (IGF-I) concentrations and a rise in SHBG levels.[56] A moderate restriction of dietary energy over a longer period (6–7 months) resulted in a 40% reduction in Ferriman–Gallway scores in women who lost more than 5% of their starting weight.[57] It has been shown that weight loss decreased ovarian P450c17α activity and reduced serum free testosterone concentration in obese women with PCOS, but not in obese ovulatory women.[58] The authors of this study suggest that the changes observed in women with PCOS only may be related to a reduction in serum insulin.

Weight loss thus decreases both hyperinsulinaemia and insulin resistance, increases SHBG and results in overall reduction of hyperandrogenism.[59] Therefore low-energy diet and exercise should be encouraged as a form of first-line therapy.

Cosmetic procedures

All forms of hormonal treatment will benefit from concurrent mechanical hair removal. This provides an immediate effect while the impact of long-term hormone treatment is awaited. Although electrolysis is advertised as a form of permanent hair removal, in many women regrowth occurs. The combination of medical therapy, to remove the stimulus for new hair growth, with electrolysis, to remove established hair, offers the best cosmetic results. Patients should be advised that plucking hairs causes irritation and stimulation of hair growth. In contrast, shaving does not cause hair to grow more rapidly. Depilatory creams should be avoided, particularly for the face, because they could cause irritation and pigmentation changes.

Antibiotic and topical therapies

Antibiotics such as tetracycline, erythromycin and minocycline are the mainstays of therapy for acne[60] and are often used in conjunction with antiandrogen therapy, at least at the start of treatment.

Improvement of acne has been achieved with the topical non-steroidal antiandrogen, oncoterone acetate.[61] Topical benzoyl peroxide can be used but in severe scarring acne 13-*cis*-retinoic acid (tretinoin) is indicated.[62] These drugs should be administered by a dermatologist.

Androgenic alopecia may respond to topical application of 2% minoxidil twice daily in addition to systemic antiandrogen therapy.[60]

Psychological interventions

In view of the limitations of existing therapies for hirsutism it is important to appreciate the social and psychological impact of this disorder in some women. While most patients will accept explanation by the physician and reassurance regarding their gender identity, some women, particularly adolescents, could have serious behaviour problems and damaged self-confidence. Hirsute women have increased levels of anxiety and depression.[63] These emotional factors may make weight reduction particularly difficult to achieve.[63] Eating disorders, bulimia in particular, are frequently present in women with PCOS.[64] In our experience psychological treatment in the form of group therapy has important beneficial effects on the management of obese women with PCOS.

REFERENCES

1   Prelevic GM. Hirsutism and the polycystic ovary syndrome. In: Ginsburg J, ed., *Drug Therapy in Reproductive Endocrinology* (Arnold: London, 1996) 67–85.

2   Randall VA. Androgens and human growth. *Clin Endocrinol* (1994) **40**: 439–58.

3   Rittmaster RS. Medical treatment of androgen-dependent hirsutism. *J Clin Endocrinol Metab* (1995) **80**: 2559–63.

4   Givens JR, Anderson RN, Wiser WL, Fish SA. Dynamics of suppression and recovery of plasma FSH and LH, androstenedione and testosterone in polycystic ovarian disease during oral contraception. *J Clin Endocrinol Metab* (1974) **38**: 727–35.

5   Jeffcoate W. Treatment of women with hirsutism. *Clin Endocrinol* (1993) **39**: 143–50.

6   Wiebe RH, Morris CV. Effect of an oral contraceptive on adrenal and ovarian androgenic steroids. *Obst Gynec* (1984) **63**: 12–14.

7   Prelevic GM, Puzigaca Z, Balint-Peric LJA. Effects of an oral contraceptive containing cyproterone acetate (Diane 35) on the symptom, hormone profile and ovarian volume of hirsute women with polycystic ovarian syndrome. *Ann NY Acad Sci* (1993) **687**: 255–62.

8   Aydinlik S, Kaufmann J, Lachnitofixon U, Lehnert J. Long-term therapy of signs of androgenisation with a low-dosed antiandrogen-oestrogen combination. *Clin Trial J* (1990) **27**: 392–402.

9   Homburg R, Weissglas L, Goldman J. Improved treatment for anovulation in polycystic ovarian disease utilising the effect of progesterone on the inappropriate gonadotrophin release and clomiphene response. *Hum Reprod* (1988) **3**: 285–8.

10 Prelevic GM, Ginsburg J, Maletic D et al. The effects of the somatostatin analogue octreotide on ovulatory performance in women with polycystic ovaries. *Hum Reprod* (1995) **10**: 28–32.

11 Prelevic GM, Wurzburger MI, Trpkovic D, Balant-Peric L. Effects of a low dose estrogen-antiandrogen combination (Diane-35) on lipid and carbohydrate metabolism in patients with polycystic ovary syndrome. *Gynecol Endocrinol* (1990) **4**: 157–68.

12 Falsetti L, Pasinetti E. Long term treatment with Diane-35 and its influence on lipid profile in patients with polycystic ovary syndrome. In: Franks S, ed., *Polycystic Ovary Syndrome* (Adis: Chester, 1993) 55–62.

13 Conway GS. Polycystic ovary syndrome: clinical aspects. *Ballière's Clinical Endocrinology and Metabolism* (1996) **10**: 263–79.

14 Miller JA, Jacobs HS. Treatment of hirsutism and acne with cyproterone acetate. *Clin Endocrinol Metab* (1986) **15**: 373–89.

15 Hammerstein J, Meckies J, Leo-Rossberg I et al. Use of cyproterone acetate (CPA) in the treatment of acne, hirsutism and virilism. *J Steroid Biochem* (1975) **6**: 827–36.

16 Jaconni VM, Bulletti E, Cappuccini F, Naldi S, Flamigni C. Treatment of hirsutism by an association of oral cyproterone acetate and transdermal 17-beta estradiol. *Fertil Steril* (1991) **55**: 742–5.

17 Belisle S, Love EJ. Clinical efficacy and safety of cyproterone acetate in severe hirsutism: results of a multicentred Canadian study. *Fertil Steril* (1986) **46**: 689–99.

18 Speed M, Godsland IF, Wynn V, Jacobs HS. The effects of cyproterone acetate and ethinyl oestradiol on carbohydrate metabolism. *Clin Endocrinol* (1984) **21**: 689–99.

19 Committee on Safety of Medicines. *Current Problems* (1995) **21**: 1.

20 Shaw JC. Spironolactone in dermatologic therapy. *J Am Acad Dermatol* (1991) **24**: 236–43.

21 Lobo RA, Shoupe D, Serafini P, Brinton D, Horton R. The effects of two doses of spironolactone on serum androgens and anagen hair in hirsute women. *Fertil Steril* (1985) **43**: 200–5.

22 Crosby PDA, Rittmaster RS. Predictors of clinical response in hirsute women treated with spironolactone. *Fertil Steril* (1991) **55**: 1076–81.

23 O'Brien RC, Cooper ME, Murray RML, Seeman E, Thomas AK, Jerums G. Comparison of sequential cyproterone acetate/estrogen versus spironolactone/oral contraceptive in the treatment of hirsutism. *J Clin Endocrinol Metabol* (1991) **72**: 1008–13.

24 Kelstimur F, Sahin Y. Comparison of Diane 35 and Diane 35 plus spironolactone in the treatment of hirsutism. *Fertil Steril* (1998) **69**: 66–9.

25 Wild RA, Demers LM, Applebaum-Rowden D, Lenker R. Hirsutism: metabolic effects of two commonly used oral contraceptives and spironolactone. *Contraception* (1991) **44**: 113–24.

26 Dollery C, ed., *Therapeutic Drugs* (Churchill Livingstone: Edinburgh, 1991).

27 Marcondes JAM, Minnani SL, Luthold WW, Wajchenberg BL, Samojlik E, Kirschner MA. Treatment of hirsutism with flutamide. *Fertil Steril* (1992) **57**: 543–7.

28 Cusan L, Dupont A, Gomez JL, Tremblay RR, Labrie F. Comparison of flutamide and spironolactone in the treatment of hirsutism: a randomised controlled trial. *Fertil Steril* (1994) **61**: 281–7.

29 Erenus M, Gurbuz O, Durmusoglu F, Demircay Z, Pekin S. Comparison of the efficacy of spironolactone versus flutamide in the treatment of hirsutism. *Fertil Steril* (1994) **61**: 613–16.

30 Venturoli S, Marescalchi O, Colombo FM et al. A prospective randomized trial comparing low dose flutamide, finasteride, ketoconazole and cyproterone acetate-estrogen regimens in the treatment of hirsutism. *J Clin Endocrinol Metab* (1999) **84**: 1304–10.

31 Moghetti P, Tosi F, Tosi A et al. Comparison of spironolactone, flutamide and finasteride efficacy in the treatment of hirsutism: a randomized, double blind, placebo-controlled trial. *J Clin Endocrinol Metab* (2000) **85**: 89–94.

32 Muderris II, Bayram F. Clinical efficacy of lower dose flutamide 125 mg/day in the treatment of hirsutism. *J Endocrinol Invest* (1999) **22**: 165–8.

33 Wysowski DK, Fourcroy. Safety of flutamide? *Fertil Steril* (1994) **62**: 1089–90.

34 Diamanti-Kandarakis E, Mitrakou A, Raptis S, Tolis G, Duleba AJ. The effect of a pure antiandrogen receptor blocker, flutamide, on the lipid profile in the polycystic ovary syndrome. *J Clin Endocrinol Metab* (1998) **83**: 2699–705.

35 Rittmaster RS. Finasteride. *N Engl J Med* (1994) **330**: 120–5.

36 Dallob AL, Sadick NS, Unger W et al. The effects of finasteride, 5-alpha-reductase inhibitor, on scalp skin testosterone and dihydrotestosterone concentrations in patients with male pattern baldness. *J Clin Endocrinol Metab* (1994) **79**: 703–6.

37 Fruzzetti F, deLorenzo D, Parrini D, Ricci C. Effects of finasteride, a 5-alpha-reductase inhibitor, on circulating androgens and gonadotrophin secretion in hirsute women. *J Clin Endocrinol Metab* (1995) **80**: 233–8.

38 Wong IL, Morris RS, Chang L, Spahn MA, Stanczyk FZ, Lobo RA. A prospective randomised trial comparing finasteride to spironolactone in the treatment of hirsute women. *J Clin Endocrinol Metab* (1995) **80**: 233–8.

39 Diani AR, Mulholland MJ, Shull KL et al. Hair growth effects of oral administration of finasteride, a steroid 5-alpha reductase inhibitor, alone and in combination with topical minoxidil in the balding macaque. *J Clin Endocrinol Metab* (1992) **74**: 345–50.

40 Moghetti P, Castello R, Magnani CM et al. Clinical and hormonal effects of the 5-alpha-reductase inhibitor finasteride in idiopathic hirsutism. *J Clin Endocrinol Metab* (1994) **79**: 1115–21.

41 Carr BR, Breslau NA, Givens C et al. Oral contraceptive pills, gonadotrophin-releasing hormone agonists, or use in combination for treatment of hirsutism: a clinical research centre study. *J Clin Endocrinol Metab* (1995) **80**: 1169–78.

42 Falsetti L, Pasinetti E. Treatment of moderate and severe hirsutism by gonadotrophin-releasing hormone agonist in women with polycystic ovary syndrome and idiopathic hirsutism. *Fertil Steril* (1994) **61**: 817–22.

43 Heiner JS, Greendale GA, Kawakami AK, Misher LM, Young D, Judd HL. Comparison of gonadotrophin-releasing hormone agonist and a low dose oral contraceptive given alone or together in the treatment of hirsutism. *J Clin Endocrinol Metab* (1995) **80**: 3412–18.

44 Carmina E, Janni A, Lobbo RA. Physiological estrogen replacement may enhance the effectiveness of the gonadotrophin-releasing hormone agonist in the treatment of hirsutism. *J Clin Endocrinol Metab* (1994) **78**: 126–30.

45 Azziz R, Ochoa TM, Bradely EL, Potter HD, Boots LR. Leuprolide and estrogen versus oral contraceptive pills for the treatment of hirsutism: a prospective randomised study. *J Clin Endocrinol Metab* (1995) **80**: 3406–11.

46 Dahlgren E, Landin K, Krotkiewski M, Holm G, Janson PO. Effects of two antiandrogen treatments on hirsutism and insulin sensitivity in women with polycystic ovary syndrome. *Hum Reprod* (1998) **13**: 2706–11.

47 Venturoli S, Fabbri R, Dal Prato L et al. Ketoconazole therapy for women with acne and/or hirsutism. *J Endocrinol Metab* (1990) **71**: 335–9.

48 Cavalho D, Pignateli D, Resne C. Ketoconazole for hirsutism. *Lancet* (1985) **ii**: 560.

49 Martikainen H, Heikinen J, Ruokonen A, Kuoppila A. Hormonal and clinical effects of ketoconazole in hirsute women. *J Clin Endocrinol Metab* (1988) **66**: 987–91.

50 Gal M, Orly J, Barr I, Algur N, Boldes R, Diamant YZ. Low dose ketoconazole attenuates serum androgen levels in patients with polycystic ovary syndrome and inhibits ovarian steroidogenesis in vitro. *Fertil Steril* (1994) **61**: 823–32.

51 Moghetti P, Castello R, Negri C et al. Metformin

effects on clinical features, endocrine and metabolic profiles and insulin sensitivity in polycystic ovary syndrome: a randomized, double-blind, placebo-controlled 6-month trial, followed by open, long-term clinical evaluation. *J Clin Endocrinol Metab* (2000) **85**: 139–46.

52 Conway GS, Honour JW, Jacobs HS. Heterogeneity of the polycystic ovary syndrome: clinical, endocrine and ultrasound features in 556 patients. *Clin Endocrinol* (1989) **40**: 459–70.

53 Balen AH, Coneway GS, Kaltas GS et al. Polycystic ovary syndrome: the spectrum of the disorder in 1741 patients. *Hum Reprod* (1995) **10**: 2107–11.

54 Pasquali R, Antenucci D, Casimirri F et al. Clinical and hormonal characteristics of obese amenorrhoeic hyperandrogenic women before and after weight loss. *J Clin Endocrinol Metab* (1989) **68**: 173–9.

55 Guzick DS, Wing R, Smith D, Berga SL, Winters SJ. Endocrine consequences of weight loss in obese, hyperandrogenic anovulatory women. *Fertil Steril* (1994) **61**: 598–604.

56 Kiddy DS, Hamilton-Fairley D, Seppala M et al. Diet-induced changes in sex hormone binding globulin and free testosterone in women with normal or polycystic ovaries: correlation with serum insulin and insulin-like growth factor. *J Clin Endocrinol* (1989) **31**: 757–63.

57 Kiddy DS, Hamilton-Fairley D, Bush A et al. Improvement in endocrine and ovarian function during dietary treatment of obese women with polycystic ovary syndrome. *Clin Endocrinol* (1992) **36**: 105–11.

58 Jakubowicz DJ, Nestler JE. 17-alpha-hydroxy-progesterone responses to leuprolide and serum androgens in obese women with and without polycystic ovary syndrome after dietary weight loss. *J Clin Endocrinol Metab* (1997) **82**: 556–60.

59 Franks S. Polycystic ovary syndrome. *N Engl J Med* (1995) **333**: 853–61.

60 Rosenfield RL, Lucky AW. Acne, hirsutism and alopecia in adolescent girls. *Endocr Metab Clin North Am* (1993) **22**: 507–32.

61 Lookingbill DP, Abrahams BB, Ellis CN et al. Inocoterone and acne. *Arch Dermatol* (1991) **127**: 210–14.

62 Drake LA, Ceilley RJ, Cornelison RL et al. Guidelines of care of acne vulgaris. *J Am Acad Dermatol* (1990) **22**: 676–9.

63 Modell E, Goldstein D, Reyes FI. Endocrine and behavioural responses to psychological stress in hyperandrogenic women. *Fertil Steril* (1990) **53**: 454–9.

64 McCluskey S, Evans C, Lacey JH, Pearce JM, Jacobs HS. Polycystic ovary syndrome and bulimia. *Fertil Steril* (1991) **55**: 287–91.

11

Ovulation induction with clomiphene citrate

Margo R Fluker

Clomiphene citrate (CC), alone or in combination with weight loss, continues to be the first line of treatment for anovulatory infertility associated with polycystic ovary syndrome (PCOS). Clomiphene is widely available and relatively well accepted in terms of safety, simplicity, side effects and cost. However, although approximately 70–90% of women will ovulate during treatment with CC, only about half of those will conceive.[1–9] This chapter reviews the conventional usage of CC and the factors associated with CC non-responsiveness. Less conventional CC protocols are also discussed as strategies for the management of non-responders.

MECHANISM OF ACTION

Clomiphene citrate is a triphenylethylene derivative which exists as a racemic mixture of two isomers: enclomiphene and the active zuclomiphene form. The drug was first synthesized in 1956 and has been commercially available in 50 mg tablets since the late 1960s.[10] Clomiphene exerts very weak estrogenic activity and appears to act predominantly as an antiestrogen. By binding to hypothalamic estro-gen receptors, CC displaces endogenous estrogen from the receptor, leading to a decrease in the negative feedback exerted by endogenous estrogen and reduced replenishment of estrogen receptors. As a result, gonadotropin releasing hormone (GnRH) secretion appears to increase, followed by GnRH-mediated luteinizing hormone (LH) and follicle-stimulating hormone (FSH) secretion. As gonadotropin levels increase, peak ovarian follicular development and estradiol secretion become evident approximately 5–10 days after the last tablet.[11] Rising estradiol levels then appear to trigger the mid-cycle LH surge and ovulation.

CONVENTIONAL CLOMIPHENE ADMINISTRATION

Clomiphene citrate treatment is usually initiated between the second and fifth day of a spontaneous or progestin-induced withdrawal bleed. Providing that therapy is commenced in the early follicular phase, prior to the selection of the dominant follicle, the outcome of treatment does not appear to be influenced by starting on day 2, 3, 4 or 5.[11] However, one recent series noted more rapid follicular growth, a longer CC-free interval prior to ovulation and better pregnancy rates when CC was started on day 1 rather than day 5 in women with unexplained infertility.[12]

The usual starting dose is 50 mg per day for 5 days, although some authors have advocated a reduced dose of 25 mg for women weighing less than 45 kg or for those who experience marked side effects on the standard 50 mg dose.[13] If anovulation persists, the dose may be increased in increments of 50 mg per day every one or two cycles until reaching a maximum dose of 250 mg for 5 days.

In view of recent concerns about the potential association between ovulation induction agents and ovarian cancer,[14,15] it would seem prudent to adopt an active approach to the treatment of anovulation.[16] This approach requires identification of the ovulatory dose of CC without undue delay. The patient can then complete a satisfactory number of ovulatory cycles of CC (usually three to six cycles)[1] or determine that she is CC-resistant and move on to more complex forms of therapy in a timely fashion (usually within six to eight cycles). As there is a significant relationship between CC dose and body weight[13,17,18] some authors have suggested starting at a daily dose of 100 mg for patients weighing more than 74 kg in order to shorten the number of treatment cycles.[13]

There appears to be little justification for persisting with an anovulatory dose of CC for more than one or two cycles. Likewise, there is little rationale for additional increases in the CC dose once a *satisfactory* ovulatory response has been documented by biphasic basal body temperature charts, luteal phase serum progesterone concentrations or secretory endometrial biopsies. However, an *unsatisfactory* ovulatory response, such as a prolonged follicular phase or a deficient luteal phase may be suggestive of suboptimal folliculogenesis secondary to a suboptimal CC dose, and may respond appropriately to dose increases.

Unlike exogenous gonadotropins, increasing doses of clomiphene are not usually associated with increasing follicular recruitment. Only three studies appear to have addressed this question directly, although they did not specifically evaluate women with PCOS. They documented no difference,[19] less than one additional follicle[13] or an average of 1.4 additional follicles larger than 15 mm,[20] respectively, as the CC dose increased from 50 mg to 150 mg or 200 mg per day. As well, conception rates and multiple birth rates do not appear to rise significantly as the CC dose is increased,[13] lending additional support to the notion that multi-follicular recruitment is not increased in a dose-dependent manner. Thus, while multifollicular ovulation appears to occur in a proportion of women taking CC, it does not appear to be markedly influenced by the dosage, and seems more likely to be a characteristic of the individual ovarian response rather than the dose of CC.

CLOMIPHENE FAILURES

As the ultimate goal of treatment is the induction of ovulation and pregnancy, CC failures must be subclassified into those who fail to ovulate (ovulation failures) and those who ovulate but fail to conceive (conception failures). While considerable overlap exists between these two subgroups, the distinction is important as the clinical management of the two problems may be quite different.

Ovulation failures

The term 'CC non-responsiveness' usually refers to ovulation failure despite maximal conventional doses, generally considered to be 250 mg for 5 days. However, the proportion of women who require more than 150 mg of CC per day is small and the proportion of their cycles that are ovulatory decreases steadily,[1,18] prompting many clinicians to use 150 mg as the cut-off value for determining non-responsiveness. Among women with various ovulatory disorders including PCOS, approximately 25% will remain anovulatory at a dose of 150 mg while up to 15% remain anovulatory despite 250 mg of CC for 5 days.[1,9] Among women who ovulate and conceive during CC therapy,

70–80% conceive during treatment with doses up to 150 mg daily while 15–28% require higher doses.[1,8,13,18] Several investigators have identified a relationship between CC dose and body weight, body mass index (BMI) or ponderal index.[9,13,17,18,21] It has been speculated that the higher estrone concentrations found in obese women necessitate higher CC doses in order to compete with the endogenous estrogens for hypothalamic receptor sites.[17]

In addition to body weight, other parameters have been investigated as predictors of CC responsiveness. Unfortunately, none has sufficient predictive power to ensure ovulation or to preclude a trial of CC even in the presence of marked abnormalities. Clomiphene non-responders tend to have significantly larger ovarian volumes with significantly more intermediate-sized follicles than CC responders and normal controls, although considerable overlap exists.[3,9] As well, increasing levels of LH,[19] elevated total or free testosterone concentrations,[9,19,20,22] fasting hyperinsulinemia or insulin resistance,[22,23] and decreasing concentrations of sex hormone binding globulin (SHBG)[23] tend to predict a poor response to CC. Although CC has been shown to have a beneficial effect on the secretion of FSH and SHBG,[24] the ovary may not be able to respond to an apparently adequate rise in serum FSH.[3] Alternately, the beneficial effects may be outweighed by a concomitant increase in the already elevated concentrations of LH and ovarian androgens,[23,24] thus perpetuating the hyperandrogenic anovulation. In general, the more severe the hormonal and ultrasonographic abnormalities, the less likely it is that ovulation will be induced with CC.

Conception failures

Considerable discrepancy exists between ovulation rates (70–90%) and conception rates (40–50%) during CC treatment.[1–9,22] Among women with PCOS, the factors that predict ovulation (obesity, hyperandrogenism and insulin resistance) differ from those that predict conception (age, severity of the menstrual cycle abnormality, and other infertility factors). Approximately 75% of the pregnancies achieved during CC treatment occur within the first three cycles of treatment.[1] Among those who do not conceive within six ovulatory cycles are couples with other infertility factors and women with a variety of potential CC- or PCOS-related factors which may account for their continuing infertility.

The antiestrogenic actions of CC may adversely affect vaginal cornification, cervical mucus and endometrial thickness, thus potentially affecting sperm transport, sperm survival and early implantation. Cervical mucus volume is reduced[25] and the postcoital test may be abnormal in approximately 15% of women taking CC.[1] Although exogenous estrogen therapy has been widely used in an attempt to improve cervical mucus quality, the efficacy of this approach remains controversial.[26,27]

The second major site of the proposed antiestrogenic actions of CC is the endometrium. Ultrasonographically determined endometrial thickness and echogenicity have been shown to be predictors of conception during ovulation induction and in vitro fertilization cycles.[28] Although endometrial thickness and glandular volume appear to be decreased in CC cycles,[29–31] there does not appear to be a deleterious effect on endometrial estrogen or progesterone receptors.[32] The endometrial thinning effect is not sufficient to preclude pregnancy in most women. A critical threshold may exist below which the occurrence of pregnancy is unlikely, but the precise cut-off value for endometrial thickness remains controversial.[28,30,33] The effect does not appear to be related to CC dose or duration of therapy,[13] but instead appears to be an idiosyncratic response which may reduce the likelihood of conception in a subgroup of women taking CC.

In addition to the potential antiestrogenic effects of CC, ovulation induction in women with PCOS occurs in an environment characterized by high basal LH and androgen concentrations, both of which may be exacerbated during CC treatment[26,27] and may have a negative impact on outcome. This suboptimal environment may affect oocyte quality and fertilization rates, as seen during in vitro fertilization cycles in women with PCOS,[34,35] or it may increase the likelihood of an early pregnancy loss.[36]

MANAGEMENT OF CLOMIPHENE FAILURES WITH NON-CONVENTIONAL CC ADMINISTRATION

Approximately 10–25% of anovulatory women will be unresponsive to maximal conventional doses of CC (200 mg or 250 mg per day for 5 days).[2] These women generally become candidates for more complex forms of ovulation induction therapy with exogenous gonadotropins (human menopausal gonadotropins, hMG). However, there are significant costs associated with hMG treatment in addition to the risk of complications, such as higher-order multiple pregnancies and ovarian hyperstimulation syndrome (OHSS). Because hMG therapy may not be available, acceptable or affordable for a number of women with PCOS and CC-resistant anovulation, several alternatives have been proposed as modifications to the conventional CC protocols.

Extended-duration CC

Ovulation has been induced by extending the duration of CC administration to 7 days or more in women who were unresponsive to the conventional 5-day administration (Table 11.1). Various regimens have been evaluated in small series, although none appears to be clearly superior to the others.[16,37–40] It has been the practice in the author's department to decrease the dose to 100 mg per day when the duration is extended to 10 days, so that the total dose per cycle does not exceed the amount that would be used in a conventional protocol of 200 mg per day for 5 days. Although the occasional patient will ovulate on a higher dose of 150 mg for 10 days, it is not yet clear whether there is an additional dose-response effect in this situation, or whether the increased duration is the most important factor. In our experience, ovulation tended to occur 5–10 days after the last tablet, as with standard CC protocols. This usually resulted in a delay of ovulation to day 18 to 22 when the CC was administered from cycle days 3 to 12.[16]

Extended-duration CC therapy appears to be

Authors	Regimen	Maximum CC dose per cycle (mg)	Ovulatory subjects	Pregnant subjects
O'Herlihy et al[40]	50–250 mg up to 25 d	3750	21/30 (70%)	8/30 (27%)
Garcia-Flores and Vazquez-Mendez[37]	50–250 mg up to 21 d	3150	77/77 (100%)*	60/77 (78%)
Lobo et al[38]	250 mg for 8 d	2000	8/13 (62%)	3/13 (23%)
Fluker et al[16]	100 mg for 10 d	1000	14/30 (47%)	5/30 (17%)
Isaacs et al[39]	100 mg or 150 mg for 7 d (plus prednisone 5 mg)	1050	19/24 (79%)	11/24 (46%)

Table 11.1 Extended-duration clomiphene citrate ovulation induction therapy

* An unspecified number of subjects also ovulated during standard CC therapy.

well tolerated, although this is probably due to patient selection, as women who attempt this form of therapy have usually tolerated higher daily doses of CC during conventional protocols. Occasionally, women who were unable to tolerate high daily doses of CC during conventional protocols (200 mg daily), were able to take lower daily doses (100 mg daily) as part of an extended-duration regimen. No factors have been identified thus far to predict which women will respond to extended-duration CC, as the occurrence of ovulation appeared to be independent of body weight, BMI, and baseline gonadotropin and androgen concentrations.[16] To date, there has been no increase in the risk of complications such as multiple pregnancies or OHSS with extended-duration CC.[16,37–40]

Addition of metformin

Accumulating evidence indicates that hyperinsulinemia is a pivotal factor in the pathogenesis of PCOS, prompting the investigation of insulin-sensitizing agents for the treatment of PCOS. Metformin is a biguanide derivative that appears to increase the cellular action of insulin and decrease hepatic gluconeogenesis, without causing hypoglycemia. Two published randomized controlled trials reported a significant increase in ovulatory cycles compared to the placebo group, both when metformin was administered alone[41,42] and in conjunction with CC.[41] Several small observational studies reported improvement in menstrual cyclicity or ovulation during metformin treatment,[43–47] while two studies reported improved ovulation rates and lower cancellation rates (due to excessive follicular growth) when metformin was combined with exogenous gonadotropins in women with CC-resistant anovulation.[48,49]

Many but not all of the studies reported improvements in hyperandrogenemia and insulin resistance, although one notable randomized controlled trial noted no additional benefit from metformin over that observed with weight loss alone.[50] Weight loss is known to improve endocrine and menstrual parameters in obese PCOS patients.[51] Some clinicians sug-

gest that weight loss during therapy may be due to the dose-related gastrointestinal side effects of metformin, including nausea, diarrhoea, loss of appetite and a metallic taste. To minimize gastrointestinal side effects, the starting dose of 500 mg daily should be gradually increased to the usual therapeutic dose of 500 mg three times daily or 850 mg twice daily with meals.

There is little information about the outcome of pregnancies conceived on metformin. Similarly, there is little information about the optimal duration of therapy, although it has been our practice to discontinue metformin when conception occurs, or after a 3-month trial if there has been no appreciable weight loss or improvement in clinical or endocrine parameters.

Addition of glucocorticoids

The administration of low doses of glucocorticoids may be of benefit to women with hyperandrogenic anovulation. The mechanism of action presumably involves a reduction in adrenal androgen secretion which may reduce total circulating androgen levels by as much as 40%.[40,52,53] As well, low-dose glucocorticoid treatment may enhance FSH synthesis and secretion.[54,55] The combination of reduced androgen concentrations and augmented FSH secretion may induce CC responsiveness in a previous non-responder (Table 11.2). While this approach appears most logical in the subset of anovulatory PCOS patients who have elevated adrenal androgen levels,[2,52–54] it has also been shown to be effective in CC-resistant women with normal levels of dehydroepiandrosterone sulfate (DHEA-S).[52,55]

Although ovulation and conception may occur with single-agent low-dose glucocorticoid therapy, most patients will also require the addition of CC. Treatment begins with dexamethasone 0.25–0.5 mg or prednisone 5 mg at bedtime together with progestin therapy to induce a withdrawal bleed prior to reinstituting CC.[56] If the DHEA-S and/or testosterone levels were elevated prior to therapy, a decrease in these levels can often be documented between

Table 11.2 Clomiphene citrate plus low-dose glucocorticoids

Authors	CC regimen	Glucocorticoid regimen	Ovulatory subjects	Pregnant subjects
Diamant and Evron[53]	50–150 mg for 5 d	Dex 0.5 mg daily	12/15 (80%)	7/15 (47%)
Lobo et al[2]	250 mg for 5 d	Dex 0.5 mg for 6 wk	6/12 (50%)	1/12 (8%)*
Daly et al[52]	50–150 mg for 5 d	Dex 0.5 mg daily	23/23 (100%)†	17/23 (74%)
Singh et al[54]	50–150 mg for 5 d	Dex 0.5 mg daily	16/18 (89%)	14/18 (78%)
Trott et al[55]	50–150 mg for 5 d	Dex 0.5 mg for 10 d	11/13 (47%)	5/13 (38%)
Isaacs et al[39]	100–150 mg for 7 d	Prednisone 5 mg daily	19/24 (79%)	11/24 (46%)

Dex, dexamethasone.
* Subjects were only treated for a single cycle.
† Subjects were anovulatory but had not yet tried standard doses of clomiphene.

days 21 and 24 of the first CC cycle. Concomitantly, serum progesterone is measured to confirm ovulation and an 0800 h serum cortisol level to ensure that adrenal function is not suppressed below the lower limit of normal for the assay. The latter test can generally only be performed in patients who are taking dexamethasone, as exogenous prednisone may cross-react in the cortisol assay.[57,58] Subsequently, the dose of CC can be increased if the patient remains anovulatory, while the glucocorticoid dose may be decreased or changed to alternate-day administration if the a.m. cortisol level is suppressed or if glucocorticoid side effects appear.[58] If androgen levels decrease and CC responsiveness is restored, we continue the glucocorticoid on a nightly basis until a sufficient number of ovulatory CC cycles or a pregnancy has occurred. Recently, Trott et al reported success with follicular phase dexamethasone (cycle days 3 to 12) in CC-resistant women with normal DHEA-S levels.[55] It is not yet clear whether intermittent follicular phase glucocorticoid administration will also be sufficient in women with elevated androgen concentrations.

Addition of human chorionic gonadotropin

Occasionally, clomiphene non-responsiveness occurs when the LH surge is delayed or absent despite apparently adequate follicular development. In such cases, normal preovulatory estradiol levels and sonographic observation of a preovulatory follicle can be used to time the administration of an ovulatory dose of human chorionic gonadotropin (hCG), 5000 or 10 000 units.[59,60] Documenting a delayed or absent LH surge is not always feasible as it may require much more monitoring than would usually be performed during a CC cycle. While the addition of a mid-cycle hCG injection is logical if the endogenous LH surge is truly delayed or absent,[3] the routine addition of a mid-cycle hCG injection does not appear to improve luteal phase parameters or conception rates when compared with cycles in which a spontaneous surge was documented with urinary LH testing.[61]

Addition of pulsatile GnRH

Pulsatile GnRH has been used for ovulation induction in women with PCOS, with reported ovulation rates of approximately 50%.[62–64] These rates are somewhat lower than those achieved with CC alone, presumably because the exogenous GnRH cannot always override the underlying disordered gonadotropin secretion which characterizes women with PCOS. However, Tan and colleagues recently reported successful ovulation in 66% (94/142) and conception in 17% of cycles in women with PCOS who received pulsatile GnRH plus CC (100 mg for 5 days) after failing to respond to pulsatile GnRH alone.[65] There were no cases of moderate or severe OHSS and no multiple pregnancies in this particular treatment group. The precise mechanism underlying the presumed synergistic action of pulsatile GnRH and CC remains unclear, but it appears to offer another less expensive and less invasive alternative to exogenous gonadotropin therapy for women with CC-resistant PCOS.

Addition of bromocriptine

The use of bromocriptine, alone or in conjunction with CC, is indicated in women with anovulation in the presence of galactorrhea and/or hyperprolactinemia.[66,67] However, the empiric use of bromocriptine in women who do not exhibit hyperprolactinemia or galactorrhea is controversial and not well supported by controlled trials.[68]

CONCLUSION

The safety and simplicity of CC continue to support its use as the first line of treatment for anovulatory women with PCOS. The drug can be administered alone or in combination with weight loss in the case of overweight women with PCOS. As well, various non-conventional CC protocols have been developed involving extended-duration CC or adjuvant medications to induce ovulation in women who were traditionally considered non-responders. Thus, using an individualized treatment protocol and active management of ovulation induction, anovulatory women can achieve a satisfactory ovulatory response or progress to more complex forms of therapy in a safe, economical and timely fashion.

REFERENCES

1   Gysler M, March CM, Mishell DR, Bailey EJ. A decade's experience with an individualized clomiphene treatment regimen including its effects on the postcoital test. *Fertil Steril* (1982) **37**: 161–7.

2   Lobo RA, Paul W, March CM, Granger L, Kletzky OA. Clomiphene and dexamethasone in women unresponsive to clomiphene alone. *Obst Gynec* (1982) **60**: 497–501.

3   Polson DW, Kiddy DS, Mason HD, Franks S. Induction of ovulation with clomiphene citrate in women with polycystic ovary syndrome: the difference between responders and nonresponders. *Fertil Steril* (1989) **51**: 30–4.

4   MacGregor AH, Johnson JE, Bunde CA. Further clinical experience with clomiphene citrate. *Fertil Steril* (1968) **19**: 616–22.

5   Gorlitsky GA, Kase NG, Speroff L. Ovulation and pregnancy rates with clomiphene citrate. *Obst Gynec* (1978) **51**: 265–9.

6   Hammond MG, Halme JK, Talbert LM. Factors affecting the pregnancy rate in clomiphene citrate induction of ovulation. *Obst Gynec* (1983) **62**: 196–202.

7   Opsahl MS, Robins ED, O'Connor DM, Scott RT, Fritz MA. Characteristics of gonadotropin response, follicular development, and endometrial growth and maturation across consecutive cycles of clomiphene citrate treatment. *Fertil Steril* (1996) **66**: 533–9.

8   Imani B, Eijkemans MJ, te Velde ER, Habbema JD, Fauser BC. Predictors of chances to conceive in ovulatory patients during clomiphene citrate induction of ovulation in normogonadotropic oligoamenorrheic infertility. *J Clin Endocrinol Metab* (1999) **84**: 1617–22.

9   Imani B, Eijkemans MJ, te Velde ER, Habbema JD, Fauser BC. Predictors of patients remaining anovulatory during clomiphene citrate induction of ovulation in normogonadotropic oligoamenorrheic infertility. *J Clin Endocrinol Metab* (1998) **83**: 2361–5.

10 Allen RE, Palopoli FP, Schumann EL, Van Campen MJ. US Patent 2,914,561, 1959.

11 Wu CH, Winkel CA. The effect of therapy initiation day on clomiphene citrate therapy. *Fertil*

Steril (1989) **52**: 564–8.

12 Biljan MM, Mahutte NG, Tulandi T, Tan SL. Prospective randomized double-blind trial of the correlation between time of administration and antiestrogenic effects of clomiphene citrate on reproductive end organs. *Fertil Steril* (1999) **71**: 633–8.

13 Dickey RP, Taylor SN, Curole DN, Rye PH, Lu PY, Pyrxak R. Relationship of clomiphene dose and patient weight to successful treatment. *Hum Reprod* (1997) **12**: 449–53.

14 Whittemore AS, Harris R, Itnyre J. Characteristics relating to ovarian cancer risk: collaborative analysis of 12 US case control studies. II. Invasive epithelial ovarian cancer in white women. *Am J Epidemiol* (1992) Vol 136 1184–203.

15 Rossing M, Daling JR, Weiss NS, Moore DE, Self SG. Ovarian tumors in a cohort of infertile women. *N Engl J Med* (1994) **331**: 771–6.

16 Fluker MR, Wang IY, Rowe TC. An extended 10-day course of clomiphene citrate (CC) in women with CC-resistant ovulatory disorders. *Fertil Steril* (1996) **66**: 761–4.

17 Shepard MK, Balmaceda JP, Leija CG. Relationship of weight to successful induction of ovulation with clomiphene citrate. *Fertil Steril* (1979) **32**: 641–5.

18 Lobo RA, Gysler M, March CM, Goebelsmann U, Mishell D. Clinical and laboratory predictors of clomiphene response. *Fertil Steril* (1982) **37**: 168–74.

19 Ficicioglu C, Api M, Ozden S. The number of follicles and ovarian volume in the assessment of response to clomiphene citrate treatment in polycystic ovarian syndrome. *Acta Obstet Gynecol Scand* (1996) **75**: 917–21.

20 Armstrong AB, Hoeldtke N, Wiess TE, Tuttle RM, Jones RE. Metabolic parameters that predict response to clomiphene citrate in obese oligo-ovulatory women. *Mil Med* (1996) **161**: 732–4.

21 Espinosa de los Monteros A, Ayala J, Sanabria LC, Parra A. Serum insulin in clomiphene responders and nonresponders with polycystic ovarian disease. *Rev Invest Clin* (1995) **47**: 347–53.

22 Murakawa H, Hasegawa I, Kurabayashi T, Tanaka K. Polycystic ovary syndrome. Insulin resistance and ovulatory responses to clomiphene citrate. *J Reprod Med* (1999) **44**: 23–7.

23 Dupon C, Rosenfield R, Cleary R. Sequential changes in total and free testosterone and androstenedione in plasma during spontaneous and clomid-induced ovulatory cycles. *Am J Obstet Gynecol* (1973) **115**: 478–53.

24 Butzow TL, Kettel LM, Yen SS. Clomiphene citrate reduces serum insulin-like growth factor I and increases sex hormone-binding globulin levels in women with polycystic ovary syndrome. *Fertil Steril* (1995) **63**: 1200–3.

25 Thompson LA, Barratt CLR, Thornton SJ, Bolton AE, Cooke ID. The effects of clomiphene citrate and cyclofenil on cervical mucus volume and receptivity over the periovulatory period. *Fertil Steril* (1993) **59**: 125–9.

26 Kokia E, Bider D, Lunenfeld B, Blankstein J, Mashiach S, Ben-Rafael Z. Addition of exogenous estrogens to improve cervical mucus following clomiphene citrate medication. Patient selection. *Acta Obstet Gynecol Scand* (1990) **69**: 139–42.

27 Bateman BG, Nunley WCJ, Kolp LA. Exogenous estrogen therapy for treatment of clomiphene citrate-induced cervical mucus abnormalities: is it effective? *Fertil Steril* (1990) **54**: 577–80.

28 Gonen Y, Casper RF. Prediction of implantation by the sonographic appearance of the endometrium during controlled ovarian stimulation for in vitro fertilization (IVF). *J In Vitro Fert Embryo Transf* (1990) **7**: 146–52.

29 Eden JA, Place J, Carter GD, Jones J, Alaghband-Zadeh J, Pawson ME. The effect of clomiphene citrate on follicular phase increase in endometrial thickness and uterine volume. *Obst Gynec* (1989) **73**: 187–90.

30 Gonen Y, Casper RF. Sonographic determination of a possible adverse effect of clomiphene citrate on endometrial growth. *Hum Reprod* (1990) **5**: 670–4.

31 Rogers PAW, Polson D, Murphy CR, Hosie M, Susil B, Leoni M. Correlation of endometrial histology, morphometry, and ultrasound appearance after different stimulation protocols for in vitro fertilization. *Fertil Steril* (1991) **55**: 583–7.

32 Hecht BR, Khan-Dawood FS, Dawood MY. Peri-implantation phase endometrial estrogen and progesterone receptors: Effect of ovulation induction with clomiphene citrate. *Am J Obstet Gynecol* (1989) **161**: 1688–93.

33 Check JH, Nowroozi K, Choe J, Lurie D, Dietterich C. The effect of endometrial thickness and echo pattern on in vitro fertilization outcome in donor oocyte-embryo transfer cycles. *Fertil Steril* (1991) **59**: 72–5.

34 Homburg R, Berkowitz D, Levy T, Feldberg D, Ashkenazi J, Ben-Rafael Z. In vitro fertilization and embryo transfer for the treatment of infertility associated with polycystic ovary syndrome. *Fertil Steril* (1993) **60**: 858–63.

35 Urman B, Fluker MR, Yuen BH, Fleige-Zahradka BG, Zouves CG, Moon YS. The outcome of in vitro fertilization and embryo transfer in women with polycystic ovary syndrome failing to conceive after ovulation induction with exogenous gonadotropins. *Fertil Steril* (1992) **57**: 1269–73.

36 Regan L, Owen EJ, Jacobs HS. Hypersecretion of luteinising hormone, infertility, and miscarriage. *Lancet* (1990) **336**: 1141–4.

37 Garcia-Flores RF, Vazquez-Mendez J. Progressive dosages of clomiphene in hypothalamic anovulation. *Fertil Steril* (1984) **42**: 543–7.

38 Lobo RA, Granger LR, Davajan V, Mishell D. An extended regimen of clomiphene citrate in women unresponsive to standard therapy. *Fertil Steril* (1982) **37**: 762–6.

39 Isaacs JD, Lincoln SR, Cowan BD. Extended clomiphene citrate (CC) and prednisone for the treatment of chronic anovulation resistant to CC alone. *Fertil Steril* (1997) **67**: 641–3.

40 O'Herlihy C, Pepperell RJ, Brown JB, Smith MA, Sandri L, McBain JC. Incremental clomiphene therapy: a new method for treating persistent anovulation. *Obst Gynec* (1981) **58**: 535–42.

41 Nestler JE, Jakubowicz DJ, Evans WS, Pasquali R. Effects of metformin on spontaneous and clomiphene-induced ovulation in the polycystic ovary syndrome. *N Engl J Med* (1998) **338**: 1876–80.

42 Pirwany IR, Yates RWS, Cameron IT, Fleming R. Effects of the insulin sensitizing drug metformin on ovarian function, follicular growth and ovulation rate in obese women with oligomenorrhea. *Hum Reprod* (1999) **14**: 2963–8.

43 Velazquez EM, Mendoza S, Hamer T, Sosa F, Glueck CJ. Metformin therapy in polycystic ovary syndrome reduces hyperinsulinemia, insulin resistance, hyperandrogenemia, and systolic blood pressure, while facilitating normal menses and pregnancy. *Metab Clin Exp* (1994) **43**: 647–54.

44 Velazquez E, Acosta A, Mendoza SG. Menstrual cyclicity after metformin therapy in polycystic ovary syndrome. *Obst Gynec* (1997) **90**: 392–5.

45 Morin-Papunen LC, Koivunen RM, Ruokonen A, Martikainen HK. Metformin therapy improves the menstrual pattern with minimal endocrine and metabolic effects in women with polycystic ovary syndrome. *Fertil Steril* (1998) **69**: 691–6.

46 Glueck CJ, Wang P, Fontaine R, Tracy T, Sieve-Smith L. Metformin-induced resumption of normal menses in 39 of 43 (91%) previously amenorrheic women with the polycystic ovary syndrome. *Metab Clin Exp* (1999) **48**: 511–19.

47 Diamanti-Kandarakis E, Kouli C, Tsianateli T, Bergiele A. Therapeutic effects of metformin on insulin resistance and hyperandrogenism in polycystic ovary syndrome. *Eur J Endocrinol* (1998) **138**: 269–74.

48 De Leo V, la Marca A, Ditto A, Morgante G, Cianci A. Effects of metformin on gonadotropin-induced ovulation in women with polycystic ovary syndrome. *Fertil Steril* (1999) **72**: 282–5.

49 Van der Spuy ZM, Dhansay R, Nugent FA. Adjuvant therapy with metformin to improve the therapeutic outcome in anovulatory hyperinsulinaemic women with polycystic ovary syndrome. *Hum Reprod* (1996) **11**: 167.

50 Crave JC, Fimbel S, Lejeune H, Cugnardey N, Dechaud H, Pugeat M. Effects of diet and metformin administration on sex hormone-binding globulin, androgens, and insulin in hirsute and obese women. *J Clin Endocrinol Metab* (1995) **80**: 2057–62.

51 Kiddy DS, Hamilton-Fairley D, Bush A et al. Improvement in endocrine and ovarian function during dietary treatment of obese women with polycystic ovary syndrome. *Clin Endocrinol* (1992) **36**: 105–11.

52 Daly DC, Walters CA, Soto-Albors CE, Tohan N, Riddick DH. A randomized study of dexamethasone in ovulation induction with clomiphene citrate. *Fertil Steril* (1984) **41**: 844–8.

53 Diamant YZ, Evron S. Induction of ovulation by combined clomiphene citrate and dexamethasone treatment in clomiphene citrate nonresponders. *Eur J Obstet Gynecol Reprod Biol* (1981) **11**: 335–40.

54 Singh KB, Dunnihoo DR, Mahajan DK, Bairnsfather LE. Clomiphene-dexamethasone treatment of clomiphene-resistant women with and without the polycystic ovary syndrome. *J Reprod Med* (1992) **37**: 215–18.

55 Trott EA, Plouffe L, Hansen K, Hines R, Brann DW, Mahesh VB. Ovulation induction in clomiphene-resistant anovulatory women with normal dehydroepiandrosterone sulfate levels: beneficial effects of the addition of dexamethasone during the follicular phase. *Fertil Steril* (1996) **66**: 484–6.

56 Ho Yuen B, Fluker MR, Urman B. Infertility: medical management of ovulation induction. In: Copeland LJ, ed., *Textbook of Gynecology* (WB Saunders: Philadelphia, 1993) 292–300.

57 Rittmaster RS, Loriaux DL, Cutler GB Jr.

Sensitivity of cortisol and adrenal androgens to dexamethasone suppression in hirsute women. *J Clin Endocrinol Metab* (1985) **61**: 462–6.

58 Avgerinos P, Cutler G, Tsokos G et al. Dissociation between cortisol and adrenal androgen secretion in patients receiving alternate day prednisone therapy. *J Clin Endocrinol Metab* (1987) **65**: 24–8.

59 Hammond MG. Anovulation and ovulation induction. In: Aiman J, ed., *Infertility: Diagnosis and Management* (Springer: New York, 1984) 101–21.

60 Blankstein J, Mashiach S, Lunenfeld B. *Ovulation Induction and In Vitro Fertilization* (Year Book: Chicago, 1984) 111–30.

61 Agarwal SK, Buyalos RP. Corpus luteum function and pregnancy rates with clomiphene citrate therapy: comparison of human chorionic gonadotropin-induced versus spontaneous ovulation. *Hum Reprod* (1995) **10**: 328–91.

62 Homburg R, Eshel A, Armar NA et al. One hundred pregnancies after treatment with pulsatile luteinizing hormone releasing hormone to induce ovulation. *Br Med J* (1989) **289**: 809–12.

63 Burger CW, Hompes PG, Korsen TJ, Schoemaker J. Ovulation induction with pulsatile luteinizing hormone-releasing hormone in women with clomiphene citrate-resistant polycystic ovary-like disease: endocrine results. *Fertil Steril* (1989) **51**: 20–9.

64 Saffan DS, Seibel MM. Value of subcutaneous and intravenous pulsatile gonadotropin releasing hormone in polycystic ovary disease. *J Reprod Med* (1992) **37**: 545–51.

65 Tan SL, Farhi J, Homburg R, Jacobs HS. Induction of ovulation in clomiphene-resistant polycystic ovary syndrome with pulsatile GnRH. *Obst Gynec* (1996) **88**: 221–6.

66 Falaschi P, Rocco A, del Pozo E. Inhibitory effect of bromocriptine treatment on luteinizing hormone secretion in polycystic ovary syndrome. *J Clin Endocrinol Metab* (1986) **62**: 348–53.

67 Homburg R, Ashkenazi J, Goldman J. Resistant cases of polycystic ovarian disease successfully treated with a combination of corticosteroids, clomiphene, and bromocriptine. *Int J Fertil* (1988) **33**: 393–7.

68 Padilla SL, Person GK, McDonough PG, Reindollar RH. The efficacy of bromocriptine in patients with ovulatory dysfunction and normoprolactinemic galactorrhea. *Fertil Steril* (1985) **44**: 695–9.

12

Treatment with chronic low-dose FSH

Joop Schoemaker

In order to understand the modern approach to induction of ovulation by gonadotropins, one should know something of the history of this type of treatment. Induction of ovulation by gonadotropins has been practiced since the 1950s. Gemzell and co-workers were the first to publish results;[1] this was in 1958, even before Greenblatt published his first paper on induction of ovulation by clomiphene citrate.[2] This therapy had early difficulties, mainly because of the lack of therapeutic material. Gemzell originally worked with human pituitary follicle-stimulating hormone (FSH), a material that was later on used almost exclusively by the British and the Australians. In Europe and especially in Israel, use was made of human menopausal gonadotropins (hMG), extracted from the urine of postmenopausal women.[3] The side effects of this therapy, i.e. the ovarian hyperstimulation syndrome and the occurrence of multiple pregnancies, soon became evident. It was Brown who was the first to conclude that because of these side effects clomiphene citrate was the drug of choice and that the use of gonadotropins should be restricted to patients who did not respond to clomiphene.[4]

Thanks to the work of pioneers, such as Lunenfeld, Gemzell, Townsend, Evans and Brown, Crooke and others,[1,3–9] new techniques were developed, particularly when daily estrogen determinations became available for careful monitoring.[10] Consensus on the use of these monitoring techniques was soon reached but remarkable differences existed with respect to the dose schedules. Standard dose schedules were rejected by all, and individualized step-up schedules became the standard. Rabau et al[3] recommended starting with one ampule and increasing by one ampule each week, while Brown and co-workers insisted that the increase in dose should never exceed a third of the preceding dose.[4]

Brown's recommendations were based on extensive analysis and careful evaluation of the many cycles, performed in their department. Townsend, then chairman of the Royal Women's Clinic in Melbourne, where Brown was the director of the endocrine laboratory, delivered the eighth John Shields memorial lecture in 1966, in which he stated: 'It has been shown that in many patients there is very little range between a dose that will fail to stimulate follicle ripening at all and one which produces ovarian enlargement or multiple pregnancies.'[5]

This was the birth of the 'threshold' concept. It was more precisely formulated by Brown in 1978, who stated:

> In gonadotropin therapy the ovary has a threshold requirement for FSH below which follicular development, as judged by oestrogen production, does not occur, even though the dose is continued indefinitely. Increasing the dose by a factor of only 10–30% above this threshold causes normal rates of follicle stimulation and further increases cause excessive stimulation. The threshold for administered FSH may differ in different individuals by a factor of up to 10 and therefore the dose must be accurately determined for each patient. The FSH requirements of an individual are usually reproducible from cycle to cycle over considerable periods of time including an intervening pregnancy.[7]

In the same paper Brown recognized the importance of the FSH level rather than the FSH dose by stating: 'This increment of 30% agrees well with the elevation of serum FSH levels seen early in the normal cycle as measured by radioimmuno-assay and reported by many workers.'[7] It is amazing that these accurate observations were neglected for such a long time outside Australia. It was only in 1987 that Polson and Franks published their first results of the low-dose step-up technique in induction of ovulation by gonadotropins.[11]

Physiology of follicular growth

The mechanism by which primordial and primary follicles are recruited into the pool of growing follicles is unknown. It takes approximately 70 days for such a follicle to develop from the primary stage to the early antral stage, where it arrives at the end of the luteal phase preceding the cycle in which it has the potential to become a Graafian or (pre)ovulatory follicle (Figure 12.1). At this point, just before the period with which that cycle begins, the follicle has a size of 2–5 mm,[12] contains a small antrum and has just become completely dependent on

FSH for further growth and development, meaning that if the follicle is not supplied with enough FSH it will become atretic. The sensitivity to FSH increases during subsequent days,[13] meaning that less and less FSH is needed to keep the follicle growing. This effect can at least in part be explained by an increase in FSH receptors on the granulosa cells.[14] This increase in receptors has long been thought to be the major event responsible for the selection of the dominant follicle. As it was known that estrogens are in part responsible for the increase in FSH receptors, a follicle that has a slight advantage over other follicles, i.e. one that produces slightly more estrogens, would increase its FSH receptor content faster, becoming more sensitive to FSH and hence producing more estrogens by virtue of FSH inducing the P450 cytochrome aromatase enzyme, which converts androgens into estrogens. More estrogens would increase the advantage and so on. It has now been shown, however, in many different papers (reviewed by Chappel and Howles[15]) that estradiol production by the follicles is not a prerequisite for proper follicle development and thus estrogens may not be needed at all to increase FSH receptors in granulosa cells. On the other hand, estradiol and inhibin-B[16] are responsible for the decrease of FSH once the follicle has started to grow. This decrease in FSH causes the demise of all follicles which are not (yet) sensitive enough to cope with the lower FSH concentrations, which are usually all growing follicles except the leading one.

The FSH threshold concept

Early antral follicles do not respond to FSH in a straightforward dose–effect relationship. This means that in order for an early antral follicle to grow the FSH concentration in the blood has to exceed a certain level, the threshold level of the follicle. Once the FSH concentration has surpassed this threshold the follicle will start to grow as if 'a switch has been thrown'[7] and will continue to grow as long as the FSH concentration remains above the threshold. The threshold of a growing follicle decreases during its fur-

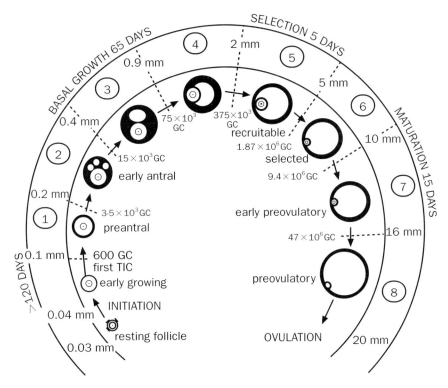

Figure 12.1 Development of the follicle from the primordial to the preovulatory stage. GC, granulosa cells; TIC, theca interna cells. From Gougeon TA. Regulation of ovarian follicular development in primates: facts and hypotheses. *Endocr Rev* (1996) **17**(2): 126–55, with permission.

ther development[13] and therefore the follicle needs less and less FSH. This is called the 'increasing sensitivity' of the follicle. It does not mean that the follicle will grow faster with the same amount of FSH but that the follicle needs less FSH to continue its development, which in itself is programmed to proceed at a certain speed. If for any reason the FSH concentration drops below the threshold of a particular follicle during its development, that follicle will eventually go into atresia.

Thus, each follicle has its own individual threshold, which changes during its development. If we speak of a 'patient's threshold', the threshold level of the most sensitive follicle is meant. It is thus the FSH concentration at which the first follicle will start its further development. This threshold level, usually, is very sta-

ble from cycle to cycle in an individual over prolonged periods, even when compared before and after a pregnancy.[7] It varies, however, considerably from woman to woman.[17] Particularly at later age, when the woman becomes climacteric, the threshold level increases dramatically, making the woman much less sensitive to gonadotropins.

The threshold originally was defined as a dose, the threshold dose, being the lowest dose of FSH to which an amenorrheic woman would respond with monofollicular growth. It was again Brown who in the late 1960s first defined the threshold dose as the dose at which normal follicular development would take place and hence mono-ovulation would occur.[4] He found that a difference as small as 10% of the dose would determine whether follicular growth would take place or not. He also found that there was at most a difference of 30% between a dose that would lead to no growth at all and one resulting in multifollicular growth. On these findings he based his advice never to increase the dose by more than 30% of the preceding dose in one step. The relative stability of the threshold dose in one patient and the tremendous variation of the threshold dose between different patients, sometimes as much as 10-fold, was, first by Brown, and later in careful studies by Ben Rafael and Benadiva (for review see reference 18), demonstrated to be caused by differences in metabolic clearance rate of FSH in individual patients. Therefore expressing the FSH threshold in terms of serum concentration seems to be more appropriate than using the number of ampules. Van Weissenbruch and co-workers[19] were the first to estimate the FSH threshold levels of individual patients, with either hypothalamic amenorrhea or polycystic ovary disease (PCOS). These studies were later extended by van der Meer in a prospective trial.[20] The interindividual variation in threshold levels appeared to range from 4.3 IU/l to 8.2 IU/l in women with normal menstrual cycles, whose endogenous FSH stimulation had been suppressed by a gonadotropin releasing hormone (GnRH) agonist, and from 4.7 IU/l to 8.2 IU/l in women with PCOS, also under pituitary GnRH agonist suppression (Figure 12.2). Administration of a GnRH agonist, however, does not seem to influence the threshold (Figure 12.2).[20]

The intraindividual variability in the dose from cycle to cycle was within a margin of not more than half an ampule in the great majority of the patients.

The threshold level changes during life. With increasing age, the thresholds of the follicles, including the most sensitive follicle, increase. It is well known that women approaching the climacteric but still having regular menstrual cycles have a higher FSH concentration on the third day of their cycle.[22] This means that to stimulate the most sensitive follicle a higher FSH level is necessary.

What determines the threshold level of the different follicles is largely unknown, although

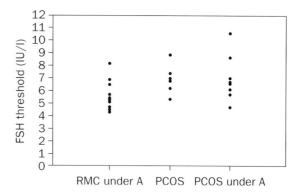

Figure 12.2 Threshold levels of FSH for monofollicular growth in volunteers with regular menstrual cycles (RMC) under pituitary suppression with a GnRH agonist (A) and in patients with polycystic ovary syndrome (PCOS) without and under pituitary suppression with a GnRH agonist.

it is likely that the number of FSH receptors on the granulosa cells of the follicle is important. Hillier found that growth factors such as insulin-like growth factor (IGF) have a synergistic effect with FSH on follicular growth;[14] IGF, or possibly growth hormone (GH), might therefore be able to influence follicular sensitivity. Indeed, de Boer et al[23] showed that in women with GH deficiency the threshold level was lower during GH substitution treatment (Figure 12.3). Also, a long-acting somatostatin analog increased[24] and GH administration decreased the threshold levels in women with PCOS (author's data), suggesting that indeed GH influences follicular sensitivity.

FSH sensitivity above the threshold level

Little is known about the dose-effect relationship between FSH concentrations and the number of follicles that will start to grow. Van der Meer et al[20] determined the threshold levels in 12 PCOS patients and 11 regularly cycling women in a first stimulation cycle. In the

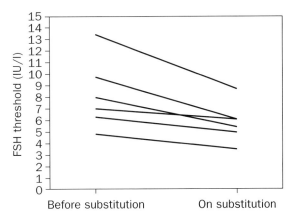

Figure 12.3 Change of FSH threshold levels for monofollicular growth before and during growth hormone substitution in GH-deficient women.

second cycle both groups were randomized to receive either half or one ampule of FSH more than their threshold dose. It appeared that there were no statistically significant differences in the number of growing follicles between the groups stimulated with half and one ampule more, either in the PCOS group or in the controls. This suggests that stimulation with only half an ampule more than the threshold dose leads to the growth of all stimulable follicles. This group of stimulable follicles is called the

cohort. The cohort cannot be determined exactly as such. McNatty found 6 to 30 antral follicles greater than 1 mm in diameter per late luteal ovary, although according to his estimation, approximately 75% of those were atretic already.[25] Van der Meer stimulated patients with PCOS and a control group with either half an ampule or one ampule more than the threshold dose and measured the number of follicles larger than 13 mm at the time the largest follicle had been stimulated to a size of 18 mm.[20] She found the number of stimulated follicles to be approximately equal under both stimulation regimens (Table 12.1). This suggests that the whole cohort had been stimulated.

The number of stimulated follicles varied from 0 to 14 in women with regular menstrual cycles (median 6) and from 6 to 25 in PCOS patients (median 12). For follicles 10–13 mm in diameter these figures were 3 (median, range 0–10) and 10 (median, range 5–23) respectively. Thus the cohort size in PCOS patients is approximately twice that of regularly cycling women. This difference explains why women with PCOS so easily develop an excessive number of follicles, and hence are so susceptible to the ovarian hyperstimulation syndrome.

The size and density of the cohort seem to diminish with advancing age, because it is difficult to stimulate an appreciable number of follicles during controlled hyperstimulation in IVF treatment in older women, particularly in those

Table 12.1 Number of follicles between 10 mm and 18 mm in diameter obtained after stimulation with half or one ampule more than the threshold dose

	Number of follicles			
	Diameter 10–13 mm		Diameter >13 mm	
	PCOS	Controls	PCOS	Controls
Half an ampule extra	13.7 (6)	4.8 (6)	14.0 (6)	5.2 (6)
One ampule extra	11.8 (6)	3.6 (5)	12.7 (6)	6.5 (5)

The number of subjects is shown in parentheses.

with an elevated FSH level on the third day of the cycle.[22]

Induction of ovulation with chronic low-dose FSH

In addition to physicians on the Australian continent, low-dose step-up regimens were advocated by the group of Seibel, Berger and Taymor in the USA.[26–28] By using this technique they hoped to invert the high luteinizing hormone (LH)/FSH ratio, in this way eliminating the deleterious effect of high LH levels. They did not use the threshold concept as such. The paper by Polson et al[11] can be considered as the birth of a new era of ovulation induction with optimal amounts of gonadotropins and a minimum of side effects, such as the ovarian hyperstimulation syndrome (OHSS) and multiple pregnancies. Franks' group, as reported by Polson, administered FSH subcutaneously in a pulsatile manner, slowly increasing the dose of FSH as long as no signs of follicular growth were observed. The initial dose was one ampule of FSH and was only increased if after 14 days of stimulation no follicular growth was visible on ultrasonography (no follicles larger than 12 mm) and no appreciable increase of endometrial thickness had been observed. Even then the increase was only half an ampule at a time. If a follicle was observed with a diameter of 12 mm or more, the dose was not increased and stimulation was continued until the largest follicle was 16 mm in diameter. A dose of 3000 IU of human chorionic gonadotropin (hCG) was then administered in order to actually induce ovulation. A maximal stimulatory dose of 225 IU of FSH was used. If no follicular growth occurred following this dose, stimulation was discontinued. In ten patients 33 cycles were induced. Of those 23 were ovulatory. Eighteen were mono-ovulatory. In another ten patients hCG was withheld because of multiple follicular growth in three, an ovarian cyst in three, and insufficient follicular growth under the maximum dose in four patients. In a subsequent study FSH was given intramuscularly once a day.[29] The same results were obtained,

showing that it was not the pulsatile administration that was responsible for the monofollicular growth. A prospective randomized comparison was made between FSH and hMG, which showed that there were no differences between the two gonadotropin preparations, excluding the possibility that the monofollicular growth had been caused by the use of a purified gonadotropin preparation.[30]

Buvat and co-workers developed their 'slow administration protocol'.[31] They started ovarian stimulation with one ampule of FSH per day without increasing the dose during the first stimulation. If stimulation was unsuccessful in this cycle, a new cycle was started using two ampules per day, and so on. In comparison with historical controls a higher number of cases of monofollicular and bifollicular growth were seen as well as a lower estradiol level and higher pregnancy rate. In view of the fact that the threshold dose hardly varies from cycle to cycle, this protocol in fact is not a low-dose step-up protocol, because the increases still are with one ampule.

Van der Meer et al induced ovulation by administering FSH intravenously.[17] After determining the FSH for three consecutive days as a baseline, FSH was administered in such a way that the FSH level increased by approximately 1 IU/l each time. Apparently because of differences in metabolic clearance rate, for this increase an average of half an ampule was needed, but the necessary dose varied from a quarter to a whole ampule. After the initial rise of 1 IU/l the dose was kept unchanged for 10 days. If follicles did not start to grow, as evidenced by ultrasound observation or by determining estradiol levels, another increment of 1 IU/l was made. The level again was kept constant for 7 days, and so on. If follicles started to grow, the level was not increased and stimulation was continued till the largest follicle had grown to a diameter of 18 mm. At that time 10 000 IU of hCG were administered to induce final maturation and ovulation. The hCG would not be given if at the time the largest follicle was 18 mm, more than three follicles greater than 16 mm or more than six follicles greater than 13 mm were present, or the estradiol level exceeded 3000 pmol/l. Of 15 first cycles, 9 (60%) were monofollicular. Of these 9, only 8 actually ovulated. Five cycles were canceled because of multifollicular growth. This relatively high number was caused by the fact that for comparison reasons the stimulation was carried on until the largest follicle had a diameter of 18 mm in all cycles. Had hCG been given earlier, e.g. on the basis of estradiol levels, more cycles would have been ovulatory. In subsequent cycles, when the experience of previous cycles could be used, only one cancellation was necessary while maintaining the same rate of ovulation (75%). Also, van der Meer found that the difference between monofollicular and multifollicular growth might be determined by a dosage change as small as a quarter of an ampule.

This technique not only relies on a slow increase of the dose of FSH but also on the integrity of the endogenous feedback which steroids and non-steroidal factors exert on the pituitary gland and hypothalamus, as shown by Scheele[21] and later on by van der Meer and co-workers.[32] They showed that using a GnRH agonist for pituitary desensitization (which blocked the feedback on the endogenous component of the FSH concentration) jeopardized the technique, making it much more difficult to obtain monofollicular growth.

Several other authors have now confirmed the efficacy and safety of low-dose gonadotropin ovulation induction in PCOS patients.[33–43] Hamilton-Fairley in 1991 and White in 1996 evaluated the results of the group of Franks in London, the group who by far has the most experience.[42,43] They evaluated 225 women with PCOS who together were treated for 934 cycles (Table 12.2). The pregnancies were evaluated separately for the whole group and for the group with a body mass index (BMI) greater than 25 kg/m² (Figure 12.4). It is clear that the cumulative pregnancy rate in the latter group, as calculated by life-table statistics, is worse than in the whole group. Whether there was a statistically significant difference between the women whose BMI exceeded 25 kg/m² and those whose BMI did not was not reported.

Table 12.2 Results of low-dose gonadotropin treatment of 225 women with anovulatory PCOS, treated at a single center	
Number of patients	225
Number of cycles	934
Number of ovulatory cycles	672 (72%)
Number of uniovulatory cycles	522 (77%)
Number of pregnancies	109 (48%)
Number of women pregnant	102 (45%)
Number of multiple pregnancies*	7 (6%)

* All multiples were twin pregnancies.
From White et al[43] with permission.

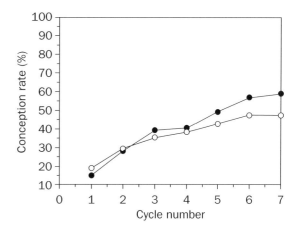

Figure 12.4 Cumulative conception rate, calculated by life-table analysis for 49 pregnancies in 91 women treated with low-dose gonadotropin (solid circles). The initial dose of FSH was 52.5 IU (0.7 of an ampule). The cumulative conception rate was recalculated for women with a body mass index greater than 25 kg/m² (open circles). From White et al[43] with permission.

A study comprising 668 cycles in 110 patients showed similar results with 85% ovulatory cycles, 13% pregnancy rate per cycle and 16% pregnancy rate per ovulatory cycle (authors data). The cumulative pregnancy rate in a subgroup of patients without additional infertility factors was 59% and 72% after 6 and 12 cycles respectively. The abortion rate was 25%. Mild OHSS occurred in 4.9% of the cycles and moderate OHSS in 1.5% of cycles. The twin pregnancy rate was 8%. No higher-order multiple pregnancies were encountered. In a multivariate analysis BMI was the most important explanatory factor determining pregnancy chance. The intercycle threshold variation was no more than 0.5 ampule in 77% of the patients. More variation occurred in women with a BMI over 26 kg/m².

Indications

Low-dose step-up induction of ovulation is the method of choice in clomiphene-resistant PCOS. What exactly clomiphene resistance is, however, is debatable. Over recent years clomiphene resistance has apparently changed from failure to ovulate on 250 mg daily for 5 days[44] to failure on 150 mg daily for 5 days[45,46] or even 100 mg daily for 5 days. Moreover, patients who have received treatment for 12 or even 6 ovulatory cycles in which they did not become pregnant, nowadays, are considered to be clomiphene-resistant. This change is probably brought about by the popularization of the use of gonadotropins through their use in assisted reproduction, as well as by reports on the increased incidence of ovarian cancer in women who have been treated with clomiphene citrate for 12 months and have not yet become pregnant.[47] The use of gonadotropins for ovulation induction is recommended here when the patient does not ovulate on clomiphene citrate, 150 mg daily for 5 days or when she has not become pregnant after 12 ovulatory cycles on clomiphene.

Protocol

Ovarian stimulation is started on the third day of either a spontaneous period or a progesterone-induced withdrawal bleed.

- Stimulation is begun with 50 IU or 75 IU of a highly purified FSH preparation, either extracted from human menopausal urine or manufactured by modern recombinant technology. Although intravenous administration is possible using a pulsatile infusion pump, subcutaneous administration is preferred for reasons of simplicity.
- Stimulation is monitored at the minimum by ultrasonography; combined monitoring with ultrasonography and estradiol determinations is preferable.
- A follicle of at least 12 mm in diameter or a doubling of the basal estradiol level constitutes a sign of follicular development. If such a sign is observed the dose should under no circumstance be increased.
- Stimulation is continued until the largest follicle is 18 mm in diameter. At that time 5000–10 000 IU of hCG are given IM for final follicle and oocyte maturation and to actually induce ovulation.
- Human chorionic gonadotropin is withheld when, at the time the largest follicle is 18 mm, more than three follicles greater than 16 mm or more than six follicles greater than 13 mm are present, or the estradiol level exceeds 3000 pmol/l. Referring the patient for in vitro fertilization under such circumstances may be a good alternative.
- If at the end of the first 10 days of stimulation no sign of follicular growth is observed, the FSH dose is increased by half an ampule. This is repeated every 7 days as long as follicular growth is absent.
- If multifollicular growth occurs during the first cycle on one ampule per day, the next cycle is started with half an ampule per day.
- When the patient does not become pregnant during the first cycle, she should begin her next cycle with a dose that is half an ampule less than the maximal dose of the previous cycle (the threshold dose). This dose is maintained for 7 days.
- No luteal support is given, either by progesterone or by hCG.
- Do not use GnRH analogs in combination with the low-dose step-up protocol.

Under this protocol results may be expected as described by White and co-workers.[43]

In conclusion it is fair to say now that where gonadotropin therapy is needed, the low-dose step-up protocol is the protocol with the highest ratio of effect to side effect.

REFERENCES

1 Gemzell CA, Diczfalusy E, Tillinger G. Clinical effect of human pituitary follicle-stimulating hormone (FSH). *J Clin Endocrinol Metab* (1958) **18**: 1333–48.

2 Greenblatt RB, Barfield WE, Junget EC, Roy AW. Induction of ovulation with MRL-41. *J Am Med Assoc* (1961) **178**: 101.

3 Rabau E, David A, Serr DM, Mashiach S, Lunenfeld B. Human menopausal gonadotropins for anovulation and sterility. *Am J Obstet Gynecol* (1967) **98**: 92–8.

4 Brown JB, Evans JH, Adey FD, Taft HP, Townsend SL. Factors involved in the induction of fertile ovulation with human gonadotrophins. *J Obst Gyn Br Comm* (1969) **76**: 289–307.

5 Townsend SL, Brown JB, Johnstone JW, Adey FD, Evans JH, Taft HP. Induction of ovulation. *J Obst Gyn Br Comm* (1966) **73**: 529–43.

6 Brown JB, Evans JH, Adey FD et al. Clinical induction of ovulation using gonadotropins. In: Scow RO, ed., *Regulation of Ovarian Function.* International Congress Series 273 (Excerpta Medica: Amsterdam, 1973) 891–6.

7 Brown JB. Pituitary control of ovarian function – concepts derived from gonadotrophin therapy. *Aust NZ J Obstet Gynaecol* (1978) **18**: 47–54.

8 Crooke AC. The clinical effects of human pituitary and urinary gonadotrophins. *Proc Roy Soc Med* (1964) **57**: 111–14.

9 Crooke AC, Butt WR, Palmer RF, Morris R, Logan Edwards R, Anson CJ. Clinical trial of human gonadotrophins. I – The effect of pituitary and urinary follicle stimulating hormone and chorionic gonadotrophin on patients with idiopathic secondary amenorrhoea. *J Obst Gyn Br Comm* (1963) **70**: 604–35.

10 Brown JB, Beischer NA. Current status of estrogen assay in gynecology and obstetrics. I. Estrogen assays in gynecology and early pregnancy. *Obstet Gynecol Surv* (1972) **27**(4): 205–35.

11 Polson DW, Mason HD, Saldahna MB, Franks S. Ovulation of a single dominant follicle during treatment with low-dose pulsatile follicle stimulating hormone in women with polycystic ovary syndrome. *Clin Endocrinol (Oxf)* (1987) **26**: 205–12.

12 Gougeon A. Rate of follicular growth in the human ovary. In: Rolland R, van Hall EV, Hillier SG, McNatty KP, Schoemaker J, eds, *Follicular Maturation and Ovulation* (Excerpta Medica: Amsterdam, 1982) 155–63.

13 Zeleznik AJ, Kubik CJ. Ovarian responses in macaques to pulsatile infusion of follicle-stimulating hormone (FSH) and luteinizing hormone: increased sensitivity of the maturing follicle to FSH. *Endocrinology* (1986) **119**: 2025–32.

14 Hillier SG. Paracrine control of follicular estrogen synthesis. *Semin Reprod Endocrinol* (1991) **9**: 332–40.

15 Chappel SC, Howles C. Reevaluation of the roles of luteinizing hormone and follicle-stimulating hormone in the ovulatory process. *Hum Reprod* (1991) **6**: 1206–12.

16 Groome NP, Illingworth PJ, O'Brien M et al. Measurement of dimeric inhibin B throughout the human menstrual cycle. *J Clin Endocrinol Metab* (1996) **81**(4): 1401–5.

17 Van der Meer M, Hompes PG, Scheele F, Schoute E, Veersema S, Schoemaker J. Follicle stimulating hormone (FSH) dynamics of low dose step-up ovulation induction with FSH in patients with polycystic ovary syndrome. *Hum Reprod* (1994) **9**: 1612–17.

18 Ben Rafael Z, Levy T, Schoemaker J. Pharmacokinetics of follicle-stimulating hormone: clinical significance. *Fertil Steril* (1995) **63**: 689–700.

19 Van Weissenbruch MM. *Gonadotrophins for induction of ovulation.* Thesis, Vrije Universiteit, Amsterdam, The Netherlands, 1989.

20 van der Meer M, Hompes PGA, de Boer JAM, Schats R, Schoemaker J. Cohort size rather than FSH threshold level determines ovarian sensitivity in polycystic ovary syndrome. *J Clin Endocrinol Metab* (1998) **83**(2): 423–6.

21 Scheele F, Hompes PG, van der Meer M, Schoute E, Schoemaker J. The effects of a gonadotrophin-releasing hormone agonist on treatment with low dose follicle stimulating hormone in polycystic ovary syndrome. *Hum Reprod* (1993) **8**: 699–704.

22 Scott RTJ, Hofmann GE. Prognostic assessment of ovarian reserve [see comments]. *Fertil Steril* (1995) **63**: 1–11.

23 de Boer JAM, van der Meer M, van der Veen EA, Schoemaker J. Growth hormone substitution in hypogonadotropic, growth hormone deficient

women decreases the follicle stimulating hormone threshold for monofollicular growth. *J Clin Endocrinol Metab* (1999) **84**(2): 590–5.

24 van der Meer M, de Boer JAM, Hompes PGA, Schoemaker J. Octreotide, a somatostatin analogue, alters ovarian sensitivity to gonadotrophin stimulation as measured by the FSH threshold in polycystic ovary syndrome. *Hum Reprod* (1998) **13**(6): 1465–9.

25 McNatty KP, Hillier SG, van den Boogaard AM, Trimbos-Kemper TC, Reichert LE, van Hall EV. Follicular development during the luteal phase of the human menstrual cycle. *J Clin Endocrinol Metab* (1983) **56**(5): 1022–31.

26 Claman P, Seibel MM, McArdle C, Berger MJ, Taymor ML. Comparison of intermediate-dose purified urinary follicle-stimulating hormone with and without human chorionic gonadotropin for ovulation induction in polycystic ovarian disease [published erratum appears in *Fertil Steril* (1987) **48**(1): 163]. *Fertil Steril* (1986) **46**: 518–21.

27 Kamrava MM, Seibel MM, Berger MJ, Thompson I, Taymor ML. Reversal of persistent anovulation in polycystic ovarian disease by administration of chronic low-dose follicle stimulating hormone. *Fertil Steril* (1982) **37**: 520–3.

28 Seibel MM, Kamrava MM, McArdle C, Taymor ML. Treatment of polycystic ovary disease with chronic low-dose follicle stimulating hormone: biochemical changes and ultrasound correlation. *Int J Fertil* (1984) **29**: 39–43.

29 Polson DW, Mason HD, Kiddy DS, Winston RM, Margara R, Franks S. Low-dose follicle-stimulating hormone in the treatment of polycystic ovary syndrome: a comparison of pulsatile subcutaneous with daily intramuscular therapy. *Br J Obstet Gynaecol* (1989) **96**: 746–8.

30 Sagle MA, Hamilton Fairley D, Kiddy DS, Franks S. A comparative, randomized study of low-dose human menopausal gonadotropin and follicle-stimulating hormone in women with polycystic ovarian syndrome. *Fertil Steril* (1991) **55**: 56–60.

31 Buvat J, Buvat Herbaut M, Marcolin G, Dehaene JL, Verbecq P, Renouard O. Purified follicle-stimulating hormone in polycystic ovary syndrome: slow administration is safer and more effective. *Fertil Steril* (1989) **52**: 553–9.

32 van der Meer M, Hompes PG, Scheele F, Schoute E, Popp-Snijders C, Schoemaker J. The importance of endogenous feedback for monofollicular growth in low-dose step-up ovulation induction with follicle-stimulating hormone in polycystic ovary syndrome: a randomized study. *Fertil Steril* (1996) **66**(4): 571–6.

33 Shoham Z, Patel A, Jacobs HS. Polycystic ovarian syndrome: safety and effectiveness of stepwise and low-dose administration of purified follicle-stimulating hormone. *Fertil Steril* (1991) **55**: 1051–6.

34 Dale PO, Tanbo T, Haug E, Abyholm T. Polycystic ovary syndrome: low-dose follicle stimulating hormone administration is a safe stimulation regimen even in previous hyperresponsive patients. *Hum Reprod* (1992) **7**: 1085–9.

35 Dale PO, Tanbo T, Lunde O, Abyholm T. Ovulation induction with low-dose follicle stimulating hormone in women with polycystic ovary syndrome. *Acta Obstet Gynecol Scand* (1993) **72**: 43–6.

36 Strowitzki T, Seehaus D, Korell M, Hepp H. Low-dose follicle stimulating hormone for ovulation induction in polycystic ovary syndrome. *J Reprod Med* (1994) **39**: 499–503.

37 Homburg R, Levy T, Ben Rafael Z. A comparative prospective study of conventional regimen with chronic low-dose administration of follicle-stimulating hormone for anovulation associated with polycystic ovary syndrome. *Fertil Steril* (1995) **63**: 729–33.

38 Herman A, Ron-El R, Golan A, Soffer Y, Bukovsky I, Caspi E. Overstimulated cycles under low-dose gonadotrophins in patients with polycystic ovary syndrome. *Hum Reprod* (1996) **8**: 30–4.

39 Grigoriou O, Antoniou G, Antonaki V, Patsouras C, Zioris C, Karakitsos P. Low-dose follicle stimulating hormone treatment for polycystic ovary disease. *Int J Gynecol Obstet* (1996) **52**: 55–9.

40 Balasch J, Tur R, Alvarez P et al. The safety and effectiveness of stepwise and low-dose administration of follicle stimulating hormone in WHO group II anovulatory infertile women: evidence from a large multicenter study in Spain. *J Assist Reprod Genet* (1996) **13**(7): 551–6.

41 Yong EL, Ng SC, Chan C, Khumar J, Teo LS, Ratnam S. Responses of polycystic ovary syndrome and related variants to low-dose follicle stimulating hormone. *Int J Gynecol Obstet* (1997) **57**: 305–11.

42 Hamilton Fairley D, Kiddy D, Watson H, Sagle M, Franks S. Low-dose gonadotrophin therapy for induction of ovulation in 100 women with polycystic ovary syndrome. *Hum Reprod* (1991) **6**: 1095–9.

43 White DM, Polson DW, Kiddy D et al. Induction of ovulation with low-dose gonadotropins in polycystic ovary syndrome: an analysis of 109 pregnancies in 225 women. *J Clin Endocrinol Metab* (1996) **81**(11): 3821–4.

44 Hoffman DI, Lobo RA, Campeau JD et al. Ovulation induction in clomiphene-resistant anovulatory women: differential follicular response to purified urinary follicle-stimulating hormone (FSH) versus purified urinary FSH and luteinizing hormone. *J Clin Endocrinol Metab* (1985) **60**(5): 922–7.

45 Fluker MR, Wang IY, Rowe TC. An extended 10-day course of clomiphene citrate (CC) in women with CC-resistant ovulatory disorders. *Fertil Steril* (1996) **66**(5): 761–4.

46 Trott EA, Plouffe L, Hansen K, Hines R, Brann DW, Mahesh VB. Ovulation induction in clomiphene-resistant anovulatory women with normal dehydroepiandrosterone sulfate levels: beneficial effects of the addition of dexamethasone during the follicular phase. *Fertil Steril* (1996) **66**(3): 484–6.

47 Bristow RE, Karlan BY. Ovulation induction, infertility, and ovarian cancer risk [review, 49 refs]. *Fertil Steril* (1996) **66**(4): 499–507.

13

Treatment with GnRH agonists

Peter GA Hompes

Gonadotrophin releasing hormone (GnRH) agonists are synthetic peptide analogues of hypothalamic GnRH with a higher biopotency and longer duration of gonadotrophin release. Paradoxically, repeated administration causes pituitary desensitization, and induces a reversible state of hypogonadotrophic hypogonadism. This effect of GnRH agonists is due to an increased binding affinity to pituitary GnRH receptors[1] and increased resistance to the proteolytic degradation which rapidly removes native GnRH.[2] The clinical applications of GnRH agonists are numerous. They extend from precocious puberty, endometriosis[3] and leiomyomas[4] to hormone-dependent tumours, male and female contraception and ovulation induction in patients suffering from polycystic ovary syndrome (PCOS)[5] and in vitro fertilization (IVF).[6] These agents have also been proposed for the treatment of hirsutism in women with PCOS.[7,8] The reduction in androgen concentrations by the GnRH agonist is accompanied by an improved insulin sensitivity.[9]

Treatment regimens with GnRH agonists for ovulation induction cover a wide dose range, and include nasal spray administration and subcutaneous injections. Up to now the nasal spray has been used in most studies concerning ovulation induction in PCOS. The patients are treated daily with supraoptimal doses, self-administered and spread out over the waking hours. This repeated administration causes pituitary desensitization and induces a reversible state of medical hypophysectomy. In PCOS this approach could be an advantage, because it decreases the luteinizing hormone (LH)/follicle-stimulating hormone (FSH) ratio and the patient becomes hypogonadotrophic. The rationale behind this is the fact that patients suffering from PCOS respond relatively poorly to ovulation induction with gonadotrophins, with fewer pregnancies than in hypogonadal patients and a high frequency of hyperstimulation, and a state of relative hypogonadotrophic hypogonadism may be beneficial in these cases. The idea of using GnRH agonists in ovulation induction in PCOS stems from the assumption that the endogenous secretion of relatively large amounts of LH may well be the cause of the higher incidence of development of the ovarian hyperstimulation syndrome (OHSS) in comparison with hypogonadotrophic amenorrhoea under stimulation with gonadotrophins. Moreover, the high tonic secretion of LH may be deleterious to the quality of the ovum as well, explaining the lower pregnancy rates under ovulation induction in PCOS compared with hypothalamic amenorrhoea, namely 40% versus 75%.[10]

Function of GnRH agonists

Continuous gonadotrophin releasing hormone stimulation of the gonadotroph may be imitated by agonistic GnRH analogues, known as GnRH agonists. By manipulation of the chemical structure of GnRH – Glu-His-Trp-Ser-Tyr-Gly-Leu-Arg-Pro-Gly-NH$_2$ – the GnRH agonists have acquired a longer half-life, a higher affinity to the receptor and an enhanced ability to activate postreceptor mechanisms compared with GnRH itself. The chemical manipulations of the GnRH molecule that have proved to be effective are an ethylamide modification at the carboxy-terminal glycine (position 10) and, more importantly, the substitution of D-amino acids containing bulky hydrophobic side groups at position 6 (Gly). The latter substitutions stabilize a spatial conformation necessary for activation of postreceptor mechanisms and block biodegradation through hydrolysis by endopeptidases.[11]

Physiologic secretion of gonadotrophins requires intermittent GnRH secretion. Upon continuous GnRH stimulation LH secretion vanishes and FSH secretion decreases. In addition to a short period of secretion, a single GnRH pulse induces a short period of refractoriness of the gonadotroph for a subsequent GnRH pulse. When GnRH is given with an infinitely small pulse interval, i.e. continuous administration, gonadotrophin secretion becomes greatly impaired. Initially, continuous stimulation results in secretion of large amounts of LH and FSH but after a while, gonadotrophin secretion declines despite the presence of GnRH.[12] This phenomenon is called desensitization.

The GnRH challenge test

Not every gynaecological indication requires the same degree of desensitization of the pituitary.[13] Therefore, for each indication, the dosage as well as the duration and route of administration of the GnRH agonist has to be established. For indications such as contraception, ovulation induction and treatment of uterine leiomyomas and hirsutism, partial desensitization may suffice. Several authors have used GnRH challenges to measure the degree of pituitary desensitization.[14,15] The level of LH and the responses of LH and FSH to the GnRH challenge showed significant dose-dependent suppression. Multiple regression indicated that the LH response to the GnRH challenge was the best way to measure pituitary desensitization. From the LH responses to the GnRH challenge a standard curve has been established for the assessment of the degree of pituitary desensitization. To quantify pituitary desensitization, the percentage of suppression of the LH response to the GnRH challenges in the third week of GnRH infusion must be plotted against the dose of GnRH infused (Figure 13.1).[16]

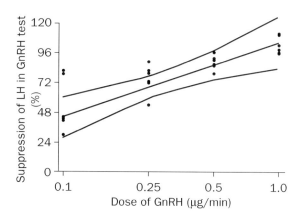

Figure 13.1 The mean suppression with 95% confidence limits of the LH response to the GnRH challenge in the third week of GnRH infusion is plotted against the dose of GnRH infused. From Scheele et al.[16]

Side effects of GnRH agonists

Allergic reactions have been described, but are rare.[17] All other effects of GnRH agonist treatment can be explained by the suppression of synthesis and secretion of biologically active pituitary gonadotrophins and the consequent decrease in gonadal activity. During the initial agonistic phase, patients may experience symptoms of increased oestrogen secretion, followed by an episode of vaginal bleeding. During the subsequent hypo-oestrogenic phase patients may experience hot flushes (80–90%), vaginal dryness (20–30%), headaches (20%), mood swings (15–20%) and decreased libido (10–20%).[18] The frequency and extent of these side effects depend on oestradiol levels: the lower the oestradiol levels, the higher the frequency of side effects. Although the increase of alkaline phosphatase is significant during GnRH agonist therapy, the level does not exceed the upper limit of the normal range. This increase is due to the activation of bone metabolism.[19] There is a significant correlation between the differences in bone mineral density changes in the lumbar spine and the post-treatment oestradiol level and the age of the patient. However, bone loss was found to be reversible after agonist therapy was discontinued.[20] In general, only a brief application of the GnRH agonist is necessary for its adjuvant role in ovulation induction. In such a short course of therapy, hypo-oestrogenaemia is not a concern. Lipid metabolism is sensitive to changes in gonadal steroid levels and may be a good indicator of overall metabolic effects. High plasma cholesterol levels are a classical risk factor for coronary heart disease. Leuprolin treatment did not, however, significantly affect either triacylglycerol or total cholesterol concentrations.

Combined treatment with GnRH agonists and gonadotrophin results in an increased incidence of the ovarian hyperstimulation syndrome.[21] It is established that the response to gonadotrophins of a pharmacologically hypophysectomized PCOS patient is not the same as in hypogonadotrophic amenorrhoea: the diagnosis-dependent predisposition to multifollicular growth persists.[22] The clinical consequences of a potential direct action of GnRH agonists on the ovary are uncertain, but may turn out to be important, especially for ovulation induction.[23] Potentially negative effects on reproductive tissues and organs and teratogenicity must therefore be excluded. Short-term GnRH agonist administration in patients with PCOS and its impact on the utero-ovarian blood flow have been studied. The resistance index of utero-ovarian blood flow is not affected by the GnRH agonist administration.[24]

The use of GnRH agonists in polycystic ovary syndrome

Studies as to the efficacy of treatments in PCOS are at least partially undermined by the variety of definitions of the syndrome. 'A disorder without identity: 'HCA', 'PCO', 'PCOD', 'PCOS', 'SLS' – what are we to call it?' For the sake of convention (not necessarily correctness) it was agreed to call it 'polycystic ovary syndrome', the syndrome traditionally associated with the finding of polycystic ovaries.[25] The full-blown-syndrome includes oligo-amenorrhoea, infertility, obesity, hirsutism, enlarged ovaries which appear polycystic on ultrasonography, raised LH levels and raised androgen levels. Homburg suggests that PCOS is a predominantly genetic disorder of ovarian androgen production induced by extraovarian factors, in particular insulin resistance, hyperinsulinaemia and their biochemical sequelae. The clinical and endocrinological expression of the syndrome is determined by the extraovarian factors present.[26,27] Moreover, the prevalence of PCOS among hyperandrogenic women who report normal menses is high (up to 74%).[28]

GnRH agonists in combination with gonadotrophins

The results of ovulation induction with gonadotrophins in hypogonadotrophic amenorrhoea are much better than in PCOS. In hypogonadotrophic amenorrhoea cumulative pregnancy rates are 91% after six cycles of gonadotrophin treatment.[29] If the response pattern of PCOS to gonadotrophin therapy is compared with hypogonadotrophic disease, it turns out that the response in PCOS patients is often unpredictable, sometimes with a severe ovarian hyperstimulation syndrome (1–2%). In hypogonadotrophic disease a more predictable response is seen and the ovarian hyperstimulation syndrome is less frequent, although it does occur. Therefore the use of GnRH agonists, in order to suppress endogenous gonadotrophin secretion in PCOS patients and to mimic hypogonadotrophic hypogonadism, seemed to be a logical approach for ovulation induction.

Administration of a GnRH agonist causes an initial 'flare-up' of LH from the already elevated pretreatment levels within a period of 3 days. Thereafter, as treatment is continued, total suppression of LH is observed within 2–3 weeks. Levels of FSH also show an abrupt surge, with a maximum on the third day. However, FSH is never totally suppressed and may even show a gradual rise after 2 weeks of pituitary suppression. Oestradiol, testosterone and androstenedione show a similar pattern; after an initial rise a gradual decline is observed.[30] If agonist treatment is stopped in a patient suffering from PCOS, the LH/FSH ratio increases after 7–10 days, and within a period of 3 weeks LH and FSH levels are back to pretreatment PCOS values.

In 1985 Fleming et al were the first to publish results of co-treatment using GnRH agonists and human menopausal gonadotrophin (hMG) for anovulatory PCOS patients.[31] The eight patients studied were first treated with hMG alone, followed by the combination of GnRH agonist plus hMG. None of the patients had conceived during conventional hMG/human chorionic gonadotrophin (hCG) treatment and in 7 out of 11 cycles ovarian enlargement was noticed. Following co-treatment with GnRH agonists, however, seven out of eight patients conceived within 2 treatment cycles. The main contribution of this co-treatment is the reduction of LH concentrations throughout the follicular phase of the cycle. This almost completely eliminates premature luteinization and the need to abandon cycles for this reason. Both the prevention of premature luteinization and promising pregnancy results by the use of GnRH agonists have been confirmed by others.[32–36] However, none of the randomized trials showed a significantly improved fecundity if GnRH agonists were used in PCOS.[33–38] The duration of the pretreatment with the GnRH agonist did not seem to affect the results either. Pretreatment with a 3-month administration of a GnRH agonist in ovulation induction with low-dose pure FSH did not improve ovulation and pregnancy rates.[39] In one of our studies it was investigated whether pretreatment with GnRH agonists led to a higher occurrence of monofollicular growth during stimulation with low-dose FSH. One group of patients (group 1) suffering from clomiphene-resistant PCOS were stimulated with low-dose FSH. The results were compared with those from another group of similar patients (group 2) subsequently stimulated with low-dose FSH combined with a GnRH agonist.

In group 1 fifteen patients had 39 stimulation cycles performed; in group 2 thirteen patients had 33 stimulation cycles performed. In the first group 44% of the cycles were monofollicular, while the corresponding figure in group 2 was 14% ($P = 0.04$). Evidence was found for postponed atresia in group 2. In both groups 1 and 2 interindividual and intraindividual variability of the FSH dose required for induction of follicular growth were observed. It was concluded that during the use of GnRH agonist, stimulation with low-dose FSH less frequently resulted in monofollicular growth, possibly owing to postponed atresia. Furthermore, the use of a GnRH agonist did not abolish the inter- and intraindividual variability of the FSH dose required to induce ongoing follicular growth.

As far as I know there are no papers published on co-treatment with GnRH agonists and a low-dose FSH step-down schedule. Nevertheless, there is mounting evidence that the ability of GnRH agonists to reduce the elevated LH concentrations serves to increase ovulation and pregnancy rates. Co-treatment reduces the prevalence of early spontaneous miscarriages, which are notoriously high in PCOS and accompanied by raised LH concentrations.[40]

GnRH agonist pretreatment for ovulation induction in the recovery phase

With regard to treatment regimens with luteinizing hormone releasing hormone (LHRH) agonists for ovulation induction there are in principle three periods during which the use of an agonist could be of some advantage. First, during the 'flare-up' period, secondly during downregulation, and finally during the recovery period after discontinuation of the analogue (Figure 13.2).

During the flare-up period the GnRH agonist is used for its direct stimulating effect. During downregulation the agonist is used for increasing fertility of ovulated oocytes, and finally for facilitation of ovulation during the recovery period. Scheele et al were the first to study the usefulness of the flare-up induced by a GnRH agonist for ovulation induction in PCOS.[41] The question was whether the flare-up of FSH and LH induced by 4 days of agonist treatment would elicit follicular growth and ovulation in polycystic ovary syndrome. The results were disappointing. The pilot study suggested that the flare-up of LH and FSH induced by 4 days of GnRH agonist treatment was ineffective for

ovulation induction in PCOS. The observed ovulation in one of the seven patients had to be judged as a placebo effect.

There are several ways in which a GnRH agonist could be useful in the recovery phase:

1. The resistance to clomiphene citrate might be broken in the recovery phase.
2. Stimulation with a fixed dose of FSH might lead to ovulation.
3. Also stimulation with pulsatile GnRH could be successful.

After discontinuation of a 17–21 day GnRH agonist treatment, ovulation induction was attempted with clomiphene citrate, or with a fixed dose of FSH in two separate trials. The group treated with clomiphene citrate was a selected group showing resistance to this agent. No clomiphene citrate-treated patient ovulated and after FSH stimulation only two patients ovulated. Endocrine measurements in the recovery phase showed an early rise of FSH compared with the rise of LH and androgens. This study could not demonstrate any effect of the recovery phase with respect to facilitation of follicular growth in PCOS.[42] Both hypotheses had to be rejected.

Pulsatile GnRH and PCOS

Pulsatile GnRH has become an accepted and highly effective treatment in patients suffering from hypothalamic amenorrhoea. This therapy can successfully induce ovulation in 90–100% of women with hypothalamic amenorrhoea.[43] Because of this success, its efficacy has also been tried in PCOS. Braat has reviewed the literature on pulsatile GnRH treatment in PCOS.[44] In this overview 17 papers concerning the results of pulsatile GnRH treatment in PCOS are described. Only papers reporting more than 10 cycles were included. The frequency of ovulatory cycles varied from 5% to 87%. Ovulation was achieved in approximately 50%. The pregnancy rate per cycle varied from 0% to 28%. In all papers together (95 pregnancies) only 5 multiple pregnancies were reported; 34 pregnancies aborted (36%). A pulse

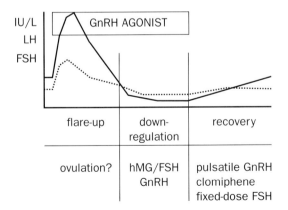

Figure 13.2 Three periods in which the use of a GnRH agonist could be of some advantage for ovulation induction in PCOS. Solid line, LH; dashed line, FSH.

interval of 90 minutes was applied in most studies. Although the endogenous LH pulse frequency is elevated in many PCOS patients, varying the interval from 60 minutes to 120 minutes did not seem to interfere with the results.[45]

First ovulatory cycles on pulsatile GnRH therapy were characterized by significantly increased mean follicular-phase LH levels compared with second cycles and controls.[46] The changes occurring between the first and second ovulatory cycles in women with PCOS resulted in a more physiological overall pattern of gonadotrophins and sex steroid secretion in the second cycles. However, women with PCOS, even when ovulatory on pulsatile GnRH, do not display entirely normal gonadotrophin and sex steroid dynamics. Pulsatile GnRH therapy in PCOS patients is particularly unsuitable for obese patients and patients with high LH and androgen levels.[47] It had to be concluded that the overall results of GnRH treatment in PCOS patients are disappointing.

GnRH agonist pretreatment and pulsatile GnRH in the recovery phase

The use of the transiently normogonadotrophic recovery phase after GnRH agonist treatment seemed to be a logical concept for ovulation induction with pulsatile GnRH. There is good evidence that high follicular-phase LH levels coincide with poor pregnancy outcome.[48–51] The recovery phase immediately after cessation of GnRH agonist therapy is characterized by low serum LH and androgen levels.[52,53] Filicori was the first to utilize the beneficial effects of the GnRH agonist, to increase its efficacy and reduce its undesired influence on multiple follicular development with the use of pulsatile GnRH in the recovery phase.[54–57] In this study a sequential use of 8 weeks of GnRH agonist and pulsatile GnRH in comparison with pulsatile GnRH alone improved the ovulatory rate, as well as the pregnancy rate per ovulatory cycle. The abortion rate was not decreased by the treatment. The increased ovulation rate in the cycles following GnRH agonist treatment was

not due to a raised follicular-phase FSH level. On the contrary, early follicular-phase FSH levels were significantly higher in cycles treated with pulsatile GnRH without GnRH agonist pretreatment.[58] However, such a long pretreatment with GnRH agonists is not attractive for clinical practice. It implies a persistent oligomenorrhoea with only about four ovulations per year. Another problem with the study from Filicori is the fact that the PCOS patients were not strictly required to be resistant to clomiphene citrate. This is important because a small study of clomiphene-resistant PCOS patients did not obtain significantly better results after GnRH agonist pretreatment.[59] Scheele et al investigated the use of pulsatile GnRH after a shorter, medium-term, period of 3 weeks of GnRH agonist pretreatment in patients.[60] Despite the fact that the LH levels during the 12 days before ovulation were lowered in cycles following GnRH agonist treatment, no significant clinical improvement could be proved in these cycles (Figure 13.3).

The effectiveness of this form of treatment in clomiphene-resistant PCOS patients is an urgent issue in clinical practice. A larger study is necessary to demonstrate whether this therapy could be counterbalanced by its advantages of safety and effectiveness.

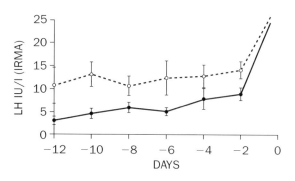

Figure 13.3 Follicular phase LH levels (median ± SEM) until day 0 (LH peak) of pre- and post-GnRH agonist cycles in PCOS patients (solid circles with, open circles without GnRH agonist). The upper limit of a normal LH level until 2 days before the LH peak is 6.5 IU/l. From Scheele et al.[60]

GnRH agonists and miscarriage rates

Two retrospective studies have suggested that the use of GnRH agonists may reduce miscarriage rates by more than 50%.[40,61] Balen et al studied the risk of miscarriage in 1060 IVF pregnancies in relation to age, cause of infertility, ovarian morphology and treatment regimen.[61] The miscarriage rate was 23.6% in women with normal ovaries compared with 35.8% in those with PCOS. When treated with a long agonist protocol these PCOS patients had a significant reduction in the rate of miscarriage: 20.3% when treated with the agonist, compared with 47.2% with gonadotropins and clomiphene citrate. Homburg et al analysed 239 women suffering from clomiphene-resistant PCOS, receiving hMG with or without a GnRH agonist.[40] Of pregnancies achieved with the GnRH agonist, there were 17.6% miscarriages compared with 39.1% of those achieved with gonadotrophins alone. Cumulative live birth rates for GnRH agonist after four cycles were 64% compared with 26% for gonadotrophins only.

A review of the literature by Shoham et al shows a correlation between raised LH levels and infertility, but a lack of proven causal relationship.[62] In support of a causal relation, however, is an IVF study in which the urinary LH output was significantly higher in women who did not conceive, compared with women who did.[63] In a group of 28 PCOS patients treated with clomiphene citrate the results were better if the follicular LH values were lower.[64] In a prospective study in which the relationship between pregnancy LH concentrations and outcome of pregnancy was studied in 193 women, it was demonstrated that high LH values correlated with a decreased fecundity and an increased risk of miscarriage.[65]

Oocytes obtained from PCOS patients had a fertilization potential equal to oocytes obtained from donors with mechanical infertility. Furthermore, because the oocytes of patients with PCOS exposed to a GnRH agonist had a significantly higher implantation rate, a detrimental role of high LH levels on oocyte quality seems probable.[66] All these data could give the impression that the correlation between high LH values and infertility is indisputable, but not all reports agree on the association of high LH values and miscarriage rates.[67–69] A randomized, prospective study is lacking to confirm these data, therefore the question whether there is a causal relationship between high LH level and miscarriage remains to be answered.

GnRH agonists and the ovarian hyperstimulation syndrome

Ovarian hyperstimulation syndrome (OHSS) and multiple pregnancies are the two main complications of ovulation induction using gonadotrophins. Severe ovarian hyperstimulation syndrome is more frequently seen in PCOS patients than in patients suffering from other anovulation problems. Stimulating protocols which include GnRH agonist downregulation together with hMG have been shown to exacerbate OHSS.[70,71] The GnRH agonist stimulation protocols prevent an endogenous LH surge, allowing hCG to be administered with more advanced follicular development. Furthermore, the 'flare-up' effect of GnRH agonist initiation also allows enhanced stimulation of the ovary, which leads to earlier and more numerous recruitment.[72] To evaluate the role of endogenous feedback in monofollicular growth during low-dose gonadotrophin therapy in PCOS we investigated FSH levels in a group of patients co-treated with a GnRH agonist compared with patients not receiving a GnRH agonist.[73] The rate of monofollicular growth was significantly higher in the group without the agonist (80%) than in the group co-treated with the agonist (22%). No significant differences in oestradiol levels or inhibin levels were found between the groups.

The use of GnRH agonists in the context of triggering ovulation has been reported by several authors.[74–76] Despite the fact that OHSS caused by GnRH agonist treatment without gonadotrophin therapy in a patient suffering from PCOS has been described, it is concluded that a GnRH agonist may be an acceptable substitute for hCG to salvage treatment cycles in patients thought to be at risk of OHSS or multiple pregnancies.[77] In a debate on the issue of ovarian hyperstimulation with GnRH agonists,[78–80] it was concluded that a controlled, randomized and masked study is needed to determine whether GnRH agonists do, in fact, prevent OHSS. It is premature to conclude that the use of GnRH agonists to trigger ovulation will protect patients against development of severe OHSS.

Other combinations with GnRH agonists in PCOS

The effect of GnRH agonist treatment on growth hormone (GH) secretion in women with PCOS shows a reduced GH response to growth hormone releasing hormone compared with normal controls. This suggests that a different level of sensitivity in the somatotrophic axis exists in PCOS.[81]

Homburg et al explored the effect of co-treatment with recombinant human growth hormone, a GnRH agonist and hMG for induction of ovulation in women with clomiphene-resistant PCOS.[82] In a randomized, double-masked, placebo-controlled trial, 30 patients were treated with a GnRH agonist and a conventional hMG dose regimen for ovulation induction. From day 1 of hMG therapy patients were randomized to receive either GH or placebo. There were no significant differences between GH and placebo groups in any of the outcomes measured. They concluded that GH does not seem likely to be of any potential clinical benefit for the treatment of PCOS. The combination of GnRH agonist plus low-dose oral contraceptive agent in PCOS seems to be more promising. This combination was already in use to improve the treatment of hirsute women with ovarian hyperandrogenism.[83] Oral contraceptive therapy failed to improve significantly the therapeutic effect of GnRH agonist treatment alone in hirsutism. In a comparison between the effects of ovarian cauterization and GnRH agonist plus oral contraceptive therapy in PCOS, it was found that both therapeutic regimens had similar effects on the endocrine profiles.[84] The

GnRH agonist plus oral contraceptive combination seems to be effective in restoring the optimal follicular environment in women with PCOS. An even better result was published by Genazzani et al,[85] who, after long-term treatment with GnRH agonist plus low-dose oral contraceptives, found ovulatory cycles during the 6 months following treatment. Their PCOS patients were selected on the basis of ultrasonography, oligo-amenorrhoea and plasma androstenedione levels above the normal range. After a treatment period of 6 months only the patients given GnRH agonist plus oral contraceptives showed a normal LH/FSH ratio and adequate plasma oestradiol and progesterone levels. This therapeutic schedule might be proposed as the ideal treatment for women whose infertility is mainly related to an ovarian hyperandrogenism-induced ovulation. Dual suppression with oral contraceptives and GnRH agonists improves IVF outcome in high-responder patients including those with PCOS. Hormonal analyses revealed that the chief mechanism may be through an improved LH/FSH ratio following dual suppression. An additional feature of this dual method is significantly lower serum androgen concentrations.[86]

Conclusion

The use of GnRH agonists in the treatment of patients suffering from PCOS for ovulation induction has become more and more a standard procedure. There is mounting evidence that GnRH agonists suppress the excessive LH levels during the follicular phase, suppress the premature LH surge, and may have a direct effect on the ovum. The combined GnRH agonist/gonadotrophin stimulation protocols produce higher pregnancy rates and smaller pregnancy wastages compared with gonadotrophin treatment alone. Especially in PCOS patients with high LH levels, this co-treatment reduces the prevalence of early spontaneous miscarriages. Stimulation protocols of low-dose FSH combined with GnRH agonists do not increase the occurrence of monofollicular growth. Different stimulation protocols using the recovery phase after GnRH agonist treatment have been studied. The resistance to clomiphene citrate appeared not to be broken by the GnRH agonist treatment. Subsequent stimulation with a fixed dose of FSH was not effective. Better results were seen with pulsatile GnRH in the recovery phase. Luteinizing hormone levels during the 12 days before ovulation were lowered in cycles following GnRH agonist treatment compared with pretreatment cycles.

This co-treatment reduces multiple follicular development and improves the ovulation rate as well as the pregnancy rate per ovulatory cycle. However, as pulsatile GnRH therapy is still a complicated method of treatment it should be reserved for clomiphene-resistant PCOS patients only. It is regrettable that most studies on GnRH agonists have not exclusively studied clomiphene-resistant PCOS patients; a larger study involving these patients is necessary to demonstrate if this therapy could be counterbalanced by its advantages of safety and efficacy. As far as OHSS is concerned it is clear that the use of GnRH agonists does not prevent the occurrence of the syndrome. It is premature to conclude that the use of GnRH agonists to trigger ovulation will protect patients from development of severe OHSS. The use of a GnRH agonist in combination with low-dose oral contraceptive seems to be effective in restoring the follicular environment in women with PCOS. The question whether it is effective in infertility patients needs to be investigated. Finally, the safety questions are still unanswered with regard to reproductive function after therapy and the risk of hormone-dependent neoplasia. Much research in this field remains to be done.

REFERENCES

1 Loumaye E, Naor Z, Catt KJ. Binding affinity and biological activity of gonadotrophin-releasing hormone agonists in isolated pituitary cells. *Endocrinology* (1982) **111**: 730–6.

2 Swift AD, Crighton DB. Relative activity, plasma elimination and tissue degradation of synthetic luteinizing hormone releasing hormone and certain of its analogues. *J Endocrinol* (1979) **80**: 141–52.

3 Hughes EG, Fedorkow DM, Collins JA. A quantitative overview of controlled trials in endometriosis-associated infertility. *Fertil Steril* (1993) **59**: 963–70.

4 Friedman AJ. Treatment of uterine myomas with GnRH agonists. *Semin Reprod Endocrinol* (1993) **11**: 154–61.

5 Fleming R, Haxton MJ, Hamilton MPR et al. Combined gonadotropin-releasing hormone analog and exogenous gonadotropins for ovulation induction in infertile women: efficacy related to ovarian function assessment. *Am J Obstet Gynecol* (1988) **159**: 376–81.

6 Hughes EG, Fedorkow DM, Daya S, Sagle MA, van de Koppel P, Collins JA. The routine use of gonadotropin-releasing hormone agonists prior to in vitro fertilization and gamete intrafallopian transfer: a meta-analysis of randomized trials. *Fertil Steril* (1992) **58**: 888–96.

7 Moghetti P, Castello R, Zamberlan N et al. Spironolactone, but not flutamide, administration prevents bone loss in hyperandrogenic women treated with gonadotropin-releasing hormone agonist. *J Clin Endocrinol Metab* (1999) **84**(4): 1250–4.

8 Motta EL, Baracat EC, Haidar MA, Juliano I, Lima GR. Ovarian activity before and after gonadal suppression by GnRH-a in patients with polycystic ovary syndrome, hyperandrogenism, hyperinsulinism and acanthosis nigricans. *Rev Assoc Med Bras* (1998) **44**(2): 94–8.

9 Dahlgren E, Landin K, Krotkiewski M, Holm G, Janson PO. Effects of two antiandrogen treatments on hirsutism and insulin sensitivity in women with polycystic ovary syndrome. *Hum Reprod* (1998) **13**: 2706–11.

10 Schoemaker J, Hompes PGA, Scheele F, Weissenbruch MM. PCOD: treatment with LHRH analogues. *Gynecol Endocrinol* (1989) **3**(suppl. 2): 51–62.

11 Karten MJ, Rivier JE. Gonadotropin-releasing hormone analog design. Structure-function studies toward the development of agonists and antagonists: rationale and perspective. *Endocr Rev* (1986) **7**: 44–66.

12 De Koning J, van Dieten JAMJ, van Rees GP. Refractoriness of pituitary gland after continuous exposure to LHRH. *J Endocrinol* (1978) **79**: 311–18.

13 Ron-El R, Herman A, Goland A, Soffer Y,

Nachum H, Caspi E. Ultrashort gonadotropin releasing hormone agonist (GnRH-a) protocol in comparison with the long acting GnRH-a protocol and menotropin alone. *Fertil Steril* (1992) **58**: 1164–8.

14 Filicori M, Flamigni C, Cognigni G et al. Comparison of the suppressive capacity of different depot gonadotropin-releasing hormone analogs in women. *J Clin Endocrinol Metab* (1993) **77**: 130–3.

15 Uemura T, Minaguchi H, Okuda K, Sugimoto O. GnRH agonist Zoladex in the treatment of endometriosis. In: Lunenfeld B, ed., *Advances in the Study of GnRH Analogues*. Proceedings of the 2nd International Symposium on GnRH Analogues in Cancer and Human Reproduction (Parthenon: Carnforth, 1992) 159–71.

16 Scheele F, Hompes PGA, Lambalk CB, Schoute E, Broekmans J, Schoemaker J. The GnRH challenge test: a quantitative measure of pituitary desensitization during GnRH agonist administration. *Clin Endocrinol* (1996) **44**: 581–6.

17 Letterie GS, Stevenson D, Shah A. Recurrent anaphylaxis to a depot form of GnRH analogue. *Obst Gynec* (1991) **78**: 943–6.

18 Leroy Heinrichs W, Monroe SE. Safety issues related to the use of GnRH agonists in gynecology. *Infert Reprod Med Clin North Am* (1993) **4**: 189–200.

19 Bühler K, Winkler U, Schindler AE. Influence on hormone levels, lipid metabolism and reversibility of endocrinological changes after leuprorelin acetate depot therapy. *Clin Therap* (1992) **14**(suppl. A): 104–13.

20 Fogelman I. Gonadotropin releasing hormones and the skeleton. *Fertil Steril* (1992) **57**: 715–17.

21 Homburg R, Eshel A, Kilborn J, Adams J, Jacobs HS. Combined luteinizing hormone releasing hormone analogue and exogenous gonadotrophins for the treatment of infertility associated with polycystic ovaries. *Hum Reprod* (1990) **5**: 32–5.

22 Scheele F, Hompes PGA, Bernardus RE, Schoemaker J. Severe ovarian hyperstimulation: a case report and essentials of prevention and management. *Eur J Obstet Gyn Reprod Biol* (1992) **45**: 187–92.

23 Jones PBC. Potential relevance of gonadotropin-releasing hormone to ovarian physiology. *Semin Reprod Endocrinol* (1989) **7**: 41–51.

24 Vrtacnik-Bokal E, Meden-Vrtovec H. Short-term GnRH-analogue administration in patients with PCOS and its impact on hemodynamics and hormonal profile. *J Assist Reprod Genet* (1997) **14**(10): 558–61.

25 Lobo RA. A disorder without identity: 'HCA', 'PCO', 'PCOD', 'PCOS', what are we to call it. *Fertil Steril* (1995) **63**(6): 1158–60.

26 Homburg R. Polycystic ovary syndrome – from gynaecological curiosity to multisystem endocrinopathy. *Hum Reprod* (1996) **11**(1): 29–39.

27 Barnes RB. The pathogenesis of polycystic ovary syndrome: lessons from ovarian stimulation studies. *J Endocrinol Invest* (1998) **21**(9): 567–79.

28 Carmina E, Lobe RA. Do hyperandrogenic women with normal menses have polycystic ovary syndrome? *Fertil Steril* (1999) **71**(2): 319–22.

29 Dor J, Itzkowic DJ, Mashiach S, Lunenfeld B, Serr DM. Cumulative conception rates following gonadotropin therapy. *Am J Obstet Gynecol* (1980) **136**: 102–5.

30 Charbonel B, Krempf M, Blanchard P, Dano F, Delage C. Induction of ovulation in polycystic ovary syndrome with a combination of luteinizing hormone-releasing hormone analog and exogenous gonadotropin. *Fertil Steril* (1987) **47**: 920–6.

31 Fleming R, Haxton MJ, Hamilton MPR et al. Successful treatment of infertile women with oligomenorrhoea using a combination of an LHRH agonist and exogenous gonadotrophins. *Br J Obstet Gynaecol* (1985) **92**: 369–73.

32 Weise HC, Fiedler K, Kato K. Buserelin suppression of endogenous gonadotropin secretion in infertile women with ovarian feedback disorders given human menopausal/human chorionic gonadotropin treatment. *Fertil Steril* (1988) **49**: 399–403.

33 Dodson WC, Hughes CL, Whitesides DB, Haney AF. The effect of leuprolide acetate on ovulation induction with human menopausal gonadotropins in polycystic ovary syndrome. *J Clin Endocrinol Metab* (1987) **65**: 95–100.

34 Dodson WC, Hughes CL, Yancy SE, Haney AF. Clinical characteristics of ovulation induction with human menopausal gonadotropins with and without leuprolide acetate in polycystic ovary syndrome. *Fertil Steril* (1989) **52**: 915–18.

35 Homburg R, Eshel A, Kilborn J, Adams J, Jacobs HS. Combined luteinizing hormone releasing hormone analogue and exogenous gonadotrophins for the treatment of infertility associated with polycystic ovaries. *Hum Reprod* (1990) **5**: 32–5.

36 Bachus KE, Hughes CL, Haney AF, Dodson WC. The luteal phase in polycystic ovary syndrome

during ovulation induction with and without leuprolide acetate. *Fertil Steril* (1990) **54**: 27–31.

37 Hompes PGA, van Weissenbruch MM, Burger CW, Schoemaker J. The additional use of busere-lin in hMG-hCG ovulation induction in PCO: a double blind controlled study. *Prog Clin Biol Res* (1986) **225**: 391–9.

38 Scheele F, Hompes PGA, van der Meer M, Schoute E, Schoemaker J. The effects of a gonadotrophin-releasing hormone-agonist on treatment with low dose follicle stimulating hormone in polycystic ovary syndrome. *Hum Reprod* (1993) **8**: 699–704.

39 Vegetti W, Testa G, Ragni G, Parazzini F, Crosignani PG. Ovarian stimulation with low-dose pure follicle-stimulating hormone in polycystic ovarian syndrome anovulatory patients: effect of long-term pretreatment with gonadotrophin-releasing hormone analogue. *Gynecol Obstet Invest* (1998) **45**(3): 186–9.

40 Homburg R, Levy T, Berkovitz D et al. Gonadotropin-releasing hormone agonist reduces the miscarriage rate for pregnancies achieved in women with polycystic ovarian syndrome. *Fertil Steril* (1993) **59**: 527–31.

41 Scheele F, Hompes PGA, van der Meer M, Schoemaker J. The use of the 'flare-up' effect of buserelin for ovulation induction in PCOD. *Gynecol Endocrinol* (1990) **4**(suppl. 2): 70.

42 Scheele F, van der Meer M, Lambalk CB, Schoute E, Schoemaker J, Hompes PGA. Exploring the recovery phase after treatment with a GnRH-agonist for ovulation induction in polycystic ovary syndrome: three pilot trials. *Eur J Obstet Gynecol Reprod Biol* (1995) **62**: 221–4.

43 Santoro NF, Wierman ME, Filicori M, Waldstreicher J, Crowley WF. Intravenous administration of pulsatile gonadotropin-releasing hormone in hypothalamic amenorrhea: effects of dosage. *J Clin Endocrinol Metab* (1986) **62**: 109–16.

44 Braat DDM. Ovulation induction with pulsatile gonadotrophin-releasing hormone in patients with PCOS. Proceedings of the symposium *The Ovary: Regulation Dysfunction and Treatment*. International Congress Series 1106 (Excerpta Medica: Amsterdam, 1996) 385–9.

45 Burger CW, Korsen TJM, Hompes PGA, van Kessel H, Schoemaker J. Ovulation induction with pulsatile luteinizing hormone-releasing hormone (LHR) in women with clomiphene resistant polycystic ovary-like disease: clinical results. *Fertil Steril* (1986) **46**: 1045–54.

46 Corenthal L, Von Hagen S, Larkins D, Ibrahim J, Santoro N. Benefits of continuous physiological pulsatile gonadotropin-releasing hormone therapy in women with polycystic ovarian syndrome. *Fertil Steril* (1994) **61**(6): 1027–33.

47 Homburg R, Eshel A, Tucker M, Mason P, Adams J. One hundred pregnancies following pulsatile hormone releasing hormone therapy for ovulation induction. *Br Med J* (1989) **298**: 809–12.

48 Stanger JD, Yovich JL. Reduced in-vitro fertilisation of human oocytes from patients with raised basal LH levels during the follicular phase. *Br J Obstet Gynaecol* (1985) **92**: 385–93.

49 Howles CM, Macnamee MC, Edwards RG, Goswamy R, Steptoe PC. Effect of high tonic luteinising hormone on outcome of in-vitro fertilisation. *Lancet* (1986) **ii**: 521–2.

50 Homburg R, Armar NA, Eshel A, Adams J, Jacobs HS. Influence of serum luteinising hormone concentrations on ovulation, conception and early pregnancy loss in polycystic ovary syndrome. *Br Med J* (1988) **297**: 1024–6.

51 Regan L, Owen EJ, Jacobs HS. Hypersecretion of luteinising hormone, infertility and miscarriage. *Lancet* (1990) **336**: 1141–4.

52 MacLeod AF, Wheeler MJ, Gordon P, Lowy C, Sonksen PH, Conaglen JV. Effect of long-term inhibition of gonadotrophin secretion by the gonadotrophin-releasing hormone agonist, buserelin, on sex steroid secretion and ovarian morphology in polycystic ovary syndrome. *J Endocrinol* (1990) **125**: 317–25.

53 De Ziegler D, Steingold K, Cedars M et al. Recovery of hormone secretion after chronic gonadotrophin-releasing hormone agonist administration in women with polycystic ovarian disease. *J Clin Endocrinol Metab* (1989) **68**: 1111–17.

54 Filicori M, Flamigni C, Campaniello E et al. Polycystic ovary syndrome: abnormalities and management with pulsatile gonadotropin-releasing hormone and gonadotropin-releasing hormone analogs. *Am J Gynecol* (1990) **163**: 1737–42.

55 Filicori M, Campaniello E, Michelacci L et al. Gonadotrophin-releasing hormone (GnRH) analog suppression renders polycystic ovarian disease patients more susceptible to ovulation induction with pulsatile GnRH. *J Clin Endocrinol Metab* (1988) **66**: 327–33.

56 Filicori M, Flamigni C, Campaniello E et al. The abnormal response of polycystic ovarian disease patients to exogenous pulsatile gonadotrophin-releasing hormone: characterization and

management. *J Clin Endocrinol Metab* (1989) **69**: 825–31.

57 Filicori M, Flamigni C, Merrigiola C et al. Endocrine response determines the clinical outcome of pulsatile gonadotropin releasing hormone ovulation induction in different ovulatory disorders. *J Clin Endocrinol Metab* (1991) **72**: 965–72.

58 Filicori M, Flamigni C, Dellai P et al. Treatment of anovulation with pulsatile gonadotropin-releasing hormone: prognostic factors and clinical results in 600 cycles. *J Clin Endocrinol Metab* (1994) **79**(4): 1215–20.

59 Surrey ES, De Ziegler D, Lu JKH, Chang RJ, Judd HL. Effects of gonadotropin-releasing hormone (GnRH) agonist on pituitary and ovarian responses to pulsatile GnRH therapy in polycystic ovarian disease. *Fertil Steril* (1989) **52**: 547–52.

60 Scheele F, Hompes PGA, van der Meer M, Schoute E, Schoemaker J. Pulsatile gonadotrophin-releasing hormone stimulation after medium term pituitary suppression in polycystic ovary syndrome. *Hum Reprod* (1993) **8**(suppl. 2): 197–9.

61 Balen AH, Tan SL, MacDougall J, Jacobs HS. Miscarriage rates following in-vitro fertilization are increased in women with polycystic ovaries and reduced by pituitary desensitization with buserelin. *Hum Reprod* (1993) **8**: 959–64.

62 Shoham Z, Jacobs HS, Insler V. Luteinizing hormone, its role, mechanism of action, and detrimental effects when hypersecreted during the follicular phase. *Fertil Steril* (1993) **59**: 1153–61.

63 Howles CM, Macnamee MC, Edwards RG. Follicular development and early luteal function of conception and non-conception cycles after human in-vitro fertilization: endocrine correlates. *Hum Reprod* (1987) **2**: 17–21.

64 Shoham Z, Borenstein R, Lunenfeld B, Pariente C. Hormonal profiles following clomiphene citrate therapy in conception and nonconception cycles. *Clin Endocrinol (Oxf)* (1990) **33**: 271–8.

65 Regan L, Owen EJ, Jacobs HS. Hypersecretion of luteinising hormone, infertility and miscarriage. *Lancet* (1990) **336**: 1141–4.

66 Ashkenazi J, Farhi J, Orvieto R et al. Polycystic ovary syndrome patients as oocyte donors: the effect of ovarian stimulation protocol on the implantation rate of the recipient. *Fertil Steril* (1995) **64**(3): 564–7.

67 McClure N, McDonald J, Kovacs GT et al. Age and follicular phase estradiol are better predictors of pregnancy outcome than luteinizing hormone in menotropin ovulation induction for anovulatory polycystic ovarian syndrome. *Fertil Steril* (1993) **59**: 729–33.

68 Quenby SM, Farquharson RG. Predicting recurrent miscarriage: what is important? *Obst Gynec* (1993) **82**: 132–8.

69 Tulppala M, Stenman UH, Cacciatore B, Ylikorkala O. Polycystic ovaries and levels of gonadotrophins and androgens in recurrent miscarriage: prospective study in 50 women. *Br J Obstet Gynaecol* (1993) **100**: 348–52.

70 Forman RG, Frydman R, Egan D. Severe ovarian hyperstimulation syndrome using agonists of gonadotropin-releasing hormone for in-vitro fertilization: a European series and proposal for prevention. *Fertil Steril* (1990) **53**: 502–9.

71 Wada I, Matson PC, Troup SA. The ovarian hyperstimulation syndrome in GnRH-agonist/HMG stimulated cycles for IVF or GIFT. *J Obstet Gynaecol* (1990) **11**: 88.

72 Dourron NE, Williams DB. Prevention and treatment of ovarian hyperstimulation syndrome. *Semin Reprod Endocrinol* (1996) **14**(4): 355–65.

73 Van der Meer M, Hompes PGA, Scheele F, Schoute E, Popp-Snijders C, Schoemaker J. The importance of endogenous feedback for monofollicular growth in low-dose step-up ovulation induction with follicle-stimulating hormone in polycystic ovary syndrome, a randomized study. *Fertil Steril* (1996) **66**(4): 571–6.

74 Itskovitz J, Boldes R, Barlev A. The induction of LH surge and oocyte maturation by GnRH analogue (buserelin) in women undergoing ovarian stimulation for in-vitro fertilization. *Gynecol Endocrinol* (1988) **2**: 165.

75 Balasch J, Tur R, Creus M et al. Triggering of ovulation by a gonadotropin releasing hormone agonist in gonadotropin-stimulated cycles for prevention of ovarian hyperstimulation syndrome and multiple pregnancies. *Gynecol Endocrinol* (1994) **8**: 7–12.

76 Lewit N, Kol S, Manor D, Itskovitz-Eldor J. The use of GnRH analogs for induction of the preovulatory gonadotropin surge in assisted reproduction and prevention of the ovarian hyperstimulating syndrome. *Gynecol Endocrinol* (1995) **4**: 13–17.

77 Jirecek S, Nagele F, Huber JC, Wenzl R. Ovarian hyperstimulation syndrome caused by GnRH-analogue treatment without gonadotropin therapy in a patient with polycystic ovarian syndrome. *Acta Obstet Gynecol Scand* (1998) **77**(9): 940–1.

78 Kol S, Lewit N, Itskovitz-Eldor J. Ovarian hyper-stimulation: effects of GnRH analogues. *Hum Reprod* (1996) **6**: 1143–4.

79 Casper RF. Does triggering ovulation with gonadotrophin-releasing hormone analogue prevent severe ovarian hyperstimulation syndrome? *Hum Reprod* (1996) **6**: 1144–6.

80 Ben-Arie A, Weissman A, Shoham Z. Triggering the final stage of ovulation using gonadotrophin-releasing hormone analogues: effective dose, prevention of ovarian hyperstimulation syndrome and the luteal phase. *Hum Reprod* (1996) **6**: 1146–8.

81 Kaltsas T, Pontikides N, Krassas GE, Seferiadis K, Lolis D, Messinis IE. Effect of gonadotrophin-releasing hormone agonist treatment on growth hormone secretion in women with polycystic ovarian syndrome. *Hum Reprod* (1998) **13**(1): 22–6.

82 Homburg R, Levy T, Ben Rafael Z. Adjuvant growth hormone for induction of ovulation with gonadotrophin-releasing hormone agonist and gonadotrophins in polycystic ovary syndrome: a randomized, double-blind, placebo controlled trial. *Hum Reprod* (1995) **10**: 2550–3.

83 Elkind-Hirsch KE, Anania C, Mack M, Malinak R. Combination gonadotropin-releasing hormone agonist and oral contraceptive therapy improves treatment of hirsute women with ovarian hyperandrogenism. *Fertil Steril* (1995) **63**(5): 970–8.

84 Taskin O, Yalcinoglu AJ, Kafkasli A, Burak F, Ozekici U. Comparison of the effects of ovarian cauterization and gonadotropin releasing hormone agonist and oral contraceptive therapy combination on endocrine changes in women with polycystic ovary disease. *Fertil Steril* (1996) **65**(6): 1115–18.

85 Genazzani AD, Petraglia F, Battaglia C, Gamba O, Volpe A, Genazzani AR. A long-term treatment with gonadotropin-releasing hormone agonist plus low-dose oral contraceptive improves the recovery of the ovulatory function in patients with polycystic ovary syndrome. *Fertil Steril* (1997) **67**(3): 463–8.

86 Damario MA, Barmat L, Liu HC, Davis OK, Rosenwaks Z. Dual suppression with oral contraceptives and gonadotrophin releasing-hormone agonists improves in-vitro fertilization outcome in high responder patients. *Hum Reprod* (1997) **12**(11): 2359–65.

14

Treatment with GnRH antagonists

Peter Platteau, Vera Haitsma and Paul Devroey

Polycystic ovary syndrome (PCOS) is the most common cause of anovulatory infertility.[1] The disorder has been attributed to primary abnormalities in the ovaries,[2] the adrenal glands,[3] and to abnormal gonadotrophin secretion.[4]

It is generally accepted that detection by ultrasound scan of polycystic ovaries provides the unifying diagnostic criterion.[5] Additional symptoms and biochemical disturbances may occur together or separately in conjunction with the finding of polycystic ovaries by ultrasound. Treatment options for PCOS are as heterogeneous as the disorder itself and depend on the initial complaint of the patient, such as cycle abnormalities, hirsutism, infertility or recurrent abortions. For the management of the patient with PCOS, many authors emphasize the hypersecretion of luteinizing hormone (LH). Though not a constant finding, hypersecretion of LH is considered a sensitive marker for PCOS and is particularly associated with menstrual disturbances and infertility. Until recently, gonadotrophin releasing hormone (GnRH) agonists have been used to suppress LH secretion in PCOS patients. With the clinical availability of potent GnRH antagonists, a new therapeutic approach to correct LH hypersecre-

tion is possible. The potential advantages of a treatment with GnRH antagonists over the current treatment with GnRH agonists are discussed in this chapter.

GONADOTROPHIN-RELEASING HORMONE ANTAGONISTS

Gonadotrophin releasing hormone regulates the secretion of follicle-stimulating hormone (FSH) and LH from the pituitary gland. It is synthesized and released in a pulsatile manner by hypothalamic neurons and acts on the GnRH receptors of the pituitary gland via the hypothalamic–hypophyseal portal system.

Gonadotrophin releasing hormone is a decapeptide, has a half-life of 2–5 minutes and undergoes rapid degradation at position 6 by peptidases. This ensures its pulsatile character as recognized by the pituitary receptors. Pulsatility is important as continuous release results eventually in a decrease in LH and FSH secretion.[6]

The hormone was isolated and its amino acid sequence determined in 1971.[7] More than 10 years later, GnRH agonists were discovered, involving the replacement of two amino acids at positions 6 and 10. These agonists have a higher binding affinity and are more stable. Agonists were initially designed to stimulate gonadotrophin secretion, but after continuous use, LH/FSH secretion becomes paradoxically suppressed. After the initial stimulatory (flare-up) effect, agonists cause desensitization of the gonadotrophic cells and a reduction in the number of GnRH receptors (downregulation), which results in suppression of the gonadotrophins. It is therefore essential to emphasize that the suppressive effect of GnRH agonists is always preceded by a stimulatory phase, which is undesirable in most clinical indications.

The GnRH antagonists were synthesized in parallel with the development of the agonists. They are GnRH-like decapeptides, which have amino acid substitutions at positions 1, 2, 3, 6 and 10. The GnRH antagonist binds to the pituitary GnRH receptor without any intrinsic activity, competing successfully against endogenous GnRH molecules for receptor occupancy and resulting in a rapid decrease in serum levels of LH, FSH and free α-subunit (FAS).[8,9] Therefore, unlike the GnRH agonists, GnRH antagonists do not induce a flare-up effect but cause an immediate decline of gonadotrophin secretion, which is easily reversible as it is dose-dependent.

The clinical development of GnRH antagonists has lagged behind that of GnRH agonists because of allergic reactions due to histamine release from mast cells with GnRH receptors.[10] The modern antagonists, the so-called third generation, are more potent, have a longer duration of action, and no systemic and only minor local side effects. Two GnRH antagonists, Cetrorelix (ASTA-Medica, Frankfurt am Main, Germany) and Ganirelix (Organon, Oss, Netherlands), are now available for clinical use. Both induce immediate and transient hypogonadism by suppressing LH and FSH secretion. They have been used successfully in spontaneous and stimulated cycles to prevent the occurrence of a spontaneous LH surge.[11,12]

The GnRH antagonists have some advantages over GnRH agonists: (1) antagonists act by the mechanism of competitive receptor binding which makes it possible to modulate the degree of hormone suppression by the dose administered; (2) they have no intrinsic activity thus avoiding a flare-up effect; and (3) in the absence of receptor downregulation gonadal function will resume almost immediately after cessation of the treatment with the antagonist; following treatment with agonists normal function may be delayed for up to 6 weeks.

TREATMENT WITH GnRH ANTAGONISTS IN PCOS

Induction of ovulation

About 25% of patients with PCOS will not respond to ovulation induction with clomiphene citrate. Treatment with exogenous gonadotrophins in conventional doses and protocols has produced poor results: a low overall pregnancy rate with a high rate of ovarian hyperstimulation syndrome (OHSS), multiple pregnancies and miscarriages.[13] An important difference from patients with hypogonadotrophic hypogonadism (World Health Organization type I anovulation), who respond strikingly better to gonadotrophin therapy, is that PCOS patients have their own endogenous gonadotrophin secretion, which is thought to contribute to the high sensitivity of the ovaries. The higher LH serum levels are thought to be responsible for the low pregnancy rates and high prevalence of miscarriage in PCOS patients.

The use of GnRH analogues to suppress serum LH concentrations remains disputable; there is a favourable effect from the adjuvant use of GnRH agonists on the pregnancy rate per cycle,[14] but the higher number of follicles during stimulation is an adverse effect. Whether GnRH antagonists used in combination with gonadotrophins in ovulation induction give better results with respect to monofollicular growth and pregnancy rate in PCOS patients has not yet been studied. Hypothetically, GnRH antagonists have some advantages over agonists. Since the antagonist suppresses LH immediately, it can be administered in the late follicular phase when the LH peak is expected. Low-dose FSH treatment is able to induce monofollicular growth by administering FSH just above the threshold dose,[15] and only after the dominant follicle has emerged will the antagonist be administered. This regimen is therefore likely to reduce the risk of OHSS and multiple pregnancy. It is difficult to predict whether GnRH antagonists will have a positive effect on the pregnancy rate or will reduce the miscarriage rate (see below).

Another therapeutic approach to ovulation induction is to induce a hypogonadotrophic state followed by pulsatile GnRH therapy. Studies of PCOS patients combining a GnRH agonist with pulsatile GnRH therapy have yielded conflicting results.[16,17] Indeed, GnRH agonists induce downregulation of the GnRH receptors, which reduces the action of pulsatile GnRH administration.

With the use of GnRH antagonists, which do not induce downregulation of the receptors, the pituitary gland remains responsive to exogenous GnRH pulses in animal models despite profound inhibition of endogenous gonadotrophin secretion.[18,19] However, co-administration of a GnRH antagonist and pulsatile GnRH therapy in two PCOS patients resistant to clomiphene citrate failed to induce follicular growth despite restoration of the LH secretion pattern.[20] These results are in contrast with the good results for pulsatile GnRH therapy in hypothalamic amenorrhoea. This may be attributed to an intraovarian factor or defect in PCOS patients.

Superovulation for IVF

In vitro fertilization (IVF) and embryo transfer (ET) have proved to be an effective therapy for PCOS patients who are refractory to ovulation induction or who have coexisting infertility factors.[21-23] The use of GnRH agonists has been firmly established as a useful adjunct in controlled ovarian hyperstimulation (COHS) protocols. Administration of GnRH antagonists in the late follicular phase has recently been applied effectively in IVF programmes to prevent a premature rise in endogenous LH and subsequent luteinization instead of extended administration of GnRH agonists.[11,24-29] The feasibility of using GnRH antagonists in PCOS patients now opens new perspectives. The occurrence of ovarian hyperstimulation syndrome is a frequent complication in these patients.[30] Its incidence in severe form is higher in patients downregulated with GnRH agonists than in those treated with human menopausal gonadotrophins (hMG) alone.[31] This observation can be explained by the rapid increase in oestradiol levels in the combined treatment schedule, as a result of the fast, synchronous development of multiple follicles. There are at least two reasons why GnRH antagonists might be more beneficial in COHS for PCOS patients: a reduced use of gonadotrophins and the potential to use the GnRH agonist instead of human chorionic gonadotrophin (hCG) for triggering ovulation.

The GnRH antagonists have the advantage that they do not need to be administered until the midfollicular phase, so that follicular recruitment can take place under low-dose step-up FSH treatment without downregulation, which reduces the number of follicles developing and the oestradiol level.[29] Lower steroid levels in the luteal phase diminish considerably the risk of OHSS.[32]

During COHS cycles, ovulation is generally induced by the administration of hCG. In spite of its close similarity to LH, hCG does not induce identical physiological reactions, since it has a longer half-life; it therefore leads to the development of multiple corpora lutea and a sustained luteotrophic effect, which are thought to contribute to the pathogenesis of OHSS.[33] Successful attempts have been made to trigger ovulation by a single administration of a GnRH agonist, using the flare-up effect to induce an endogenous surge of LH and FSH, which may reduce the risk of OHSS.[34,35] This can be done only when the preceding ovarian stimulation is carried out without suppression by GnRH agonists. Since GnRH antagonists preserve pituitary responsiveness in ovarian superovulation, GnRH agonists can be used for induction of ovulation. The use of GnRH antagonists could even offer the possibility of other options for inducing ovulation such as native GnRH or recombinant LH.

Although a small study seems to confirm these beneficial effects of GnRH antagonists,[36] properly controlled, randomized studies are urgently required to confirm these preliminary observations. The right dosage and time of administration of the antagonist in COHS for PCOS patients are also still a matter of debate.

Treatment of hirsutism

Hirsutism in patients with PCOS is caused by adrenal and ovarian hyperandrogenism. Administration of GnRH agonists for at least 6 weeks is known to suppress circulating testosterone and androstenedione in PCOS patients, resulting in a decrease in hirsutism.[37–40] Treatment with GnRH agonists for several months leads to concern about mineral bone loss and causes subjective symptoms such as hot flushes and vaginal dryness as a result of the hypo-oestrogenic state. Hormone replacement therapy should be added to the treatment.[41,42]

Moreover, it appears that GnRH agonist therapy is not able to alter the primary change in PCOS patients, whether it is at the ovarian, pituitary or hypothalamic level.[43] After cessation of treatment plasma androgen levels rise virtually immediately, despite a normal pattern of gonadotrophin release and a normal LH/FSH ratio over the first 4 weeks.[44] Using a GnRH antagonist for this indication would, again, have the advantage of immediately suppressing LH. In addition, a normal LH/FSH ratio can be established, since LH is suppressed more than FSH. Another possible advantage over GnRH agonists is that the extent of inhibition of the antagonist can be triggered via its dosage. This allows the physician to retain defined oestradiol levels and to avoid side effects such as mineral bone loss and hot flushes.[45]

Reducing miscarriage rate

Patients with PCOS have an increased risk of early spontaneous abortion.[46] Several studies have indicated that high concentrations of LH may be responsible for the high miscarriage rate.[47,48] This endocrinological feature results in reduced conception rates and increased rates of miscarriage in both natural and assisted conceptions.[49] Serum concentrations are higher, particularly during the follicular phase, in women with polycystic ovaries who suffer an early pregnancy loss than in those with an ongoing pregnancy.[50] Regan et al found that a serum LH concentration above 10 IU/l on day 8 of a regular menstrual cycle was associated with a significant impairment of fertility and an increase in the rate of miscarriage to 65% in this group.[47]

A possible therapeutic approach to this problem is the suppression of serum LH in the follicular phase. Indeed, pituitary suppression before ovulation induction significantly reduces the risk of spontaneous abortion in women with PCOS.[48] Similarly, Homburg et al demonstrated that co-treatment with GnRH agonists in hMG cycles reduces the miscarriage rate in a large group of PCOS patients undergoing ovulation induction or IVF.[51] However, Clifford et al found no improvement in conception or live birth rates in a randomized, controlled trial of LH suppression in ovulatory women with recurrent miscarriage and LH hypersecretion,[52] and suggested that LH might be a downstream marker of some other endocrinopathy associated with PCOS.

Future studies must investigate the use of GnRH antagonists in this context. When a high preovulation LH serum level is diagnosed, a single dosage of the antagonist in the midfollicular phase of the menstrual cycle is possibly enough to counteract the deleterious effect of LH on conception and pregnancy. On the other hand, Homburg et al put forward the theory that protection of oocytes by suppression of the high concentrations of endogenous LH will prevent early pregnancy loss. For this reason, a longer period of LH suppression might be necessary during ovulation induction in PCOS patients.[53]

CONCLUSION

The development of GnRH antagonists has been a long process owing to the unwanted histamine side effects. The third-generation GnRH antagonists Cetrorelix and Ganirelix are new drugs that have proved their safety and efficacy in IVF protocols with selected patients. They are easier, safer and theoretically more advantageous to use than GnRH agonists in PCOS patients, owing to their different pharmacodynamics. However, because of limited experience with these new drugs a careful attitude should be adopted.

REFERENCES

1 Hull MGR. Epidemiology of infertility and polycystic ovarian disease: endocrinological and demographic studies. *Gynecol Endocrinol* (1987) **1**: 235–45.

2 Jacobs HS. Polycystic ovaries and polycystic ovary syndrome. *Gynecol Endocrinol* (1978) **1**: 113–31.

3 Oake RJ, Davies SJ, MacLachlan MS, Thomas JP. Plasma testosterone in adrenal and ovarian vein blood of hirsute women. *Quart J Med* (1974) **43**: 603–13.

4 McArthur JW, Ingersall FM, Worcester J. The urinary excretion of interstitial cell and follicle-stimulating hormone activity by women with disease of the reproductive system. *J Clin Endocrinol* (1985) **18**: 1202–15.

5 Ardaens Y, Robert Y, Lemaitre L, Fossati P, Dewailly D. Polycystic ovarian disease: contribution of vaginal endosonography and reassessment of ultrasonic diagnosis. *Fertil Steril* (1991) **55**: 1062–8.

6 Conn PM. The molecular mechanism of gonadotropin-releasing hormone action in the pituitary. In: Knobil E, Neill JD, eds, *The Physiology of Reproduction*, 2nd edn (Raven Press: New York, 1994) 1815–32.

7 Schally AV, Arimura A, Baba Y. Isolation and properties of the FSH and LH-releasing hormone. *Biochem Biophys Res Commun* (1971) **43**: 393–9.

8 Leal JA, Williams RG, Danforth DR, Gordon K, Hodgen GD. Prolonged duration of gonadotropin inhibition by a third generation GnRH antagonist. *J Clin Endocrinol Metab* (1988) **67**: 1325–7.

9 Hall JE, Whitcomb RW, Rivier JE, Vale WW, Crowley WF. Differential regulation of luteinizing hormone, follicle stimulating hormone, and free a-subunit secretion from the gonadotrope by gonadotropin-releasing hormone (GnRH): evidence from the use of two GnRH antagonists. *J Clin Endocrinol Metab* (1990) **70**: 328–35.

10 Morgan JE, O'Neil CE, Coy DH, Hocart SJ, Nekola MV. Antagonistic analogs of luteinizing hormone-releasing hormone are mast cell secretagogues. *Int Arch Allerg Appl Immunol* (1986) **80**: 70–5.

11 Albano C, Smitz J, Camus M, Riethmuller-Winzen H, Van Steirteghem A, Devroey P. Comparison of different doses of gonadotrophin-releasing hormone antagonist cetrorelix during controlled ovarian hyperstimulation. *Fertil Steril* (1997) **67**: 917–22.

12 Felberbaum R, Diedrich K. Ovarian stimulation for in-vitro fertilization/intracytoplasmic sperm injection with gonadotrophins and gonadotrophin-releasing hormone analogues: agonists and antagonists. *Hum Reprod* (1999) **14**(suppl. 1): 207–21.

13 Wang CF, Gemzell C. The use of human gonadotrophins for the induction of ovulation in women with polycystic ovarian disease. *Fertil Steril* (1980) **33**: 479–86.

14 Scoot DC, Pijlman B, Stijnen T, Fauser BCJM. Effects of gonadotrophin releasing hormone agonist addition to gonadotrophin induction of ovulation in polycystic ovary syndrome patients. *Eur J Obstet Gynecol Reprod Biol* (1992) **45**: 53–8.

15 Hamilton-Fairley D, Kiddy D, Watson H, Sagle M, Franks S. Low dose gonadotrophin therapy for induction of ovulation in 100 women with polycystic ovary syndrome. *Hum Reprod* (1991) **6**: 1095–9.

16 Filicori M, Flamigni C, Campaniello E et al. The abnormal response of polycystic ovarian disease patients to exogenous pulsatile gonadotropin-releasing hormone: characterization and management. *J Clin Endocrinol Metab* (1989) **69**: 825–31.

17 Surrey ES, De Ziegler D, Lu JKH, Chang RJ, Judd HL. Effects of gonadotropin-releasing hormone agonist on pituitary and ovarian responses to pulsatile GnRH therapy in polycystic ovarian disease. *Fertil Steril* (1989) **52**: 547–52.

18 Chillik CF, Itskovitz J, Hahn DW, McGuire JL, Danforth DR, Hodgen GD. Characterizing pituitary response to a gonadotropin releasing hormone (GnRH) antagonist in monkeys: tonic

follicle-stimulating hormone/luteinizing hormone secretion versus acute GnRH challenge tests before, during, and after treatment. *Fertil Steril* (1987) **48**: 480–5.

19 Lahlou N, Delivet S, Bardin CW, Roger M, Spitz IM, Bouchard O. Changes in gonadotropin and alpha-subunit secretion after a single administration of gonadotropin-releasing hormone antagonist in adult males. *Fertil Steril* (1990) **53**: 898–905.

20 Dubourdieu S, Le Nestour E, Spitz IM, Charbonnel B, Bouchard P. The combination of gonadotrophin-releasing hormone (GnRH) antagonist and pulsatile GnRH normalizes luteinizing hormone secretion in polycystic ovarian disease but fails to induce follicular maturation. *Hum Reprod* (1993) **8**: 2056–60.

21 Homburg R, Berkowitz D, Levy T, Feldberg D, Ashkenazi J, Ben-Rafael Z. In vitro fertilization and embryo transfer for the treatment of infertility associated with polycystic ovary syndrome. *Fertil Steril* (1993) **60**: 858–63.

22 Dor J, Shulman A, Levran D, Ben-Rafael Z, Rudak E, Mashiach S. The treatment of patients with polycystic ovary syndrome by in-vitro fertilization and embryo transfer: a comparison of results with those patients with tubal infertility. *Hum Reprod* (1990) **5**: 816–18.

23 MacDougall MJ, Tan SL, Balen A, Jacobs HS. A controlled study comparing patients with and without polycystic ovaries undergoing in-vitro fertilization. *Hum Reprod* (1993) **2**: 233–7.

24 Diedrich K, Diedrich C, Santos E et al. Suppression of the endogenous LH-surge by the GnRH-antagonist Cetrorelix during ovarian stimulation. *Hum Reprod* (1994) **9**: 788–91.

25 Olivennes F, Fanchin R, Bouchard P, Taieb J, Selva J, Frydman R. Scheduled administration of a gonadotrophin-releasing hormone antagonist (Cetrorelix) on day 8 of in-vitro fertilization cycles: a pilot study. *Hum Reprod* (1995) **10**: 1382–6.

26 Albano C, Smitz J, Camus M et al. Hormonal profile during the follicular phase in cycles stimulated with a combination of human menopausal gonadotropin and gonadotropin-releasing hormone. *Hum Reprod* (1996) **11**: 2114–18.

27 Felberbaum R, Reissmann T, Kupker W et al. Hormone profiles under ovarian stimulation with human menopausal gonadotropin (hMG) and concomitant administration of the gonadotropin releasing hormone (GnRH)-antag-onist cetrorelix at different dosages. *J Assist Reprod Genet* (1996) **13**: 216–22.

28 Rongières-Bertrand C, Olivennes F, Righini C et al. Revival of the natural cycles in in-vitro fertilization with the use of a new gonadotrophin-releasing hormone antagonist (Cetrorelix): a pilot study with minimal stimulation. *Hum Reprod* (1999) **3**: 683–8.

29 Albano C, Felberbaum RE, Smitz J et al, on behalf of the European Cetrorelix study group. Ovarian stimulation with HMG: results of a prospective randomised phase III European study comparing the luteinizing hormone-releasing hormone (LHRH)-antagonist cetrorelix and the LHRH-agonist buserelin. *Hum Reprod* (2000) **15**: 526–31.

30 MacDougall MJ, Tan SL, Jacobs HS. In-vitro fertilization and the ovarian hyperstimulation syndrome. *Hum Reprod* (1992) **7**: 597–600.

31 Smitz J, Camus M, Devroey P, Erard P, Wisanto A, Van Steirteghem AC. Incidence of severe ovarian hyperstimulation syndrome after GnRH-agonist/HMG superovulation for in-vitro fertilization. *Hum Reprod* (1990) **5**: 933–7.

32 Scott RT, Neal GS, Bailey SA, Hofmann GE, Kost ER, Illions EH. Comparison of leuprolide acetate and human chorionic gonadotropin for the induction of ovulation in clomiphene citrate-stimulated cycles. *Fertil Steril* (1994) **61**: 872–9.

33 Itskovitz J, Boldes R, Levron J, Erlik Y, Kahana L, Brandes JM. Induction of preovulatory luteinizing hormone surge and prevention of ovarian hyperstimulation syndrome by gonadotropin-releasing hormone agonist. *Fertil Steril* (1991) **56**: 213–20.

34 Shalev E, Geslevich Y, Ben-Ami M. Induction of pre-ovulatory luteinizing hormone surge by gonadotrophin-releasing hormone agonists for women at risk for ovarian hyperstimulation syndrome. *Hum Reprod* (1994) **9**: 417–19.

35 Olivennes F, Fanchin R, Bouchard P, Taieb J, Frydman R. Triggering of ovulation by a gonadotropin-releasing hormone (GnRH) agonist in patients pretreated with a GnRH antagonist. *Fertil Steril* (1996) **66**: 151–3.

36 Craft I, Gorgy A, Hill J, Menon D, Podsiadly B. Will GnRH antagonists provide new hope for patients considered 'difficult responders' to GnRH agonist protocols? *Hum Reprod* (1999) **12**: 2959–62.

37 Cedars MI, Steingold KA, de Ziegler D, Lapolt PS, Chang RJ, Judd HL. Long-term administration of gonadotropin-releasing hormone agonist

and dexamethasone: assessment of the adrenal role in ovarian dysfunction. *Fertil Steril* (1992) **57**: 495–500.

38 Chang RJ, Laufer LR, Meldrum DR et al. Steroid secretion in polycystic ovarian disease after ovarian suppression by a long-acting gonadotropin-releasing hormone agonist. *J Clin Endocrinol Metab* (1983) **56**: 897–903.

39 Couzinet B, Le Strat N, Brailly S, Schaison G. Comparative effects of cyproterone acetate or a long-acting gonadotropin-releasing hormone agonist in polycystic ovarian disease. *J Clin Endocrinol Metab* (1986) **63**: 1031–5.

40 Andreiko JL, Monroe SE, Jaffe RB. Treatment of hirsutism with a gonadotropin-releasing hormone agonist (nafarelin). *J Clin Endocrinol Metab* (1986) **63**: 854–9.

41 Falsetti L, Pasinetti E. Treatment of moderate and severe hirsutism by gonadotropin-releasing hormone agonists in women with polycystic ovary syndrome and idiopathic hirsutism. *Fertil Steril* (1994) **61**: 817–22.

42 Coitta L, Cianci A, Giuffrida G, Marletta E, Agliano A, Palumbo G. Clinical and hormonal effects of gonadotropin-releasing hormone agonist plus an oral contraceptive in severely hirsute patients with polycystic ovary disease. *Fertil Steril* (1996) **65**: 61–7.

43 Williams IA, Shaw RW, Burford G. An attempt to alter pathophysiology of polycystic ovarian syndrome using a gonadotrophin hormone releasing hormone agonist – nafarelin. *Clin Endocrinol* (1989) **31**: 345–53.

44 Macleod AF, Wheeler MJ, Gordon P, Sonkson PH, Conaglen JV. Effect of long-term inhibition of gonadotrophin secretion by the gonadotrophin-releasing hormone agonist, buserelin, on sex steroid secretion and ovarian morphology in polycystic ovary syndrome. *J Endocrinol* (1990) **125**: 317–25.

45 Reissman T, Felderbaum R, Diedrich K, Engel J, Comaru-Scally AM, Schally AV. Development and applications of luteinizing hormone antagonists in the treatment of infertility: an overview. *Hum Reprod* (1995) **10**: 1974–81.

46 Yen SSC. The polycystic ovary syndrome. *Clin Endocrinol* (1980) **12**: 177–208.

47 Regan L, Owen EJ, Jacobs HS. Hypersecretion of luteinising hormone, infertility and miscarriage. *Lancet* (1990) **336**: 1141–4.

48 Johnson P, Pearce MJ. Recurrent spontaneous abortions and polycystic ovarian disease: comparison of two regimens to induce ovulation. *Br Med J* (1990) **300**: 154–6.

49 Balen AH, Conway GS, Kaltsas G et al. Polycystic ovary syndrome: the spectrum of the disorder in 1741 patients. *Hum Reprod* (1995) **10**: 2107–11.

50 Homburg R, Armar NA, Eshel A, Adams J, Jacobs HS. Influence of serum luteinising hormone concentrations on ovulation, conception and early pregnancy loss in polycystic ovary syndrome. *Br Med J* (1988) **297**: 1024–6.

51 Homburg R, Levy T, Berkovitz D et al. Gonadotropin-releasing hormone agonist reduces the miscarriage rate for pregnancies achieved in women with polycystic ovarian syndrome. *Fertil Steril* (1993) **59**: 527–31.

52 Clifford K, Rai R, Watson H, Franks S, Regan L. Does suppressing luteinising hormone secretion reduce the miscarriage rate? Results of a randomised controlled trial. *Br Med J* (1996) **312**: 1508–11.

53 Homburg R, Eshel A, Kilborn J, Adams J, Jacobs HS. Combined luteinizing hormone analogue and exogenous gonadotrophins for the treatment of infertility associated with polycystic ovaries. *Hum Reprod* (1990) **5**: 32–5.

15

Laparoscopic ovarian puncture

Howard S Jacobs

Although the classic procedure of bilateral wedge resection of the ovaries was abandoned long ago because of problems associated with postoperative adhesions, the operation was in fact remarkably efficacious in terms of inducing ovulation. The development of less traumatic procedures performed through the laparoscope has therefore been a welcome addition to our therapeutic repertoire. Although the very patients most resistant to endocrine methods of induction of ovulation – the obese – are those least likely to be selected for surgical treatment, an operative approach has certain theoretical advantages over endocrine therapy. This is particularly the case with regard to the intrinsic and most serious problems of ovarian stimulation therapy, namely multiple pregnancy and ovarian hyperstimulation syndrome (OHSS). Ovarian hyperstimulation is particularly common in women with polycystic ovary syndrome, whether they are undergoing treatment with fertility drugs or by in vitro fertilization. A serious condition which may threaten the patient's life, OHSS pales in significance when compared with the problems of multiple pregnancy. Quite apart from the extraordinary increase in perinatal mortality, the physical,

psychological and social morbidity of multiple pregnancy can be appalling. Multiple pregnancy is not a feature of the outcome of treatment by ovarian diathermy. In my opinion that single observation should feature very highly in any evaluation of the procedure.

BILATERAL WEDGE RESECTION OF THE OVARIES

In their classic paper Stein and Leventhal described resection of half to three-quarters of both of the enlarged ovaries of seven patients with what we now recognize to be the polycystic ovary syndrome.[1] The women resumed regular menstrual cycles and at the time of the report two of them had conceived three pregnancies. Subsequent attempts to summarize the prodigious quantities of literature reporting the outcome of this form of surgical therapy have been bedevilled by different criteria for diagnosis of the polycystic ovary syndrome, different indications for operations which themselves have varied, different periods and intensity of follow-up, and an almost universal description of crude pregnancy rates rather than of cumulative rates based on life-table analysis. Acknowledging these limitations, Donesky and Adashi assembled information on outcome in 1766 patients whose results were published between 1935 and 1983: there was an overall pregnancy rate of 58.8%, with results ranging from Stein's high of 86.7% to a low of 25%.[2] Stein, who had stringent selection criteria for surgery, considered the restoration of fertility permanent.[3]

In terms of induction of ovulation, ovarian wedge resection is clearly efficacious. The problem is that postoperative periovarian adhesions frequently cause tubal infertility. In theory less severe adhesions may cause an increase in the rate of ectopic pregnancy. The use of microsurgical techniques reduces the problem of adhesions but does not apparently eliminate the risk. For these reasons, and no doubt also for reasons of cost (i.e. duration of hospital stay), the operation has fallen from use and laparoscopic methods have been developed.

ENDOSCOPIC PROCEDURES

The methods described range from multiple ovarian biopsy to remove 0.5–1 ml of tissue,[4] to electrocautery using a unipolar coagulating current[5] or puncture of the ovarian surface with a laser. With KTP and carbon dioxide lasers,[6] as with electrocautery, the ovarian cortex over follicles is vaporized; the number of punctures is however increased compared with electrocautery. With the Nd:YAG laser, coagulation rather than vaporization is the goal and a wedge of ovarian tissue is coagulated to a depth of 4–10 mm without opening the ovarian cortex.[7]

The method of ovarian electrocautery we have used was adapted from that described by Gjønnæss in 1984.[5] The following account is taken from the papers of Armar and Balen.[8,9] Laparoscopy is performed under general anaesthesia, careful inspection of the pelvic organs being followed by transcervical injection of methylene blue to establish tubal patency. About 300 ml of sodium chloride 0.9% solution is instilled through a suprapubic Verres needle

into the pouch of Douglas to enhance ovarian cooling after diathermy. Each ovary is lifted in turn on to the anterior surface of the uterus and unipolar diathermy is applied, usually for 4 seconds in four separate places (machine setting 4, i.e. 40 W). The ovary is then lowered into the pool of saline, which is left in the peritoneal cavity at the end of the procedure. A special probe, developed by Armar in collaboration with Rocket of London (Watford, UK), is used to apply the diathermy. It has a spring-loaded 8 mm central spike projecting from an insulated solid cone of 6 mm maximum diameter. The spike, which penetrates the ovarian capsule with the aid of a short burst of diathermy, prevents the probe from slipping on the surface of the ovary. The insulated cone further minimizes the risk of electrical damage outside the ovary.

There is no agreement on the optimum 'dose' of diathermy to apply. Our group has kept the dose (particularly the number of sites) low,[8,9] but we are not yet certain which amount of diathermy is most efficacious and which is most commonly associated with postoperative adhesions. The report of unilateral ovarian atrophy following the operation serves to remind us that the operation does have its hazards.[10]

OUTCOME OF OVARIAN ELECTROCAUTERY

The provisos mentioned earlier concerning measurement of the outcome of ovarian wedge resection are equally true for the endoscopic techniques. The most recent compilation of figures by Donesky and Adashi analysed 35 reports of 947 patients who had infertility treatment by various endoscopic procedures.[11] Following the operation, 82% ovulated either spontaneously or after treatment with medications to which previously they had been resistant; the mean time to first ovulation was 23 ± 6 days (SD). One or more pregnancies occurred in 561 patients (59.2%, range 20–88%). When the outcomes in 648 patients who had electrocautery were analysed, the pregnancy rate was 63.2%.

There are two main reasons why some

patients do not conceive after the operation. The first is the presence of coexistent disease such as endometriosis or pelvic adhesions. Thus in the 50 patients whose results were described by Armar and Lachelin,[12] the proportion conceiving was 86% in the presence of a laparoscopically normal pelvis at the time of the operation (22 cases), 70% when there were minor adhesions (10 cases), and 43% when endometriosis was detected (mild in 11, moderate in 3 cases). Of course, adhesions may also develop as a consequence of the operation (see below). The second reason is failure to induce ovulation. The important factors predicting a favourable ovulatory response are described below but here we note that one of the effects of the operation is to sensitize the ovaries to ovarian stimulation by gonadotrophin therapy. Thus 22 of 43 of patients who had been referred for surgery did not resume ovulatory cycles postoperatively.[13] They then underwent ovulation induction with gonadotrophins. Compared with the same protocol of ovarian stimulation that had been used before surgery, we found a significant increase in the proportion who ovulated and conceived, despite a significant reduction in the dose and duration of gonadotrophin administration (Table 15.1).

Table 15.1 Characteristics of gonadotrophin ovulation induction treatment cycles before and after laparoscopic ovarian electrocautery in patients with polycystic ovary syndrome

Characteristic	Before laparoscopic ovarian electrocautery	After laparoscopic ovarian electrocautery	*P* value
No. of gonadotrophin cycles*	74	59	
No. of ovulatory cycles†	27 (36)	46 (78)	<0.01
No. of pregnancies per total number of cycles†	3 (4.0)	14 (23.7)	<0.01
hMG			
No. of cycles	48	38	
No. of ampoules‡	23.7 ± 8.2	14.8 ± 6.9	<0.01
Daily effective dose (ampoules)‡	2.0 ± 0.8	1.2 ± 0.3	<0.05
Days of treatment per cycle (ampoules)‡	16.0 ± 4.2	10.1 ± 3.4	<0.01
Ovulations per cycle (%)	48 (23/48)	71 (27/38)	<0.05
Pregnancy rate per cycle (%)	2 (1/48)	23 (9/38)	<0.01
FSH			
No. of cycles	26	21	
No. of ampoules‡	12.5 ± 8.3	11.8 ± 6.0	NS
Daily effective dose (ampoules)‡	2.4 ± 0.5	1.1 ± 0.3	<0.01
Days of treatment per cycle‡	13.2 ± 6.2	12.0 ± 4.8	NS
Ovulations per cycle (%)	50 (13/26)	71 (15/21)	NS
Pregnancy rate per cycle (%)	7 (2/26)	23 (5/21)	NS

FSH, follicle-stimulating hormone; hMG, human menopausal gonadotrophin; NS, not significant.
* Gonadotrophin, hMG or FSH.
† Values in parentheses are percentages.
‡ Values are means ± SD.

The main endocrine changes caused by ovarian electrocautery are a fall in serum luteinizing hormone (attributed to a fall in pulse amplitude rather than frequency) and a small rise in serum follicle-stimulating hormone (FSH) concentrations.[2,10] A small fall in serum testosterone and androstenedione concentrations was noted in some studies. These results are similar to those that follow wedge resection.

Miscarriage rates have been reported in only a few of the studies but were lower than those usually observed in women with polycystic ovary syndrome following induction of ovulation. For example, the overall miscarriage rate in the 58 pregnancies reported by Armar and Lachelin was 14%,[11] compared with the 30–40% usually seen in women with polycystic ovary syndrome. The explanation is uncertain but may relate to the fall in concentration of luteinizing hormone (LH) noted above.[14]

The complications of ovarian electrocautery mainly concern the issue of postoperative adhesions. Where sought, adhesions have been detected in about 20% of cases. The problem, however, is the lack of systematic studies. Second-look laparoscopies tend to be performed only in cases in which conception is delayed. Nonetheless we must conclude that adhesions do occur, that they are usually mild, and that they are likely to be more frequent and severe the more intense the procedure.[9] It should be borne in mind, however, that adhesions are not infrequently discovered at the 'first look'.[8]

How does the operation work? An answer to this question must accommodate the ability of the procedure to induce ovulation, to reduce serum LH concentrations and to sensitize the ovaries to gonadotrophic stimulation. A tempting speculation is that the growth factor cascade that follows injury, in so far as it involves local activation of insulin-like growth factor-I,[15] sensitizes the ovaries to the small increase of FSH that has been recorded to follow surgery. Follicular development and ovulation then follow and normal ovarian–pituitary feedback is re-established. The latter then involves normal ovarian secretion of gonadotrophin surge attenuating factor, deficiency of which in women

with polycystic ovary syndrome has been hypothesized to be an important contributor to the hypersecretion of LH that characterizes this condition.[16] To investigate this hypothesis, Balen performed unilateral ovarian diathermy to determine whether local factors within the ovary were responsible for the return of ovulation.[9] The first postoperative ovulation was found to be randomly distributed between the operated and the non-operated sides, suggesting that the mechanism of action of the procedure must involve some aspect of ovarian–pituitary feedback independent of the laterality of the lesion.

BENEFITS OF OVARIAN ELECTROCAUTERY

The most striking benefit of ovarian electrocautery in women with polycystic ovary syndrome is that, in contrast to medical induction of ovulation,[17] there is no increased risk of multiple pregnancy. This one observation makes it a very attractive procedure, particularly since it also means that the need for intensive monitoring of ovulation is obviated. Since many ovulations result from a single operation, the operation is efficient as well as efficacious. Some have found the outcome so impressive that, not withstanding the complications discussed above, its use instead of gonadotrophin treatment in clomiphene-resistant patients is proposed. In my opinion decisions of this sort have to be made in the context of locally available skills and resources. The indications for its use in my clinic are detailed below.

INDICATIONS AND CONTRAINDICATIONS

The best results have been obtained in clomiphene-resistant women who are slim,[18] anovulatory and who have raised serum LH concentrations.[2] These are the features currently sought before the operation is recommended. It is not recommended for the management of hirsutism. The fall in serum LH concentrations after the operation makes it tempting to recommend the procedure for women with recurrent miscarriage and hypersecretion of LH,[19] but it must be recognized there are no published reports evaluating this approach. The operation is also recommended to women undergoing medical induction of ovulation who get a recurrent multifollicular response or who develop recurrent solitary cyst formation. Contraindications to the operation are obesity (body mass index exceeding 30 kg/m²) and infertility that cannot be accounted for by anovulation.

References

1   Stein IF, Leventhal ML. Amenorrhoea associated with bilateral polycystic ovaries. *Am J Obstet Gynecol* (1935) **29**: 181–91.

2   Donesky BW, Adashi EY. Surgically induced ovulation in the polycystic ovary syndrome: wedge resection revisited in the age of laparoscopy. *Fertil Steril* (1995) **63**: 439–63.

3   Stein IF. Ultimate results of bilateral ovarian wedge resection: twenty five years follow-up. *Int J Fertil* (1956) **1**: 333–44.

4   Neuwirth RS. A method of bilateral ovarian biopsy at laparoscopy in infertility and chronic anovulation. *Fertil Steril* (1972) **23**: 361–6.

5   Gjønnæss H. Polycystic ovary syndrome treated by electrocautery through the laparoscope. *Fertil Steril* (1984) **41**: 20–5.

6   Daniell KF, Miller W. Polycystic ovaries treated by laser vaporization. *Fertil Steril* (1989) **51**: 232–6.

7   Kojima E, Yanagibori A, Otaka K, Hirakawa S. Ovarian wedge resection with contact Nd:Yag laser irradiation used laparoscopically. *J Reprod Med* (1989) **34**: 444–6.

8   Armar NA, McGarrigle HHG, Honour JW, Holownia P, Jacobs HS, Lachelin GCL. Laparoscopic ovarian diathermy in the management of anovulatory infertility in women with polycystic ovaries: endocrine changes and clinical outcome *Fertil Steril* (1990) **53**: 45–9.

9   Balen AH, Jacobs HS. A prospective study comparing unilateral and bilateral laparoscopic ovarian diathermy in women with the polycystic ovary syndrome. *Fertil Steril* (1994) **62**: 921–5.

10   Dabirashrafi H. Complications of laparoscopic ovarian electrocautery. *Fertil Steril* (1989) **52**: 878–9.

11   Donesky BW, Adashi EY. Surgical ovulation induction: the role of ovarian diathermy in polycystic ovary syndrome. *Baillière's Clinical Endocrinology and Metabolism* (1996) **10**: 293–310.

12   Armar NA, Lachelin GCL. Laparoscopic ovarian diathermy: an effective treatment for anti-oestrogen resistant anovulatory infertility in women with the polycystic ovary syndrome. *Br J Obstet Gynaecol* (1993) **100**: 161–4.

13   Farhi J, Soule S, Jacobs HS. Effect of laparoscopic ovarian electrocautery on ovarian response and outcome of treatment with gonadotropins in clomiphene citrate-resistant patients with polycystic ovary syndrome. *Fertil Steril* (1995) **64**: 930–5.

14   Balen AH, Tan SL, Jacobs HS. Hypersecretion of luteinising hormone: a significant cause of infertility and miscarriage. *Br J Obstet Gynaecol* (1993) **100**: 1082–9.

15   Adashi EY, Resnick CE, D'Ercole AJ. Insulin-like growth factors as intraovarian regulators of granulosa cell growth and function. *Endocr Rev* (1985) **6**: 400–20.

16   Balen AH, Jacobs HS. Gonadotrophin surge attenuating factor: a missing link in the control of LH secretion? *Clin Endocrinol* (1991) **35**: 399–402.

17   Farhi J, West C, Patel A, Jacobs HS. Treatment of anovulatory infertility: the problem of multiple pregnancy. *Hum Reprod* (1996) **11**: 429–34.

18   Gjønnæss H. Ovarian electrocautery in the treatment of women with polycystic ovary syndrome (PCOS). Factors affecting results. *Acta Obstet Gynecol Scand* (1994) **73**: 1–5.

19   Regan L, Owen EJ, Jacobs HS. Hypersecretion of LH, infertility and spontaneous abortion. *Lancet* (1990) **336**: 1141–2.

16

In vitro fertilization

Juan A García-Velasco, Pilar Gaitán, José Navarro, José Remohí, Carlos Simón and Antonio Pellicer

Polycystic ovary syndrome (PCOS) is the most frequent cause of infertility in anovulatory patients and the most prevalent endocrinological condition.[1,2] Although the pathogenesis of PCOS is not completely understood, high circulating levels of luteinizing hormone (LH), chronic hyperandrogenemia, and insulin resistance with compensating hyperinsulinemia are associated with this syndrome.[3–6] There is a heterogeneous clinical spectrum, from a simple sonographic diagnosis of polycystic ovaries (PCO) with normal phenotype to a full expression of the classic Stein–Leventhal syndrome.

In spite of the different therapeutic options offered for the infertility and anovulatory status associated with PCO, there is a group of patients in whom pregnancy is not achieved in the absence of any other infertility cause.

When clomiphene citrate (CC) is used, the cumulative pregnancy rate reaches around 40–50%.[7,8] That this rate is not higher is probably due to CC resistance in 20–25% of women treated,[9] or possibly to a deleterious effect on human oocytes,[10] or a low ovarian response.[11] A hypothetical antiestrogenic effect on cervical mucus and endometrium may also contribute to the low pregnancy rate achieved with CC.

The pregnancy rate that follows the use of human gonadotropins at regular doses as treatment for ovulation induction in these patients is lower than 30%, with a high rate of multiple pregnancies (30%), and a high risk of ovarian hyperstimulation syndrome (OHSS).[12,13] Low-dose protocols based on the theory of the follicle-stimulating hormone (FSH) threshold, needed to initiate and maintain follicular growth without reaching supraphysiological levels with exogenous FSH,[14,15] reduce the multiple pregnancy rate and OHSS risk, but do not improve pregnancy rate. These protocols include the *step-up* protocol, with low starting levels of FSH that gradually increase according to the ovarian response, and the *step-down* protocol, with progressively lower doses of FSH. The *step-down* protocol imitates more closely the physiological profile of FSH, achieving shorter treatment cycles with lower peak estradiol levels.[16]

Pulsatile gonadotropin releasing hormone (GnRH) administration did not achieve the expected results, as it increased LH blood levels in amenorrheic women with PCO,[17] reaching low rates of ovulatory cycles (50%) and pregnancy rate per initiated cycle (14.6%).[18]

Surgical treatment with bilateral wedge resection, even though it restores ovulation in a high percentage of patients, may induce intraperitoneal adhesions. Laparoscopic electrocoagulation of the ovarian surface causes mild and unilateral adhesions in only 20% of the cases.[19–21] Ovulation was restored in 70–90% of the cycles after this procedure.[19,22,23] Patients who underwent in vitro fertilization (IVF) after laparoscopic electrocoagulation had better pregnancy rates than women who did not have surgery (28.6% vs 7.3%), and also showed lower serum estradiol levels, and a tendency towards a lower miscarriage rate.[20]

The different assisted reproductive techniques offer an attractive therapeutic alternative for women with PCO, obtaining similar pregnancy rates to those in patients with other infertility causes.[24] Interestingly, there are some intrinsic characteristics of these patients that may characterize their ovarian stimulation as well as the results, such as a high sensitivity to gonadotropins resulting in an increased ovarian response with extremely high estradiol levels that may compromise embryo implantation,[25,26] and a low oocyte quality.[27]

OVARIAN STIMULATION PROTOCOLS FOR IVF IN WOMEN WITH PCOS

Clomiphene citrate

Clomiphene citrate is an antiestrogen that replaces endogenous estrogens from their receptors, thus blocking the negative feedback on gonadotropin secretion.[28] As a consequence, there is a rise in FSH and LH blood levels. In control subjects; CC increases the frequency of the gonadotropin pulses more than the pulse width,[29] but in PCOS it only increases the pulse width.[30]

Different explanations are given for the limited success obtained with CC:

1. Up to 25% of the patients are CC resistant.[7,9]
2. Some authors have shown deleterious effects of CC on human oocytes, with a higher rate of chromosomic anomalies[10]

and a lower developmental potential of human embryos.[31] These effects may partially explain the higher miscarriage rate observed in patients undergoing treatment with CC.

3. A small number of embryos are obtained because a limited number of follicles are recruited.[11]

Urinary gonadotropins

Human menopausal gonadotropin (hMG), either alone or in combination with CC, was used at the beginning for ovulation induction. Dor et al compared a group of 16 PCOS patients stimulated with hMG or hMG–CC, with 37 patients with tubal infertility.[32] The PCOS patients showed a higher follicle number (19.4 versus 5.4), and a lower fertility rate (40.4% vs 67.7%) and cleavage rate (34.4% vs 65.5%) than control patients. However, a similar number of embryos and pregnancy rate per cycle was obtained (30.7% vs 29.7%). In a case–control study in 152 patients, MacDougall et al obtained similar results.[33] These investigators also described a higher multifetal pregnancy rate and a higher OHSS rate.[33] Several reports confirmed these findings, showing a tendency towards a lower fertility rate in PCOS patients (56% vs 75%) and a similar pregnancy rate (24% vs 25%), with fewer hMG ampules required.[34] Thus, a similar pregnancy rate was obtained in women with PCOS compared with other infertile couples, although a lower fertility rate was found, something that could be compensated for with a higher number of oocytes obtained in these patients.

When pure FSH was introduced, the absence of LH (a contaminant of hMG) created high expectations for this molecule. It was believed that it would increase the ovulatory cycles and the pregnancy rate, diminishing the deleterious effects of hMG. In fact, FSH alone is sufficient for granulosa cells to have aromatase activity.[35] This was a very promising hypothesis.

Since then, several reports have been published and their conclusions are shown in Table 16.1.[36–41] Experience has overcome the initial

Table 16.1 Comparison of ovulation induction outcome in women with PCO treated with FSH or hMG

Reference	N	Follicle number	Estradiol (pg/ml)	Fertilization rate (%)	Pregnancy rate (%)
Tanbo et al[37]	31	20.1 vs 19.6	1565 vs 1103	77.5 vs 77.5	23.5 vs 37.5
McFaul et al[38]	49	3.1 vs 6.1	5555 vs 6799	NA	17.6 vs 35.7
Larsen et al[39]	12	NA	NS	NA	13.3 vs 6.6
Sagle et al[40]	30	NA	1115 vs 1136	NA	33.3 vs 33.3
Seibel et al[41]	23	1.4 vs 1.2	–	NA	10 vs 30.7
Turhan et al[36]	35	10.6 vs 9.9	2265 vs 1961	63.2 vs 62.6	20.8 vs 25

NA, not applicable; NS, not significant.
First figures quoted correspond to data obtained with FSH while second figures correspond to hMG.

enthusiasm, showing that FSH does not improve ovulation rates when compared with hMG.[36–41] Even more importantly, FSH does not reduce the incidence of OHSS. When FSH was compared with hMG in women who were non-responders to clomiphene citrate, no significant differences were found in ovulation rate, days of stimulation or number of ampules required.[36,38,39,41,42]

Two reports have compared FSH with hMG in ovulation induction in PCOS patients in an IVF program.[36,42] Turhan and co-workers compared these two treatments in a prospective, randomized trial and could not show any statistically significant differences in days of stimulation, number of ampules used, number of oocytes retrieved, mature oocyte percentage, fertility rate, cleavage rate, pregnancy rate, OHSS rate or cancellation rate.[36] Similar results were obtained by Tanbo et al.[37] The only benefits obtained with FSH were a better synchronization in follicular growth and a higher oocyte maturity in PCOS patients treated with GnRH.[37]

Recombinant gonadotropins

In 1992 Germond et al[43] described for the first time a clinical pregnancy with recombinant gonadotropins and since then several reports have been published describing the usefulness of recombinant FSH (rFSH) in PCOS patients.[44,45,46,47,48,49]

Fisch et al randomized 20 IVF patients to receive either rFSH or urinary FSH; they found no significant differences in estradiol levels or in the number of oocytes retrieved, which suggested that both the synthetic and the natural compounds may be administered at similar doses.[49]

Shoham et al reported a similar study in three cycles of IVF in PCOS patients and did not show any significant differences in doses of gonadotropins needed, days of stimulation required, number of follicles observed on ultrasound scan, pregnancy rate or multiple pregnancy rate.[44]

However, the use of recombinant gonadotropins may have advantages that are not reflected in these clinical results.[44,49] These advantages are the chance to use pure gonadotropins free from contamination with other hormones (FSH free of LH activity), no variability among batches, a production method that is independent of postmenopausal urine availability, low immunogenic capacity of the protein due to its high purity, and a reduction in the amount of protein given to the patient, facilitating the subcutaneous administration.[50,51]

GnRH analogs

The use of GnRH analogs (GnRHa) in IVF programs is routine nowadays. Several reports have specifically addressed the issue of GnRHa usefulness in PCOS patients.[52,53,54,55,56,57] Generally speaking, greater amounts of gonadotropin and a longer duration of treatment are required in patients receiving GnRHa.

In a prospective trial by Dor et al the results of GnRHa in ovarian response and the results of IVF in PCOS patients were evaluated.[58] Thirty patients were randomized to receive GnRHa triptorelin (De-capeptyl, Ipsen, Maidenhead, UK) or not in order to achieve pituitary downregulation. The authors did not find any significant differences in the mean number of oocytes retrieved, fertilization rate or pregnancy rates. Steroid levels in follicular fluid were similar in both groups. However, granulosa cell cultures obtained from follicular aspiration in patients who did not receive GnRHa produced higher levels of progesterone (P) and androstenedione (A), while aromatase activity remained similar in both groups. The authors concluded that GnRHa administration to PCOS patients in an IVF program reduces P and A production by granulosa cells while preventing early luteinization, but does not influence IVF results. These findings are similar to those described by Homburg et al,[59] who found similar results in patients receiving either GnRHa plus gonadotropins or gonadotropins alone for ovulation induction.

Studies with a larger number of participants show conflicting results. Homburg et al reviewed 208 treatment cycles performed in 68 women with PCOS undergoing IVF after failure of conventional treatment.[60] Patients with PCOS received gonadotropins either alone or combined with GnRHa, and tubal infertility patients served as controls. Use of GnRHa improved the fertilization rate (62.2% vs 50.6%, $P < 0.002$) and pregnancy rate per transfer (27.4% vs 15.5%, $P < 0.005$) in PCOS patients. Moreover, the use of GnRHa reduced the miscarriage rate and increased the cumulative 'take-home-baby' rate in PCOS patients but not in the control group.

Nowadays, it is considered that with the use of GnRHa multiple mature and synchronic follicles are obtained.[61]

Patients with PCOS have elevated androgen levels in follicular fluid and high basal serum LH levels. The androgenic milieu inside the follicle may be associated with atretic follicles and the use of GnRHa may increase the fertilization rate.[62,63] Interestingly, when androgens, estradiol and progesterone levels are evaluated in follicular fluid of women with PCOS or controls, no differences are found between those who received GnRHa and those who did not.[64] However, granulosa cell cultures obtained from women who received GnRHa showed lower levels of androgens and progesterone while aromatase activity remained the same.[65] Administration of GnRHa to these patients may yield a higher number of oocytes, partly because of its effect in decreasing the intrafollicular androgen levels, which may induce atresia in some oocytes. The use of GnRHa does not modify insulin resistance, hyperinsulinemia, or levels of insulin-like growth factor I (IGF-I) and IGF binding protein 1 (IGFBP-1).[66,67]

A great benefit of GnRHa use in PCOS women is the capacity of these agents to reduce LH levels during the follicular phase of the menstrual cycle. This effect diminishes the cancellation and miscarriage rate, and contributes to improved embryo quality in these patients.

Increased LH levels during the follicular phase induce early luteinization of the follicles, starting the second oocyte meiosis, so that the cycle has to be cancelled.[52,53] A meta-analysis clearly showed that GnRHa use significantly reduces the cancellation rate.[54]

When progesterone is present in the follicular fluid – an early luteinization marker – morphology of both the oocyte and the embryo may be altered,[55,56] and also fertilization and cleavage rates may be reduced.[57] Patients with elevated urine levels of LH show lower implantation rates.[68]

Patients with PCOS have a higher risk of miscarriage, partly due to the elevated LH levels.[69,70] These women have an increased frequency and length of LH pulses.[71] If serum LH levels are elevated, even with regular menses, there is a five-fold increase in miscarriage rate.[69,70,71,72] Premature LH peaks induce early luteinization of the follicle, which is also associated with a higher miscarriage rate.[73] It therefore seems reasonable to speculate that pituitary blockage with GnRHa, by eliminating the erratic LH pulsatility, should improve the clinical outcome in these patients by reducing spontaneous abortion and cancelled cycles (Table 16.2).

Fleming and co-workers were the first to describe the advantages of the combined use of gonadotropins with GnRHa.[74] The main contribution of this treatment is to reduce the LH levels achieved during the follicular phase of the menstrual cycle,[70] which mainly eliminates the risk of premature luteinization and reduces the miscarriage rate. Homburg et al randomized 239 patients with PCOS treated with hMG to receive GnRHa or not.[75] They found a significant decrease in miscarriage rate in women who received GnRHa (38.5% vs 18.2%, $P < 0.05$). In a later study by the same authors they found consistent results.[76] Other investigators have corroborated these findings.[77]

If, as these publications suggest, miscarriage rate is significantly reduced when GnRHa is incorporated in ovulation induction protocols, we may speculate that it may be due to a reduction in LH levels during the follicular phase of the menstrual cycle, a characteristic finding in these patients.

An interesting hypothetical approach to reducing the incidence of OHSS is to use GnRHa in these patients instead of hCG to induce the LH peak, but this is not practicable in IVF patients who use GnRHa to desensitize the hypophysis. Maybe in the future, when FSH and LH pituitary secretion are inhibited by GnRH antagonists, this protocol could be used.[78]

Adjuvant therapies

Growth hormone

It is known that growth hormone (GH) has an effect on the ovary. Granulosa cells show GH receptors,[79] and one of this hormone's mediators, insulin-like growth factor-I, regulates granulosa cell function and growth.[80] However, the clinical indication of the use of GH or GH-releasing hormone (GHRH) in reproduction is still under investigation.

Although women with PCOS show a high sensitivity to gonadotropin stimulation and tend to develop OHSS, there is a subgroup of women who exhibit altered GH pharmacokinetics. Women with PCOS who are overweight (and some of those within the normal weight range) show lower GH levels when compared with control mature women,[81,82] and a reduced GH secretory capacity.[83] This condition is generally associated with insulin

Table 16.2 Relationship between miscarriage rate and GnRH use					
Reference	**Year**	**Polycystic ovaries (%)**		**Non-PCO with high LH levels (%)**	
		GnRH	**No GnRH**	**GnRH**	**No GnRH**
Homburg et al[69]	1988	–	33	–	–
Homburg et al[75]	1993	17.6	39.1	–	–
Homburg et al[76]	1993	17.6	38.5	38.1	35.3
Balen et al[77]	1993	20.3	35.8	20.3	23.6

Values are percentages.

resistance, hyperinsulinemia and a reduced IGFBP-1 level.[84] The treatment with GnRHa diminishes GH secretion further,[85] and ovarian hyperstimulation with gonadotropins reduces IGF-I levels in follicular fluid of PCOS patients compared with normo-ovulatory patients.[86]

Owen et al studied the effect of giving GH to 18 PCOS patients with a low response in a previous cycle with hMG plus GnRHa.[87] They found that lower hMG doses were needed, more oocytes were retrieved, and similar fertilization and cleavage rates were obtained when compared with women not receiving GH.

Later, Cano et al studied the effect of GRF and gonadotropins in PCOS patients with low oocyte quality in previous cycles and low fertilization rates with normal semen samples. These authors found a higher number of oocytes retrieved and significantly higher fertilization rates when compared with previous cycles without GRF (57.3% vs 29%).[88]

Interestingly, in a report that evaluated the role of GH in ovulation induction with GnRHa and gonadotropins in PCOS patients resistant to CC,[67] no clinical benefit was found with this treatment as no changes were evident in follicular growth or ovarian response.

RESULTS OF IVF IN PCO PATIENTS

Good results in IVF are based on gamete quality, endometrial receptivity and a perfect synchronization between these two. It has been questioned whether patients with PCO have a similar outcome in IVF programs to that of other patients. Both oocyte quality and endometrial receptivity – with high estradiol levels achieved by these patients – may be compromised.

The frequency of PCOS is increasing as a cause of infertility in couples undergoing assisted reproduction. Different studies have evaluated the outcome in these patients and compared it with tubal infertility patients. Most of these studies lacked proper design and the small number of patients recruited yielded a lower than needed statistical power (Table 16.3).

Salat-Baroux et al studied 19 women with this disease, and compared the use of FSH alone with FSH after GnRHa, using tubal infertility patients as a control group.[89] The authors found no significant differences.

Later, Dor and co-workers published a similar study in which no GnRHa was used.[32] They found in PCO patients a higher number of oocytes retrieved per cycle (19.4 vs 5.4, $P < 0.004$), and significantly lower fertilization and cleavage rates (40.4% vs 67.6%, $P < 0.001$, and 34.4% vs 65.6%, $P < 0.001$) when compared with tubal infertility patients. However, no differences in pregnancy rate per cycle could be found (30.7% vs 29.7%).[32]

Homburg et al reviewed the IVF results of 208 cycles performed in 68 women with PCOS who previously failed to conceive after six cycles of ovulation induction with gonadotropins.[60] The control group consisted of an age-paired group of women with tubal infertility. The number of oocytes retrieved was significantly higher in the PCOS group, but a lower fertilization rate was achieved (57.3% vs 65.7%, $P < 0.002$). Nevertheless, a similar mean number of embryos was transferred in both groups, and no significant differences were found in pregnancy rates (22.6% vs 26.5%). Consistent findings were reported by other investigators.[33,35,87,90]

In conclusion, we can agree that IVF is a valid and feasible alternative for infertile women with PCOS.

PROBLEMS IN IVF TREATMENT

Oocyte quality

Many patients with PCO show a high response to ovarian gonadotropin stimulation; this is associated with a lower fertilization rate when compared with control subjects.[32,33,89] Other studies of high-responder patients have reported similar findings,[27,91] although different results were observed when only the ultrasonographic ovary appearance was taken into consideration.[33,92] However, when we expanded our experience to our oocyte donation program, in which PCO patients may donate some of

Table 16.3 Outcome of IVF in patients with PCO

Reference	n	No. of cycles	Protocol	Transfer	No. of pregnancies	No. of miscarriages	OHSS
Turhan et al[36]	21	24	CC/hMG	19	5	2	–
	22	23	FSH/hMG	23	8	2	–
	24	28	GnRH/FSH/hMG	22	7	1	–
Taríbo et al[37]	17	17	Buserelin/hMG	16	4	2	5
	14	14	Buserelin/FSH	13	5	0	6
Dale et al[90]	15	21	Triptorelin/FSH	13	6	0	0
	12	12	Buserelin/FSH	11	4	1	2
Cano et al[88]	6	6	FSH	6	4	0	1
	11	11	Buserelin/FSH	10	5	0	0
Salat-Beroux et al[89]	44	58	Buserelin/hMG	39	13	6	28
Homburg et al[15]	55	106	Triptorelin/FSH/hMG	?	33	6	?
	46	84	FSH/hMG	?	13	5	?
Homburg et al[60]	68	124	Triptorelin/FSH/hMG	?	34	6	?
	–	84	FSH/hMG	?	13	5	?
Homburg et al[59]	14	30	Buserelin/hMG	?	2	?	5
	11	27	–	?	3	?	3
	11	42	Buserelin/FSH	?	3	?	3
	10	23	hMG/FSH	?	3	?	2
MacDougall et al[33]	76	76	Buserelin/hMG	63	16	4	8
Owen et al[87]	?	58	Buserelin/hMG	33	0	–	–
	58	58	–	47	12	?	?
Urman et al[34]	9	19	Buserelin/hMG	17	4	1	2
Dor et al[32]	16	26	CC/hMG	24	8	5	5

CC, clomiphene citrate; FSH, follicle-stimulating hormone; GnRH, gonadotropin releasing hormone; hMG, human menopausal gonadotropin; OHSS, ovarian hyperstimulation syndrome.

their oocytes, we observed similar results to those in the control group.

In a retrospective study by Remohí et al,[93] oocytes donated by PCO patients had similar fertilization, implantation and pregnancy rates to those from control women. Other investigators found similar results.[94] In oocyte donation programs endometrial preparation of oocyte receptors is similar and male factor (sperm quality) barely affects the results, which means that oocyte quality in most PCO patients remains unaltered.

This does not mean that we can include every PCO patient in the same group. From the frequent (23%) and unexpected finding in a routine ultrasound scan of polycystic ovaries[95] to the full clinical expression of PCOS, there is a wide spectrum of possibilities. If the only finding that we have is a polycystic ovary on the ultrasonography, with normal phenotype and no menstrual alterations or hyperandrogenic signs, this patient will show a similar oocyte quality to normal women, probably because the intrafollicular milieu may be unaltered. This concept changes when the patient expresses the full clinical PCOS, with echographic, clinical and biochemical characteristics.

Cano and co-workers studied the endocrine milieu in women with PCO diagnosed by the echographic pattern of the ovaries.[96] These patients underwent IVF cycles and donated some of their oocytes. The patients were divided in two groups: (1) patients whose embryos repeatedly failed to implant in the women themselves or in the oocyte recipients, and (2) patients who conceived after the IVF cycle or after the oocyte donation of these patients. A control group (3) consisted of patients undergoing IVF with apparently normal ovaries on ultrasonography. No significant differences were found in levels of serum FSH, LH, androstenedione, testosterone or dehydroepiandrosterone. Group 1 showed higher glucose levels in the oral glucose tolerance test than group 2 or 3, and similar results were obtained with insulin levels (Figure 16.1), which confirms insulin resistance in this particular group of women, who had a higher body mass index. When IVF results were analyzed, group 1 showed a lower fertilization rate, and implantation and pregnancy rates were zero in both PCO patients and their recipients. These findings allow us to identify a particular subgroup of PCO women with low-quality oocytes and embryos.

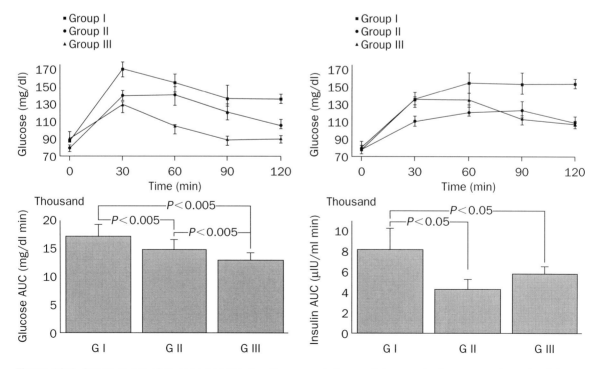

Figure 16.1 Serum levels of glucose and insulin after an oral glucose tolerance test, expressed as absolute values and as area under the curve (AUC) in the three groups studied (see text).

Implantation

Ovarian hyperstimulation reduces the implantation rate in a murine model[97] as well as in humans[27,98,99] by altering uterine receptivity. In high-responder patients such as PCO patients this is more relevant.[27,99] This may be related to altered levels of ovarian steroids, high estradiol or progesterone levels, or both.

In a retrospective analysis, Valbuena et al[100] investigated the effect of serum estradiol the day of human chorionic gonadotropin (hCG) administration on embryo implantation and if this effect was due to an endometrial defect, comparing IVF cycles of high responders (among whom some PCO patients were included), normoresponders and oocyte recipients of the oocyte donation program.[100] They found higher serum estradiol and progesterone levels in the high-responder group, with significantly lower implantation and pregnancy rates than in normoresponders. When oocyte recipients were compared according to the source of oocytes, no differences were found in fertilization, implantation or pregnancy rates: this means that embryo quality from high responders is adequate but endometrial receptivity is affected by high levels of estradiol. These investigators also found that implantation and pregnancy rates were significantly reduced when serum estradiol levels were over 2500 pg/ml.

A prospective analysis from the same group[26] described significantly higher ovarian steroid values during the peri-implantation period in high responder patients when compared with normoresponders. On days 4, 5 and 6 after hCG administration, when embryo implantation takes place, the ratio of estradiol to progesterone is elevated, based on higher estradiol levels. During these days, both normal and high responders showed no implantation or pregnancy if estradiol levels were above 1500 pg/ml. This suggests that patients previously identified as high responders may initiate an individualized ovarian stimulation protocol in order to reduce the number of oocytes retrieved and optimize their reproductive outcome.

This individualized treatment is based on the step-down principle described by Fauser et al.[101] Using the step-down regimen we have obtained fertilization and implantation rates similar to normoresponder women who were stimulated with a standard protocol.[102]

Ovarian hyperstimulation

Ovarian hyperstimulation is a frequent complication of ovulation induction in PCO patients.[103] In some cases it may induce severe complications – the ovarian hyperstimulation syndrome – with ovarian enlargement, ascites, hydrothorax with breathing difficulty, low blood pressure, hemoconcentration, oliguria which may end in renal failure, liver dysfunction and thrombotic episodes.[104]

The clinical profile of a patient at high risk of developing OHSS is a young women with a low BMI who recruits multiple small follicles and high estradiol levels with a few hMG ampules.[105] There is a strong correlation between BMI and the dose of hMG necessary to achieve an adequate follicular growth.[106] Basal levels (early follicular phase) of estradiol and prolactin in these patients are higher than in control women, which suggests that there are follicles in different maturity stages, and this asynchronic maturation favorable to OHSS is similar to that found in PCO patients.[106]

Ovarian hyperstimulation syndrome may be related to FSH accumulation at the end of the follicular phase: ovarian response is better in patients with higher FSH levels on the day of hCG administration.[107] The pathogenesis remains to be elucidated, but peripheral vasodilation together with the ovarian renin–angiotensin–aldosterone system and high estradiol levels play a decisive role.[108–110]

To prevent OHSS there are several approaches such as alternative ovarian stimulation protocols that try to emulate physiologic levels of FSH, lower in mid and late follicular phase, such as the aforementioned step-down regimen.[101,102,111] This protocol only uses FSH, and it is especially useful in patients with high LH levels. Theoretically, it may recruit a smaller group of follicles that would grow synchronously, achieving lower estradiol levels.

As pregnancy aggravates the severity of OHSS, some investigators offered elective freezing of all the embryos in patients at high risk of developing OHSS.[112] The objective was to reduce the severity and incidence of this syndrome while avoiding transfer of embryos to a non-receptive endometrium due to high estradiol levels which reduces implantation rates.[25,26] However, thawing recovers only 70–80% of the embryos, which are usually of lower quality than fresh embryos, so pregnancy rates are slightly lower.

Another alternative is to avoid hCG administration and cancel the cycle in patients at high risk of presenting with OHSS (generally with a history of OHSS) and in whom this risk does not justify the hypothetical benefits of a transfer, or if the patient decides so.

FUTURE PERSPECTIVES

Oral contraceptives combined with GnRHa

Irregular follicular maturation is a frequent event in women with PCO. It seems that these patients require more time to inhibit the pituitary stimulus of the ovary with GnRHa than non-PCO patients, so late luteal suppression may not be enough.[113] Based on this premise,[114,115] Rosenwaks et al[116] described a protocol for ovarian hyperstimulation in PCO women with the combined use of oral contraceptives and GnRHa. They started the administration of GnRHa together with the last four pills of the oral contraceptives in order to downregulate the pituitary secretions and ovarian function. This was followed by a low-dose protocol with FSH or hMG (150 IU), modifying the dose in half-ampule increments every 3–4 days according to the follicular growth. The results of the first 51 patients stimulated with this protocol have recently been published, with an outstanding 51.9% pregnancy rate per initiated cycle, and 66.7% pregnancy rate per embryo transferred.[115] The cancellation rate was only 13%. The mean number of oocytes retrieved was acceptable (15.3) with a 43.4% fertilization rate. Interestingly, mean LH concentration at the beginning of the cycle was significantly lower in the study group compared with controls (12.4 vs 19.7 IU/mL, $P < 0.01$). This suggests that the combined use of oral contraceptives with GnRHa may avoid the initial flare-up induced by the latter, which enhances LH levels and worsens the intraovarian milieu. Also, it is more cost-effective to administer oral contraceptives than to extend GnRHa administration. This protocol provides high pregnancy rates with low miscarriage and cancellation rates.

Immature oocyte retrieval

As stated before, in patients with a high response to gonadotropins a greater number of immature oocytes are obtained.[27,48,56] Although the use of GnRHa, by synchronizing follicular growth, can partially reduce this immaturity,[48,56] it is still relatively common to obtain a large number of immature oocytes in these patients.

A new approach has been proposed to solve this inconvenient problem. Instead of trying to grow as many synchronous follicles as possible up to metaphase II stage, Trounson and colleagues retrieved immature human oocytes 2–10 mm in diameter using a narrow-gauge needle and ultrasound-guided transvaginal puncture.[117] The oocytes obtained were matured in vitro, with a 34% fertilization rate, resulting in the first pregnancy in the world with this technique.[117] Fertilization and cleavage rates of these oocytes are similar to mature oocytes, although a high percentage of polyploidy has been described.[118] This interesting alternative may offer a new option for the immature oocytes that are retrieved when they grow asynchronically from the rest of the batch, or even lead to questions about the usefulness of ovulation induction, avoiding by this method the risk of OHSS and substantially reducing the cost of the drugs.

GnRH antagonists

Although GnRH antagonists have been available for several years, no clear clinical indication was established because of their relatively short half-life, which necessitated multiple administrations, and also because they caused allergic reactions by inducing histamine secretion from mast cells. New molecules with a longer half-life and minimal or even no effects on mast cells have now been clinically assayed. Gonadotropin releasing hormone antagonists bind to pituitary GnRH receptors, competing with endogenous GnRH and preventing LH secretion. Opposed to GnRHa, the antagonists do not stimulate endogenous gonadotropin secretion and induce rapid downregulation of gonadotropin secretion.

Different reports describe their effect on the normal menstrual cycle in a control group of women.[119–121] In midfollicular phase, the antagonist cetrorelix immediately decreased LH and estradiol levels, with a less pronounced FSH decrease, and postponed the endogenous LH peak from 6 days to 17 days.[121] Gonadotropin levels remain low when several doses of the antagonist are administered. In vitro fertilization programs could benefit from GnRH antagonist to prevent the endogenous LH peak and premature luteinization.[122] However, high doses of FSH would be required to induce follicular growth and development, as shown in monkeys.[123]

CONCLUSION

The available evidence indicates that IVF offers women with PCO attractive possibilities of achieving a pregnancy when other techniques have failed. Cumulative pregnancy rates in these patients are comparable to those in patients with other fertility problems such as tubal factors, which may be explained by the multifollicular growth approach.

The protocol that offers the best results in these women, as in most IVF patients, is based on pituitary downregulation to inhibit endogenous FSH and LH secretion, thus reducing the deleterious effects of elevated LH levels characteristic in these patients prior to ovarian hyperstimulation.

The two determining factors for these patients to achieve a pregnancy are hyperinsulinemia and circulating LH levels. Correcting these factors not only improves ovarian response to hyperstimulation but also reduces the miscarriage rate.

These patients are at high risk of OHSS, and GnRHa administration does not reduce this risk. However, different approaches allow us to reduce its severity or its incidence.

In the near future, new recombinant gonadotropins free of contaminating hormones and better tolerated, the use of GnRH antagonists, and the attractive possibility of in vitro oocyte maturation, may simplify the therapeutic alternatives in these patients.

REFERENCES

1 Adams J, Polson DW, Franks S. Prevalence of polycystic ovaries in women with anovulation and idiopathic hirsutism. *Br Med J* (1986) **293**: 355–9.

2 Hull MG. Epidemiology of infertility in polycystic ovaries disease: endocrinological and demographic studies. *Gynaecol Endocrinol* (1987) **1**: 235–45.

3 Goldzieher JW, Green JA. The polycystic ovary. Clinical and histological features. *J Clin Endocrinol Metab* (1962) **22**: 325–38.

4 Buyalos RP, Geffner ME, Bersch N et al. Insulin and insulin growth factor-1 responsiveness in polycystic ovarian syndrome. *Fertil Steril* (1992) **57**: 796–803.

5 Dunaif A, Segal K, Futterweit W, Dobrjansky A. Profound peripheral insulin resistance independent of obesity in polycystic ovarian syndrome. *Diabetes* (1987) **38**: 1165–74.

6 Kazer RR, Kessel B, Yen SSC. Circulating luteinizing hormone pulse frequency in women with polycystic ovarian syndrome. *J Clin Endocrinol Metab* (1987) **65**: 233–6.

7 Lobo RA, Gysler M, March CM, Goebelsmann U, Mishell DR. Clinical and laboratory predictors of clomiphene response. *Fertil Steril* (1982) **37**: 168–74.

8 Harrimond MG, Halme JK, Talbert LM. Factors

affecting the pregnancy rate in clomiphene citrate induction of ovulation. *Obst Gynec* (1983) **62**: 196–202.

9 Franks S. Induction of ovulation. In: Templeton AA, Drife JO, eds, *Infertility* (Springer: London, 1992) 237–50.

10 Wrarnsby H, Fredga K, Liedholm P. Chromosome analysis of human oocytes recovered from preovulatory follicles in stimulated cycles. *N Engl J Med* (1987) **316**: 120–4.

11 Lechmann F, Baban N, Webber B. Ovarian stimulation for in vitro fertilization: clomiphene and hMG. *Hum Reprod* (1988) **3**(suppl. 2): 11–21.

12 Wang DE, Gemzell C. The use of human gonadotropins for induction of ovulation in women with polycystic ovarian disease. *Fertil Steril* (1980) **33**: 479–86.

13 Hamilton-Fairley D, Franks S. Common problems in induction of ovulation. *Baillière's Clinical Obstetrics and Gynaecology* (1990) **4**: 609–25.

14 Hamilton-Fairley D, Kiddy D, Watson H, Sagle M, Franks S. Low-dose gonadotropin therapy for induction of ovulation in 100 women with polycystic ovary syndrome. *Hum Reprod* (1991) **6**: 1095–9.

15 Homburg R, Levy T, Ben-Rafael Z. A comparative prospective study of conventional regimen with chronic low dose administration of follicle stimulation hormone for anovulation associated with polycystic ovary syndrome. *Fertil Steril* (1995) **63**: 729–33.

16 Van Santbrink EJ, Fauser BC. Urinary follicle-stimulating hormone for normogonadotropic clomiphene-resistant anovulatory infertility: prospective, randomized comparison between low dose step-up and step-down dose regimens. *J Clin Endocrinol Metab* (1997) **82**: 3597–602.

17 Abdulwahid NA, Adams J, Van der Spuy ZM, Jacobs HS. Gonadotrophin control of follicular development. *Clin Endocrinol* (1985) **23**: 613–26.

18 Shoham Z, Homburg R, Jacobs HS. Induction of ovulation with pulsatile LHRH. *Baillière's Clinical Obstetrics and Gynaecology* (1990) **4**: 589–608.

19 Naether OG, Fischer R, Weise HC, Geiger Kotzler L, Delfs T, Rudolf K. Laparoscopic eletrocoagulation of the ovarian surface in infertile patients with polycystic ovarian disease. *Fertil Steril* (1993) **60**: 88–94.

20 Colacurci N, Zullo F, De Francis P et al. IVF after ovarian electrocautery through laparoscopy in patients with polycystic ovary syndrome. *Acta Obstet Gynecol Scand* (1997) **76**: 555–8.

21 Dabirasbrafi H, Mohamad K, Behjatnia Y, Moghadami-Tabrizi N. Adhesion formation after ovarian electrocauterization on patients with polycystic ovarian syndrome. *Fertil Steril* (1991) **55**: 1200–1.

22 Kovacs G, Buckler H, Bangah M et al. Treatment of anovulation due to polycystic ovarian syndrome by laparoscopic ovarian electrocautery. *Br J Obstet Gynaecol* (1992) **98**: 30–5.

23 Aakvaag A. Hormonal response to electrocautery of the ovary in patients with polycystic ovarian disease. *Br J Obstet Gynaecol* (1985) **92**: 12 458–64.

24 Buyalos RP, Lee CT. Polycystic ovary syndrome: pathophysiology and outcome with in vitro fertilization. *Fertil Steril* (1996) **65**: 1–10.

25 Simón C, Cano F, Valbuena D, Remohí J, Pellicer A. Clinical evidence for a detrimental effect on uterine receptivity of high serum oestradiol concentrations in high and normal responder patients. *Hum Reprod* (1995) **10**: 2432–7.

26 Pellicer A, Valbuena D, Cano F, Remohí J, Simón C. Lower implantation rates in high responders: evidence for an altered endocrine milieu during the preimplantation period. *Fertil Steril* (1996) **65**: 1190–5.

27 Pellicer A, Ruiz A, Castellví RM, Calatayud C, Ruiz M, Tarín JJ. Is the retrieval of high number of oocytes desirable in patients treated with gonadotrophin-releasing hormone analogues (GnRHa) and gonadotrophins? *Hum Reprod* (1989) **4**: 536–40.

28 Adashi EY. Clomiphene citrate: mechanism(s) and site(s) of action hypothesis revisited. *Fertil Steril* (1984) **42**: 331–44.

29 Kerin JE, Liu JH, Phillipou G, Yen SSC. Evidence for a hypothalamic site of action of clomiphene citrate in women. *J Clin Endocrinol Metab* (1985) **61**: 265–8.

30 Kettel LM, Roseff SL, Berga SL et al. Hypothalamic-pituitary-ovarian response to clomiphene citrate in women with polycystic ovary syndrome. *Fertil Steril* (1993) **59**: 532–8.

31 Oelsner G, Barnea ER, Admon D et al. Letter to the editor. *N Engl J Med* (1987) **316**: 318.

32 Dor J, Shultnan A, Levran D, Ben-Rafael Z, Rudak E, Mashiach S. The treatment of patients with polycystic ovarian syndrome by in vitro fertilization and embryo transfer: a comparison of results with those of patients with tubal infertility. *Hum Reprod* (1990) **5**: 816–18.

33 MacDougall MJ, Tan SL, Balen A, Jacobs HS. A controlled study comparing patients with and

without polycystic ovaries undergoing in vitro fertilization. *Hum Reprod* (1993) **2**: 233–7.

34 Urman B, Flukes MR, Then BH, Fleige-Zabra BG, Zouves CG, Moon YS. The outcome of in vitro fertilization and embryo transfer in wornen with polycystic ovary syndrome failing to conceive after ovulation induction with exogenous gonadotropins. *Fertil Steril* (1992) **57**: 1269–73.

35 Erickson OF, Hsueh AJW, Quigley ME, Rebar RW, Yen SSC. Functional studies of aromatase activity in human granulosa cells from normal and polycystic ovaries. *J Clin Endocrinol Metab* (1979) **49**: 514–20.

36 Turhan NO, Artini PG, D'Ambrogio GD et al. A comparative study of three ovulation induction protocols in polycystic ovarian disease patients in an in vitro fertilization embryo transfer program. *J Assist Reprod Genet* (1993) **10**: 15–20.

37 Taríbo T, Dale PO, Kjekshus E, Hau E, Abyholm T. Stimulation with human menopausal gonadotropin versus follicle-stimulating hormone after pituitary suppression in polycystic ovarian syndrome. *Fertil Steril* (1990) **53**: 798–803.

38 McFaul PB, Traub AL, Thompson W. Treatment of clomiphene citrate-resistant polycystic ovarian syndrome with pure follicle-stimulating hormone or human menopausal gonadotropin. *Fertil Steril* (1990) **53**: 792–7.

39 Larsen T, Larsen JE, Schioler V, Bostofte E, Felding C. Comparison of urinary human follicle-stimulating hormone and human menopausal gonadotropin for ovarian stimulation in polycystic ovarian syndrome. *Fertil Steril* (1990) **53**: 426–31.

40 Sagle MA, Hamilton-Fairley D, Kiddy DS, Franks S. A comparative, randomized study of low-dose human menopausal gonadotropin and follicle-stimulating hormone in women with polycystic ovarian syndrome. *Fertil Steril* (1991) **55**: 56–60.

41 Seibel MM, McArdle C, Smith D, Taymor ML. Ovulation induction in polycystic ovary syndrome with urinary follicle-stimulating hormone or human menopausal gonadotropin. *Fertil Steril* (1985) **43**: 703–8.

42 Hoffman DI, Lobo RA, Campeau JD et al. Ovulation induction in clomiphene-resistant anovulatory women: differential follicular response to purified urinary follicle-stimulating hormone (FSH) versus purified urinary FSH and luteinizing hormone. *J Clin Endocrinol Metab* (1985) **60**: 922–7.

43 Germond M, Dessole S, Senn A, Lournaye E, Howles C, Beltrami V. Successful in vitro fertilization and embryo transfer after treatment with recombinant human FSH. *Lancet* (1992) **339**: 1170.

44 Shoham Z, Patel A, Jacobs HS. Polycystic ovarian disease syndrome: safety and effectiveness of stepwise and low-dose administration of purified follicle-stimulating hormone. *Fertil Steril* (1991) **55**: 1051–6.

45 Donderwinkel PF, Schoot DC, Coelingh Bennink HF, Fauser BC. Pregnancy after induction of ovulation with recombinant human FSH in polycystic ovary syndrome. *Lancet* (1992) **340**: 981.

46 Hornnes P, Giroud D, Howles C, Lournaye E. Recombinant human follicle-stimulating hormone treatment leads to normal follicular growth, estradiol secretion, and pregnancy in World Health Organization group II anovulatory woman. *Fertil Steril* (1993) **60**: 724–6.

47 Devroey P, Steirteghem A, Mannaerts B, Coelingh Bennink H. Successful in vitro fertilization and embryo transfer after treatment with recombinant human FSH. *Lancet* (1992) **1**: 1170–1.

48 Van Dessel HJ, Donderwinkel PF, Coelingh-Bennink HJ, Fauser BC. First established pregnancy and birth after induction of ovulation with recombinant human follicle-stimulating hormone in polycystic ovary syndrome. *Hum Reprod* (1994) **9**: 55–6.

49 Fisch B, Avrech OM, Pinkas H et al. Superovulation before IVF by recombinant versus urinary FSH (combined with a GnRH analog protocol): a comparative study. *J Assist Reprod Genet* (1995) **12**: 26–31.

50 Recombinant Human FSH Study Group. Clinical assessment of recombinant human follicle stimulating hormone in stimulating ovarian follicular development before in vitro fertilization. *Fertil Steril* (1995) **63**: 77–86.

51 Shoham Z, Insler V. Recombinant technique and gonadotropins production: new era in reproductive medicine. *Fertil Steril* (1996) **66**: 187–201.

52 Wildt L, Diedrich K, Van der Yen H, Al Hasani S, Hubner H, Klasen R. Ovarian hyperstimulation for in vitro fertilization controlled by GnRH agonist administered in combination with human menopausal gonadotrophins. *Hum Reprod* (1986) **1**: 15–19.

53 Lournaye E. The control of endogenous secretion during ovarian hyperstimulation for in vitro fertilization and embryo transfer. *Hum Reprod* (1990) **5**: 357–76.

54 Hughes KG, Fedorkow DM, Daya S, Sagle MA, Van de Koppel P, Collins JA. The routine use of gonadotropin-release hormone agonists to in vitro fertilization and gamete intrafallopian transfer: a meta-analysis of randomized controlled trials. *Fertil Steril* (1992) **58**: 888–98.

55 Eibscitz I, Belaisch-Allatt JC, Frydman R. In vitro fertilization management and results in stimulated cycles with spontaneous luteinizing hormone discharge. *Fertil Steril* (1986) **45**: 231–6.

56 Hartshorne GM. Steroid production by the cumulus: relationships to fertilization in vitro. *Hum Reprod* (1989) **4**: 742–5.

57 Ben-Rafael Z, Kopf FS, Blasco L et al. Follicular maturation parameters associated with the failure of oocyte retrieval, fertilization, and cleavage in vitro. *Fertil Steril* (1986) **45**: 51–7.

58 Dor J, Schulman A, Patiente C et al. The effect of gonadotrophin-releasing hormone agonist on the ovarian response and in vitro fertilization results in polycystic ovarian syndrome: a prospective study. *Fertil Steril* (1992) **57**: 366–71.

59 Homburg R, Eshel A, Kilborri J, Adams J, Jacobs HS. Combined luteinizing hormone releasing hormone analogue and exogenous gonadotrophins for the treatment of infertility associated with polycystic ovaries. *Hum Reprod* (1990) **5**: 32–5.

60 Homburg R, Berkovitz D, Levy T, Ferldberg D, Ashkenazi J, Ben-Rafael Z. In vitro fertilization and embryo transfer for the treatment of infertility associated with polycystic ovary syndrome. *Fertil Steril* (1993) **60**: 858–63.

61 Takuze S, Polan MIL. Análogos de la GnRH en reproducción asistida. In: Remohí J, Simón C, Pellicer A, Bonilla-Musoles F, eds, *Reproducción Humana* (McGraw Hill Interamericana: Madrid, 1996) 278–89.

62 Smitz J, Ronet R, Tarlatzis BC. The use of gonadotrophin releasing hormone agonists for in vitro fertilization and other assisted procreation techniques: experience from three centers. *Hum Reprod* (1992) **7**(suppl. 11): 49–66.

63 Dor J, Shulman A, Levran D, Ben-Rafael Z, Rudak E, Mashiach S. The treatment of patients with polycystic ovarian syndrome by in vitro fertilization and embryo transfer: a comparison of results with those of patients with tubal infertility. *Hum Reprod* (1990) **5**: 816–18.

64 Tavrnergen E, Tavrnergen EN, Capanoglu R. Do analogues of gonadotrophin releasing hormone influence follicular fluid steroid levels, oocyte maturity and fertilization rates? *Hum Reprod* (1992) **7**: 479–82.

65 Dor J, Schulman A, Patiente C et al. The effect of gonadotrophin-releasing hormone agonist on the ovarian response and in vitro fertilization results in polycystic ovarian syndrome: a prospective study. *Fertil Steril* (1992) **57**: 366–71.

66 Dale PO, Tanbo T, Djoseland O, Jetvell J, Abyholm T. Persistence of hyperinsulinemia in polycystic ovary syndrome after ovarian suppression by gonadotropin-releasing hormone agonist. *Acta Endocrinol* (1992) **126**: 132–6.

67 Homburg R, Levy T, Ben-Rafael Z. Adjuvant growth hormone for induction of ovulation with gonadotropin releasing-hormone agonist and gonadotropins in polycystic ovary syndrome: a randomized, double-blind, placebo controlled trial. *Hum Reprod* (1995) **10**: 2550–3.

68 Howies CM, McNamee MC, Edwards RG. Follicular development and early luteal function of conception and nonconception cycles after human in vitro fertilization: endocrine correlates. *Hum Reprod* (1987) **2**: 17–19.

69 Homburg R, Armar NA, Eshel A, Adams J, Jacobs HS. Influence of serum luteinising hormone concentrations on ovulation, conception, and early pregnancy loss in polycystic ovary syndrome. *Br Med J* (1988) **297**: 1024–6.

70 Homburg R. Polycystic ovary syndrome – from gynecological curiosity to multisystem endocrinopathy. *Hum Reprod* (1996) **11**: 29–39.

71 Kazer RR, Kessel B, Yen SSC. Circulating luteinizing hormone pulse frequency in women with polycystic ovary syndrome. *J Clin Endocrinol Metab* (1987) **65**: 233–6.

72 Regan L, Owen EJ, Jacobs HS. Hypersecretion of luteinising hormone, infertility, and miscarriage. *Lancet* (1990) **336**: 1141–4.

73 Hunter RHE, Cook B, Baker TO. Dissociation of response to injected gonadotrophin between the Graafian follicle and oocyte in pigs. *Nature* (1976) **260**: 156–8.

74 Fleming R, Haxton MJ, Hamilton MPR et al. Succesful treatment of infertile women with oligomenorrhea using a combination of a GnRH agonist and exogenous gonadotropins. *Br J Obstet Gynaecol* (1985) **92**: 369–73.

75 Homburg R, Levy T, Berkovitz D et al. Gonadotropin-releasing hormone agonist reduces the miscarriage rate for pregnancies achieved in women with polycystic ovary syndrome. *Fertil Steril* (1993) **59**: 527–31.

76 Homburg R, Berkovitz D, Levy T, Ferldberg D, Ashkenazi J, Ben-Rafael Z. In vitro fertilization and embryo transfer for the treatment of infertil-

ity associated with polycystic ovary syndrome. *Fertil Steril* (1993) **60**: 858–63.

77 Balen AH, Tan SL, MacDougall J, Jacobs HS. Miscarriage rates following in vitro fertilization are increased in women with polycystic ovaries and are reduced by pituitary desensitization with buserelin. *Hum Reprod* (1993) **8**: 959–64.

78 Koi S, Lewit N, Itskovitz-Eldor J. Ovarian hyper-stimulation syndrome after using gonadotrophin-releasing hormone analogue as a trigger of ovulation: causes and implications. *Hum Reprod* (1996) **11**: 1143–4.

79 Carlsson B, Bergh C, Bentham J et al. Expression of functional growth hormone receptors in human granulosa cells. *Hum Reprod* (1992) **7**: 1205–9.

80 Adhashi EY, Resnick CE, D'Ercole AJ, Svoboda ME, Van Wyk JJ. Insulin like growth factors as intraovarian regulators of granulosa cell growth and function. *Endocr Rev* (1985) **6**: 400–20.

81 Prelevie GM, Wurzburger MI, Balint-Peric L, Ginsburg J. Twenty four hour serum growth hormone, insulin, C-peptide and blood glucose profiles and serum insulin growth factor-I concentrations in women with polycystic ovaries. *Horm Res* (1996) **37**: 125–31.

82 Insler V, Shoham Z, Barash A et al. Polycystic ovaries in non-obese and obese patients: possible patho-physiological mechanism based on new interpretation of facts and findings. *Hum Reprod* (1993) **8**: 379–84.

83 Ovesen P, Moller J, Moller N, Christiansen JS, Jorgenson JOL, Orskov H. Growth hormone secretory capacity serum insulin-like growth factor-I levels in primary infertile, anovulatory women with regular menses. *Fertil Steril* (1992) **57**: 97–101.

84 Homburg R, Pariente C, Lunenfeld B, Jacobs HS. The role of insulin growth factor-1 and IGF binding protein-I in the pathogenesis of polycystic ovary syndrome. *Hum Reprod* (1992) **7**: 1379–83.

85 Word RA, Odom MI, Byrd W, Carr BR. The effect of gonadotrophin releasing hormone agonists on growth hormone secretion in adult pre-menopausal women. *Fertil Steril* (1990) **54**: 73–8.

86 Volpe A, Artini PG, Barreca A, Minuto F, Coukos G, Genazzani AR. Effects of growth hormone administration in addition to gonadotrophins in normally ovulating women and polycystic ovary patients. *Hum Reprod* (1992) **7**: 1347–52.

87 Owen E, Shoham Z, Mason B, Ostergaard ND, Jacobs H. Cotreatment with growth hormone, after pituitary suppression, for ovarian stimulation in in vitro fertilization: a randomized, double-blind, placebo-control trial. *Fertil Steril* (1991) **56**: 1104–10.

88 Cano A, Simón C, Ruiz A, Gutiérrez A, Tarín JJ, Remohí J, Pellicer A. The use of growth hormone-releasing factor in IVF: possible effects on quality of the human oocytes. *Hum Reprod* (1994) **9**: 44.

89 Salat-Baroux J, Alvarez S, Antoine JM et al. Results of IVF in the treatment of polycystic ovary disease. *Hum Reprod* (1988) **3**: 331–5.

90 Dale PO, Taríbo T, Abyholm T. In vitro fertilization in infertile women with polycystic ovarian syndrome. *Hum Reprod* (1991) **6**: 238–41.

91 Testart J, Belaisch-Allart J, Forman R et al. Influence of different stimulation treatments on oocyte characteristics and in vitro fertilization. *Hum Reprod* (1989) **4**: 192–7.

92 Wong IL, Morris RS, Lobo RA, Paulson RI, Sauer MV. Isolated polycystic morphology in ovum donors predicts response to ovarian stimulation. *Hum Reprod* (1995) **10**: 524–8.

93 Remohí J, Vidal A, Pellicer A. Oocyte donation in low responders to conventional ovarian stimulation for in vitro fertilization. *Fertil Steril* (1993) **59**: 1208–15.

94 Ashkenazi J, Farhi J, Orvieto NR et al. Polycystic ovary syndrome patients as oocyte donors: the effect of ovarian stimulation protocol on the implantation rate of the recipient. *Fertil Steril* (1995) **64**: 564–7.

95 Polson DW, Wadsworth J, Adams J, Franks S. Polycystic ovaries a common finding in normal women. *Lancet* (1988) **2**: 870–2.

96 Cano F, García-Velasco JA, Millet A, Remohí J, Simón C, Pellicer A. Oocyte quality in polycystic ovaries revisited: identification of a particular subgroup of women. *J Assist Reprod Genet* (1997) **14**: 254–61.

97 Fossum GT, Davidson A, Paulson JR. Ovarian hyperstimulation inhibits embryo implantation in the mouse. *J in Vitro Fertil Embr Transf* (1989) **6**: 7–10.

98 Paulson RJ, Sauer MV, Lobo RA. Embryo implantation after human in vitro fertilization: importance of endometrial receptivity. *Fertil Steril* (1990) **53**: 870–4.

99 Toner J, Bryski R, Oehninger S, Veeck L, Simonetti S, Muasher S. Impact of the number of preovulatory oocytes and cryopreservation on in vitro fertilization outcome. *Hum Reprod* (1991) **6**: 284–9.

100 Valbuena D, Gaitán P, García-Velasco JA, Simón C. Implicación de los niveles de estradiol sobre la implantación embrionaria. In: Pellicer A, Simón C, eds, *Implantación embrionaria* (Médica Panamericana: Madrid, Spain 1997) 103–18.

101 Fauser BCJM, Donderwinkl P, Schoot DC. The step-down principle in gonadotrophin treatment and the role of GnRH analogues. *Baillière's Clinical Obstetrics and Gynaecology* (1993) **7**: 309–30.

102 Simón C, García-Velasco JA, Valbuena D et al. Increased uterine receptivity by decreasing estradiol levels during the preimplantation period in high responder patients by using an FSH step-down regimen. *Fertil Steril* (1998) **70**: 234–9.

103 MacDougall MI, Tan SL, Jacobs IS. In vitro fertilization and the ovarian hyperstimulation syndrome. *Hum Reprod* (1992) **7**: 597–600.

104 Pride SM, James CST, Ho Yuen B. The ovarian hyperstimulation syndrome. *Semin Reprod Endocrinol* (1990) **8**: 247–60.

105 Navot D, Relon A, Birkenfels A et al. Risk factors and prognostic variables in the ovarian hyperstimulation syndrome. *Am J Obstet Gynecol* (1988) **159**: 210–15.

106 McClure N, McQuinn B, McDonald J, Kovacs GT, Healy DL, Burger HG. Body weight, body mass index, and age: predictors of menotropin dose and cycle outcome in polycystic ovarian syndrome? *Fertil Steril* (1992) **58**: 622–4.

107 Ben-Rafael Z, Strauss JF, Mastroianni L, Flickinger GL. Differences in ovarian stimulation in human menopausal gonadotropin treated woman may be related to follicle stimulating hormone accumulation. *Fertil Steril* (1986) **46**: 586–92.

108 Pellicer A, Palumbo A, DeChemey AH, Naftolin E. Blockage of ovulation by an angiotensin antagonist. *Science* (1988) **240**: 1661–2.

109 Naftolin F, Palumbo A, Pepperell SR. Potential role of the renin angiotensin system in polycystic ovaries. In: Chang RJ, ed., *Polycystic Ovary Syndrome,* Serono Symposia (Springer: New York, 1996) 59–70.

110 Balasch J, Arroyo V, Carmona F et al. Severe ovarian hyperstimulation syndrome: role of peripheral vasodilation. *Fertil Steril* (1991) **26**: 1077–83.

111 Mizunuma H, Takagi T, Yarnada K, Andoh K, Ibuki Y, Igarashi M. Ovulation induction by step-down administration of purified urinary follicle-stimulating hormone in patients with polycystic ovarian syndrome. *Fertil Steril* (1991) **55**: 1195–6.

112 Awonuga AO, Pittrof RJ, Zaidi J, Dean N, Jacobs HS, Tan SL. Elective cryopreservation of all embryos in women at risk of developing ovarian hyperstimulation syndrome may not prevent the condition but reduces the live birth rate. *J Assist Reprod Genet* (1996) **13**: 401–6.

113 Harnuri M, Zwírner M, Cledon P, Tinneberg HR. Androgen response in polycystic ovarian syndrome to FSH treatment after LHRH agonist suppression. *Int J Fertil* (1992) **37**: 171–5.

114 Salat-Baroux J, Álvarez S, Antoine JM et al. Comparison between long and short protocols of LHRH agonist in the treatment of polycystic ovary disease by in vitro fertilization. *Hum Reprod* (1988) **3**: 535–9.

115 Taribo T, Abyholm T, Magnus O, Henriksen T. Gonadotropin and ovarian steroid production in polycystic ovarian syndrome during suppression with a gonadotropin-releasing hormone agonist. *Gynecol Obstet Invest* (1989) **28**: 147–51.

116 Rosenwaks Z, Davis OK, Damario MA. In vitro fertilization in polycystic ovary syndrome. In: Chang RJ, ed., *Polycystic Ovary Syndrome*, Serono Symposia (Springer: New York, 1996) 71–88.

117 Trounson A, Wood C, Kausch A. In vitro maturation and fertilization and developmental competence of oocytes recovered from untreated polycystic ovarian patients. *Fertil Steril* (1994) **62**: 456–60.

118 Toth TL, Baka SG, Veeck LL, Jones HW, Muasher S, Lanzendorf SE. Fertilization and in vitro development of cryopreserved human prophase I oocytes. *Fertil Steril* (1994) **61**: 891–4.

119 Fluker MR, Marshal LA, Monroe SE, Jaffe RB. Variable ovarian response to GnRH antagonists induced gonadotrophin deprivation during different phases of the menstrual cycle. *J Clin Endocrinol Metab* (1991) **72**: 912–18.

120 Hall JE, Bharta N, Adams JM et al. Variable tolerance of the developing follicle and corpus luteum to gonadotropin withdrawal in the human. *J Clin Endocrinol Metab* (1991) **72**: 993–1001.

121 Leroy Y, Acremont MF, Brailly-Tabard S et al. A single injection of a GnRH antagonist (cetrorelix) postpones the luteinizing hormone surge: further evidence for the role of GnRH during the LH surge. *Fertil Steril* (1994) **62**: 461–7.

122 Frydman R, Cornel C, de Ziegler D et al. Prevention of premature luteinizing hormone and progesterone rise with a gonadotropin

releasing hormone antagonist, Nal-Glu, in controlled ovarian hyperstimulation. *Fertil Steril* (1991) **56**: 923–7.

123 Zelinsku-Wooten MB, Hutchison JS, Hess DL et al. Follicle stimulating hormone alone supports follicle growth and oocyte development in gonadotropin-releasing hormone antagonist-treated monkeys. *Hum Reprod* (1995) **10**: 1658–66.

17

Long-term sequelae

Mary Birdsall

Although polycystic ovary syndrome (PCOS) has been diagnosed since the 1930s, the natural history of polycystic ovaries (PCO) or PCOS and any sequelae remain a mystery. The ability to diagnose PCO using a non-invasive and repeatable method – ultrasonography – was only developed in 1981[1] and to date there have been no long-term studies using ultrasound. Two studies that followed women for some years after ovarian wedge resection are discussed in this chapter, but it should be emphasized at the outset that these studies may not answer questions about long-term sequelae or the natural history of PCO. A wedge biopsy procedure may alter the ovary's function as well as producing significant adhesions. It is also worthy of mention that follow-up of women after wedge biopsy only includes cases at the severe end of the PCO spectrum and may not be relevant to the asymptomatic majority of women with PCO. Obese women may not have been offered a wedge biopsy, which may further bias the data. The long-term sequelae of PCO are important because this condition has been diagnosed in more than 20% of premenopausal women by ultrasound scan.[2-4] More and more women are having the diagno-

sis of PCO made and want to know its significance on their lives. This chapter is an attempt to answer this question; however, it is based on limited data and perhaps in five years' time it could be rewritten with much more fact and far less theory.

THE NATURAL HISTORY OF PCO

The cause of polycystic ovaries is unknown. Although exposure to high androgen levels from a variety of sources will cause the typical ultrasonographic appearance of polycystic ovaries, in most instances it is the ovary itself which is the source of these increased androgens.[5] Defects at the hypothalamus, pituitary gland and ovary have all been described in women with polycystic ovaries. Because of the heterogeneous nature of the disorder,[6] it may be that there is more than one cause. A genetic basis for the condition has also been proposed, possibly with an autosomal dominant mode of inheritance.[7]

The natural history of PCO is unknown. The ultrasound appearances of PCO have been described in young girls and adolescents,[8] and at times of ovarian quiescence during the reproductive years, such as lactation,[4] oral contraceptive use,[4] gonadotrophin releasing hormone analogue use,[9] and hypothalamic hypogonadism.[10] It has also been described in postmenopausal women.[11]

POLYCYSTIC OVARIES IN POSTMENOPAUSAL WOMEN

A study to determine whether polycystic ovaries exist in postmenopausal women investigated two groups of participants. Group 1 consisted of 18 postmenopausal volunteers who took part in a small pilot study prior to the larger group study. The entry criteria were age greater than 50 years as well as absence of menses for 1 year or more, no major gynaecological surgery, and no prior diagnosis of PCO. Group 2 comprised 142 women who had recently undergone coronary angiography, of whom 94 were postmenopausal.

Transabdominal and transvaginal ultrasound scans were performed and measurements made of uterine area, endometrial thickness and ovarian volume. The morphological appearance of the ovaries was also noted. Fasting blood samples were taken (Table 17.1). Medical and menstrual questionnaires were completed.

Polycystic ovaries were found in 8 out of 18 patients (44%) in group 1 and 60 out of 142 (42%) in group 2. Polycystic ovaries were detected in 35 of 94 (37%) of postmenopausal women in group 2. Postmenopausal women with polycystic ovaries had larger ovaries which contained more follicles compared with postmenopausal women with normal ovaries.

Table 17.1 Laboratory findings in postmenopausal women with polycystic ovaries and normal ovaries (group 2, see text)

	Polycystic ovaries Mean (SD) $n = 35$	Normal ovaries Mean (SD) $n = 59$	*P* value
Follicle stimulating hormone (IU/l)	47.48 (15.57)	47.30 (20.19)	NS
Luteinizing hormone (IU/l)	22.14 (7.29)	22.24 (10.83)	NS
Testosterone (nmol/l)	1.25 (0.59)	0.96 (0.54)	0.02
Free testosterone (pmol/l)	28.3(14.3)	21.8 (13.7)	0.03
SHBG (nmol/l)	67.7 (22.4)	67.8 (20.6)	NS
Fasting glucose (mmol/l)	5.06 (2.20)	5.37 (2.05)	NS
Fasting insulin (MIU/l)	9.97 (4.35)	9.68 (5.40)	NS
Fasting C-peptide (nmol/l)	0.51 (0.14)	0.46 (0.17)	NS
Cholesterol (mmol/l)	5.90 (1.76)	5.86 (1.48)	NS
Triglyceride (mmol/l)	1.99 (1.28)	1.48 (0.81)	0.02
HDL (mmol/l)	1.11 (0.55)	1.30 (0.56)	NS
LDL (mmol/l)	3.20 (1.92)	3.48 (1.50)	NS

HDL, high-density lipoprotein cholesterol; LDL, low-density lipoprotein cholesterol; NS, not significant; SHBG, sex hormone binding globulin.

Table 17.2 Ultrasonographic findings according to menopausal status and ovarian appearance (group 2)						
	Premenopausal women N = 48			Postmenopausal women N = 94		
	PCO n = 25	Normal ovaries n = 23	P value	PCO n = 35	Normal ovaries n = 59	P value
Ovarian volume (cm³)	9.19 ± 3.49*	5.34 ± 2.39	0.0001	6.38 ± 3.26*	3.7 ± 2.14	0.0001
Number of follicles	9.66 ± 0.99†	2.68 ± 1.51	0.0001	9.01 ± 1.09†	1.7 ± 1.4	0.0001
Uterine size (cm³)	42.1 ± 13.7‡	40.7 ± 14.9	NS	29 ± 13.9‡	26.9 ± 10.2	NS
Endometrial thickness (mm)	6.6 ± 2.6§	5.9 ± 3.3	NS	4.2 ± 2.5§	5.0 ± 2.6	NS

* Polycystic ovaries in premenopausal women were significantly larger than polycystic ovaries in postmenopausal women ($P = 0.002$).
† More follicles were seen in premenopausal women with PCO compared with postmenopausal women with PCO ($P = 0.02$).
‡ Premenopausal women with PCO had significantly larger uterus than postmenopausal women with PCO ($P = 0.0001$).
§ Premenopausal women with PCO had thicker endometrium than postmenopausal women with PCO ($P = 0.0001$).

The ultrasound findings are shown in Table 17.2. Postmenopausal women with polycystic ovaries had higher serum concentrations of testosterone and triacylglycerols compared with postmenopausal women with normal ovaries (Table 17.1). Postmenopausal women with PCO were found to require lipid-modifying drugs more frequently than postmenopausal women with normal ovaries (13/35 vs 8/59, $P = 0.02$) and were more hirsute (5.3, $P = 0.005$) but otherwise no significant clinical differences were observed. There was no significant difference in the number of postmenopausal women with PCO currently taking hormone replacement therapy compared with postmenopausal women with normal ovaries (11/35 vs 13/48).

This study describes polycystic ovaries, as diagnosed by ultrasound, in postmenopausal women. Women with polycystic ovaries after the climacteric were more hirsute, had higher serum concentrations of testosterone and triacylglycerols, and had larger ovaries compared with postmenopausal women with normal ovaries. These findings are similar to those in premenopausal women.[6] Hysterectomy was

performed more frequently, suggesting that menstrual disturbance (the most frequent reason for hysterectomy) may occur more commonly in women with PCO. The high prevalence of polycystic ovaries found is almost certainly due to the populations studied, most of whom were undergoing coronary angiography for investigation of chest pain.

It is unclear what the cystic areas seen on ultrasound scan may be, as the postmenopausal ovary is thought to be devoid of follicles.[12] The 'cysts' may be follicles that are slowly resolving, or be variations in the echotexture of the ovaries consistent with stromal and hilar cell hyperplasia. An ultrasound study examining postmenopausal women prior to oophorectomy correlating the ultrasonographic and histologic findings might clarify this question. An explanation for these findings may be that the women studied were 'perimenopausal' and that the ovarian ultrasound appearances would return to normal with time. A follow-up study in 5 years' time would resolve this issue. It is possible that these appearances may be typical of ovaries in the early years of the menopause before the depletion of the follicles is complete.

What is the importance of the finding of postmenopausal women with polycystic ovaries? First, this observation provides an interesting insight into the natural history of PCO, as the condition is unlikely to arise de novo after the menopause and it is therefore likely that 'once a polycystic ovary, always a polycystic ovary'. Postmenopausal PCO implies that folliculogenesis is not a prerequisite for the condition and that the problem within the ovary may be associated with the ovarian stroma.

CARDIOVASCULAR RISK FACTORS

There have been many reports of metabolic abnormalities in women with polycystic ovaries. These include raised serum concentrations of triacylglycerol and low-density lipoprotein cholesterol, lowered serum concentrations of high-density lipoprotein (HDL) cholesterol[13] and evidence of insulin resistance,[14] which are all recognized cardiac risk factors. Conway et al examined risk factors for coronary artery disease in premenopausal women with PCOS attending an endocrinology clinic and reported hyperinsulinaemia and adverse lipid profiles in both lean and obese women with PCOS, with the obese women with PCOS tending to have higher systolic blood pressure measurements as well.[15] They concluded that hyperinsulinaemic women with PCOS had an increased risk of developing cardiovascular disease, and recommended metabolic screening.

The first long-term follow-up study on women with PCO came from Sweden. Dahlgren reported on a group of 33 women with PCOS who had had an ovarian wedge biopsy performed 22–31 years earlier.[16] They compared the women with PCOS with a group of 130 age-matched controls. One woman in the PCOS group had sustained a myocardial infarct compared with none in the control group (not significant). Risk factors for coronary artery disease (high triacylglycerol levels, diabetes and hypertension) were found more commonly in the women with PCOS. The conclusions from this study were similar to those of studies on

premenopausal PCO, i.e. that PCO was a definite risk factor for myocardial infarction, and indeed Dahlgren's group estimated that myocardial infarcts would be seven times more common in women with PCOS compared with the general population.

Interested by Dahlgren's paper and wishing to investigate coronary artery disease in a more quantitative manner, my colleagues and I performed a study of women in the Auckland region who were aged 60 years or less and who had had coronary angiography performed in the preceding 2 years. One hundred and forty-two women agreed to participate and all had pelvic ultrasonography. The extent of coronary artery disease was assessed by quantitative angiography; this technique allows the amount of stenosis due to plaque in the coronary artery tree to be scored in a cumulative way. Polycystic ovaries were diagnosed in 42% of the women and were associated with hirsutism, previous hysterectomy, higher free testosterone, triacylglycerol and C-peptide levels and lower HDL cholesterol levels. Women with PCO had more extensive coronary artery disease than women with normal ovaries: the number of segments with more than 50% stenosis was 1.7 (95% CI, 1.1 to 2.3) compared with 0.82 (CI, 0.54 to 1.1); $P < 0.01$. On logistic regression analysis, the extent of coronary artery disease ($P = 0.032$) and family history of heart disease were predictors of the presence of coronary artery disease.[17] We concluded that the presence of PCO on ultrasonography was associated with more extensive coronary artery disease and that women with PCO had distinct metabolic abnormalities, as previously reported. This study did not, however, answer the question as to whether women with PCO died more frequently of cardiovascular causes.

Another study examined causes of mortality in women with PCO. Pierpoint et al found a group of 842 British women with a diagnosis of PCOS made between 1930 and 1979, who had been followed until the age of 75 years or to the end of 1994 (an average of 25 years of follow-up).[18] Seventy-five per cent of the cohort had been treated by wedge resection of the ovaries. Over 80% of these women were traced. In this cohort there were fewer deaths than expected in women with PCOS (51 vs 55.9, 95% CI 0.66 to 1.18), less circulatory disease as a cause of death (12 vs 14.8, CI 0.41 to 1.42), and fewer neoplasms causing death (24 vs 25.8, CI 0.6 to 1.38), but more cases of diabetes were recorded (2 vs 0.4, CI 0.62 to 18.5). These surprising findings led the authors to conclude that PCOS may be protective against cardiac disease. While they acknowledged that women with PCOS had unfavourable profiles of cardiovascular risk, they proposed that the polycystic ovary produced more oestrogen and this meant women with PCOS were not at increased risk of death from circulatory disease.

OSTEOPOROSIS

Women with PCO may have amenorrhoea or oligomenorrhoea during their reproductive years. There have been concerns that these women may be at increased risk of osteoporosis like other groups of women with anovulation, such as those with anorexia nervosa, hypothalamic amenorrhoea, exercise-induced amenorrhoea or hyperprolactinaemia. Reassuring evidence shows that women with PCO do not have an increased risk of osteoporosis.[19] This is thought to be because women with menstrual disturbances secondary to PCO secrete significant quantities of testosterone, oestrone and oestradiol, all of which are protective against bone loss.

CANCER

Often the first question a woman asks after being told of the diagnosis of polycystic ovaries is whether there is any association with cancer. With regards to endometrial cancer, there is an increased risk associated with chronic anovulation, although the exact risk is probably small. Amenorrhoeic women with PCO should be encouraged to have exogenous progesterones every 3 months or so to induce a withdrawal bleed, or else to take the combined oral contraceptive pill. The endometrial cancers that are

reported in association with PCO tend to occur in women at the severe end of the PCO spectrum and are generally associated with a favourable prognosis.[20]

There has been one report of an association between epithelial ovarian cancer and polycystic ovaries. In a population-based case–control study 476 women with epithelial ovarian cancer were identified from eight tumour registers. Four thousand controls were recruited by random-digit telephone dialling. Seven of the women with ovarian cancer and 24 controls reported they had been diagnosed with PCOS before the study period. Ovarian cancer risk was found to be increased 2.5-fold (95% CI, 1.1 to 5.9) among women with PCOS.[21] This study is subject to recall bias, and unfortunately did not use a histological definition of PCOS, which would have made the results far more valuable. More research is needed to confirm or refute any association between PCO and ovarian cancer.

Breast cancer is the most common female malignancy and risk factors for breast cancer include infertility, obesity and hyperandrogenicity. Because this phenotype describes women with PCO, a study has examined the association between breast cancer and PCO.[2] A cohort of 34 835 cancer-free women aged 55–69 years was assembled in 1986 and followed until 1992. A total of 472 (1.35%) women reported a history of PCOS at baseline. During the follow-up period 883 women developed breast cancer, 14 of whom had PCOS. Women with PCOS were not found to develop breast cancer any more frequently than women without PCOS (relative risk 1.2, 95% CI 0.7 to 2). This study is reassuring but does not entirely answer the question as to whether any association exists between breast cancer and PCO, because premenopausal women were not included and the prevalence of PCOS was found to be only 1%.

CONCLUSION

The evidence is scanty and confused with regards to the long-term sequelae of PCO. The association of PCO and cardiac risk factors would make advice about diet, exercise and cigarettes sensible. We can be reassuring with regards to breast cancer and PCO. Endometrial cancer is probably preventable with the use of progestogens or the oral contraceptive pill. The jury is still out on any association between ovarian cancer and PCO. Osteoporosis in amenorrhoeic women with PCO would seem to be less of a concern than originally thought.

A long-term register of women with PCO is desperately needed so that all the questions raised in this chapter may be answered. Only then will we know what the prognosis for women with PCO and PCOS really is.

Advice to women with PCO

- Polycystic ovaries are associated with metabolic abnormalities such as diabetes, therefore maintaining a normal body mass index and a low-fat diet along with a regular exercise programme seems sensible.
- No association with breast or ovarian cancer has been proved. Long episodes of amenorrhoea should be managed with combined oral contraceptives or 3-monthly progestogens to minimize the risk of endometrial cancer.
- Amenorrhoea associated with PCO is not associated with osteoporosis.
- No increase in mortality rate has been shown.

REFERENCES

1. Swanson M, Sauerbrei EE, Cooperberg PL. Medical implications of ultrasonically detected polycystic ovaries. *J Clin Ultrasound* (1981) **9**: 219–22.
2. Polson DW, Adams J, Wadsworth J, Franks S. Polycystic ovaries – a common finding in normal women. *Lancet* (1988) **1**: 870–2.
3. Clayton RN, Ogden V, Hodgkinson J et al. How common are polycystic ovaries in normal women and what is their significance for the fertility of the population? *Clin Endocrinol* (1992) **37**: 127–34.
4. Farquhar CM, Birdsall MA, Manning P, Mitchell J, France JT. The prevalence of polycystic ovaries on ultrasound scanning in a population of randomly selected women. *Aust NZ J Obstet Gynaecol* (1994) **34**(1): 67–72.
5. Wajchenberg BL, Achando SS, Okada H et al. Determination of the source(s) of androgen overproduction in hirsutism associated with polycystic ovary syndrome by simultaneous adrenal and ovarian venous catheterisation: comparison with the dexamethasone suppression test. *J Clin Metab* (1986) **63**: 1204–10.
6. Balen AH, Conway GS, Kaltsas G et al. Polycystic ovary syndrome: the spectrum of the disorder in 1741 patients. *Hum Reprod* (1995) **10**: 2107–11.
7. Carey AH, Chan KL, Short F, White D, Williamson R, Franks S. Evidence for a single gene causing polycystic ovaries and male pattern baldness. *Clin Endocrinol* (1993) **38**: 653–8.
8. Bridges NA, Hindmarsh PC, Cooke A, Brook CGD, Healy MJR. Standards for ovarian volume in childhood and puberty. *Fertil Steril* (1993) **60**: 456–60.
9. MacDougall MJ, Tan SL, Balen AH, Jacobs HS. A controlled study comparing patients with and without polycystic ovaries undergoing in vitro fertilisation. *Hum Reprod* (1993) **8**: 233–7.
10. Shoham Z, Conway GS, Patel A, Jacobs HS. Polycystic ovaries in patients with hypogonadotropic hypogonadism: similarity of ovarian response to gonadotrophin stimulation in patients with polycystic ovarian syndrome. *Fertil Steril* (1992) **58**: 37–45.
11. Birdsall MA, Farquhar CM. Polycystic ovaries in pre and post-menopausal women. *Clin Endocrinol* (1996) **44**: 269–76.
12. Richardson SJ, Senikas V, Nelson JF. Follicular depletion during the menopausal transition: evidence for accelerated loss and ultimate exhaustion. *J Clin Endocrinol Metab* (1987) **65**: 1231–7.
13. Wild RA, Alaupovic P, Parker IJ. Lipid and apolipoprotein abnormalities in hirsute women. 1. The association with insulin resistance. *Am J Obstet Gynecol* (1992) **166**: 1191–7.
14. Barbieri RL. Polycystic ovarian disease. *Annu Rev Med* (1991) **42**: 199–204.
15. Conway GS, Agrawai R, Betteridge DJ, Jacobs HS. Risk factors for coronary artery disease in lean and obese women with polycystic ovary syndrome. *Clin Endocrinol* (1992) **37**: 119–25.
16. Dahlgren E, Janson PO, Johansson S, Lapidus L, Oden A. Polycystic ovary syndrome and the risk

for myocardial infarction. *Acta Obstet Gynecol Scand* (1992) **71**: 599–604.

17 Birdsall MA, Farquhar CM, White H. Association between polycystic ovaries and extent of coronary artery disease in women having cardiac catherization. *Ann Intern Med* (1997) **126**: 32–5.

18 Pierpont T, McKeigue PM, Isaacs AJ, Jacobs HS. Mortality of women with polycystic ovary syndrome at long term follow-up. *J Clin Epidemol* (1998) **51**: 581–6.

19 Di Carlo C, Shoham Z, MacDougall J, Patel A, Hall ML, Jacobs HS. Polycystic ovaries as a relative protective factor for bone mineral loss in young women with amenorrhoea. *Fertil Steril* (1992) **57**: 314–19.

20 Jafari K, Javaheri G, Ruiz G. Endometrial adenocarcinoma and the Stein–Leventhal syndrome. *Obst Gynec* (1978) **51**: 97–100.

21 Schildkraut JM, Schwingl PJ, Bastos E, Evanoff A, Hughes C. Epithelial ovarian cancer risk among women with polycystic ovary syndrome. *Obst Gynec* (1996) **88**: 554–9.

22 Anderson KE, Sellers TA, Chen PL, Rich SS, Hong CP, Folsom AR. Association of Stein Leventhal syndrome with the incidence of postmenopausal breast cancer in a large prospective study of women in Iowa. *Cancer* (1997) **79**: 494–9.

18

Future directions for research

Ghanim Almahbobi and Alan O Trounson

The term 'polycystic ovary' (PCO) – formerly 'Stein–Leventhal ovary'[1] – is now consistently used to describe the main phenotypic features of the clinical state known as polycystic ovarian syndrome (PCOS) in the human.[2] Despite the accumulated literature and remarkable advances in the understanding of PCOS, the aetiology of the syndrome is still not clear and the primary mechanism is not known.[3–5] Indeed, PCOS is a complex and heterogeneous disease,[6,7] but the data obtained (mostly from clinical studies) and the many hypotheses and suggestions regarding its aetiology are largely conflicting and therefore contribute further to the complexity of the syndrome. Part of this complexity may be due to underestimation of the overall functioning of the ovaries. For example, treatment of patients with PCOS has always aimed to stimulate ovarian function, mainly follicular development, a strategy that may not be ideal to correct the syndrome. In fact, a PCO by definition contains numerous follicles most of which are healthy when compared with normal ovary.[8,9] We believe that a new direction in research into the cause of PCOS and its treatment is required in which the hyperactivity of the PCO should be addressed

as the main concern. Molecular genetics techniques may prove valuable.

AETIOLOGY

The importance of the PCOS as a major contributor to female infertility has attracted considerable research interest into the primary causes of this disease. Several hypotheses have been proposed, although convincing evidence in their support has been difficult to obtain. This chapter summarizes the current state of knowledge and suggests new directions for the investigation of PCOS.

Follicular development and atresia

The universal morphological changes that have been associated with PCOS are often exaggerations in development and function of the ovaries rather than failure and regression. The processes of follicular recruitment, growth and degeneration are more active in PCO than in the normal ovary,[10] leading to the bilaterally enlarged ovaries[1] with numerous follicles. Both the density and morphology of primordial follicles are normal in PCO,[2,11] which excludes an intrinsic defect in early folliculogenesis. Indeed, the growing and Graafian (antral) follicles of PCO are doubled in number when compared with normal ovaries and they are found in all stages of development.[2,11–13] This led to the suggestion that in PCO a regulatory process may be acting to reduce the rate of follicular atresia.[14] Furthermore, both the granulosa and theca cells of Graafian follicles appear histologically normal[2,13] with no sign of pyknosis.[14] While granulosa cells of PCO do not show signs of active proliferation,[14] the theca interna displays hyperplasia with hypertrophic cells.[1,6,15,16] Finally, PCO granulosa cells are healthy, with a low percentage (approximately 7%) of apoptosis (a marker of atresia) comparable with those of normal ovaries.[9] Because PCO contain more growing follicles and the increase in the number of developing follicles must be followed by an increase in the incidence of follicular atresia, it is therefore not abnormal that the number, but not the proportion,[8] of atretic follicles is relatively increased in PCO.[1,2,11–13] It has been suggested that the increase in ovarian mass in PCO, which includes the increased number of Graafian follicles[12] and increased androgen production,[6] may be due to chronic stimulation by gonadotrophins, rather than a regressive process leading to the polycystic ovarian condition. Based on these results together with other functional features of follicle cells and oocytes[17] from PCO, it appears that follicles of PCO are largely healthy and functional.[9]

The key element inducing ovulatory cycles is the selection of dominant follicles undergoing high rates of growth and activity leading to maturation. While the selection of a dominant follicle is controlled mainly by follicle-stimulating hormone (FSH), both FSH and luteinizing hormone (LH) are important for late follicular maturation and ovulation. In PCOS, follicles can reach 8–10 mm in diameter. Because the process of follicle selection starts at a time when the follicles are around 5 mm in diameter,[18] it appears that this process is perhaps intact in PCOS but the maturation of the selected follicle is blocked. Moreover, it is also possible that the

degeneration of the cohort unselected follicles is inhibited,[14] leading to the blockade of the selected follicle to become dominant.[19] It is interesting to recall that the elimination of multiple follicles in PCO by electrocautery or wedge resection results in the recovery of the menstrual cycle and ovulation. This may indicate that, within a defined intraovarian hormonal milieu, the numerous growing follicles in PCO may suppress the selection and/or maturation of a dominant follicle. The mechanism by which the physiological (atresia) or mechanical (surgery) elimination of the numerous follicles in PCO results in the maturation of an ovulatory dominant follicle is not known. However, it is possible that the elimination of the persistent follicles leads to a reduction in intraovarian levels of an unknown inhibitory factor.

FSH action and aromatase activity

In early follicular development, preantral follicles possess FSH receptors but not LH receptors, hence FSH is the major hormone responsible for the transition from preantral to antral stage. Later on, FSH induces cell differentiation by induction of the granulosa cell aromatase enzyme responsible for conversion of androgens to oestrogens. This hormone is also responsible for the selection of a dominant follicle which undergoes an accelerated rate of growth and steroidogenesis. Finally, FSH induces LH cell surface receptors on granulosa cells and the enzymes responsible for conversion of cholesterol to progesterone.

Polycystic ovary syndrome is characterized by the inhibition of ovarian FSH-induced oestradiol production.[20] The intrafollicular levels of oestradiol in PCO are lower than in size-matched follicles of normal ovaries, indicating an aberration in follicular aromatization.[20–23] It was reported that little or no aromatase activity was found in cultured ovarian slices from PCO, confirming the reduction of oestradiol levels in vivo and suggesting a lack of the aromatase enzyme.[10,24] However, the intrafollicular levels of FSH were within the normal range[8] or higher than in follicular fluid of normal ovaries.[20] More specifically, freshly prepared granulosa cells from patients with anovulatory PCO express more FSH receptors than granulosa cells of size-matched follicles from normal ovaries and large preovulatory follicles from normal women.[9] In vivo, patients with PCOS usually respond excessively to exogenous gonadotrophin stimulation.[3,4,25] In fact, it is patients with PCO, not those with normal ovaries, who are most susceptible to hyperstimulation syndrome after in vivo gonadotrophin stimulation for the induction of superovulation.[4] The gonadotrophin-induced hyperstimulation syndrome is caused, in part, by multiple follicular maturation and is accompanied by excessive production of ovarian oestrogens. In vitro, dispersed granulosa cells from PCO retain their steroidogenic capacity in culture, including their responsiveness to FSH and LH. More surprisingly, granulosa cells from PCO produce much more oestradiol in culture than do granulosa cells from normal ovaries, in terms of both basal and FSH-stimulated production.[5,8,9,20,26–29] The high levels of FSH binding in freshly prepared granulosa cells from unstimulated anovulatory PCO patients may indicate a hyperfunctional characteristic of these cells before treatment with gonadotrophins.[9] In support of this, the excessive production of oestradiol by cultured granulosa cells of anovulatory PCO was not a result of in vitro-induced differentiation and luteinization, rather an inherent hypersensitivity to FSH.[9]

The absence of follicular growth and stimulation by endogenous FSH,[20] the responsiveness of ovarian follicles to exogenous FSH in vivo[3,25] and the responsiveness of granulosa cells to FSH in vitro,[5,8,9,20,26–29] raise questions about the normality of aromatase enzyme in follicles of PCO.[9,20] It has been reported that within the range of PCO follicles the bioactivity and mRNA of aromatase enzyme are not normally expressed[30,31] and that the production in vitro of oestradiol by PCO granulosa cells is due to cell differentiation in long-term (48 hours) culture.[30] In contrast, the aromatase enzyme is immunolocalized in human granulosa cells within the same range of follicle size[32] and also in those less than 1 mm in diameter.[33] The response in vivo of PCO granulosa cells after the administration of gonadotrophins may be due to the differentiation of granulosa cells, or even development of new growing follicles.[34] However, it is not clear why differentiation of the PCO granulosa cells, but not those from normal ovaries, leads to excessive oestradiol production as previously reported.[5,9,34,35] Interestingly, freshly prepared granulosa cells from PCO follicles incubated for short periods (3 hours) without added serum or gonadotrophins, contain high levels of aromatase activity comparable with that seen in preovulatory follicles of superovulated patients and 13 times more activity than those of size-matched follicles from normal ovary.[36] Another report showed that PCO granulosa luteal cells, after treatment with gonadotrophins for the induction of superovulation, also had higher levels of aromatase activity in vitro when compared with non-PCO cells.[35] These data indicate that the expression, activity and responsiveness of the aromatase system are not only intact in PCOS but also are present in much higher magnitude than in normal ovaries. The inhibition in vivo of aromatization in PCOS may be due to inhibition of aromatase activity,[10,30] induced by intraovarian inhibitor,[28,37] rather than an intrinsic deficiency in aromatase activity. In support of this, it has been shown that follicular fluid from PCO caused a significant dose-related inhibition of oestradiol production by cultured granulosa cells.[37]

Action of LH and P450c17α hydroxylase activity

The thecal cells of small antral follicles develop LH receptors and synthesize androgens (androstenedione and testosterone) from cholesterol, via progesterone, in response to basal levels of LH. In PCOS, the circulating levels of LH and androgens are constantly higher than the normal condition.[3,26,38] Hyperandrogenaemia caused by the chronic hyperfunction of LH,[15,39] together with some modulators of LH actions,[40] is the most common feature of PCOS.

In fact, it is under the chronic action of LH that the PCO produce high levels of androgens leading to what is termed functional ovarian hyperandrogenism (FOH).[15,39] Obesity and hyperinsulinaemia are also universal features of the PCOS which may play a central role in the pathogenesis of the disease.[15,41] This suggestion is based mainly on the fact that insulin and some other functionally similar insulin-like growth factors (IGFs) positively modulate the action of LH on ovarian cells, particularly the increase of androgen production. However, the fundamental question is always whether hyperandrogenaemia is the primary cause of PCOS or simply a consequence of a preceding abnormality. This may require experimental studies, particularly at the cellular level.

Few studies have been carried out using thecal and stromal tissues of PCO. Nevertheless, it is commonly agreed that thecal and stromal tissues, which are the only sources of ovarian androgens, produce a large amount of androgens in culture.[27,42] Gilling-Smith and collaborators cultured isolated thecal cells and found that the cells from PCO produce greater amounts of androgens compared with the same number of cells from size-matched follicles of normal ovaries.[43] Moreover, PCOS cells produced six times more basal progesterone than cells from normal ovaries.[43] Although thecal cells of PCO are hypertrophic[1,6,15,16] and hyperfunctional when compared with cells from size-matched follicles of normal ovaries, the authors concluded that purified thecal cells of PCO have an intrinsic increased ability to produce androgens in culture.[43] In contrast to the thecal and stromal compartments, LH receptor binding in granulosa cells from PCO is significantly reduced when compared with cells from normal ovaries.[36] This may explain the impaired responsiveness of PCO granulosa cells to LH leading to the blockade of the selected follicles to achieve dominance.

Intraovarian growth factors

Follicular growth and steroidogenesis are regulated mainly by the gonadotrophins FSH and LH, and ovarian steroid hormones. However, intraovarian growth factors play an important part in modulating gonadotrophin effects on ovarian function,[44] both stimulatory and inhibitory.[34,45] Investigations into the effects of intraovarian regulators and growth factors known to modulate granulosa cell function found that all the factors studied in relation to PCOS were either normally expressed or even hyperexpressed in PCO. Growth factors included epidermal growth factor (EGF), transforming growth factor alpha (TGFα) fibroblast growth factor (FGF) and inhibin. Because EGF and TGFα (an EGF analogue working through EGF receptors[46]) are potent inhibitors of aromatization in granulosa cells,[3,26,27,47–49] it was suggested that these factors may be involved in the aetiology of PCOS and deserved further attention by investigators.[34] In support of this is evidence that EGF and TGFα suppress both follicular growth and aromatization in cultured mouse follicles,[49] two similar characteristics found in PCOS.

In human ovary, EGF, TGFα and EGF receptors are present.[3,47,48,50–52] More interestingly, Volpe and collaborators reported that EGF levels in the follicular fluid of patients with PCO, subjected to gonadotrophin stimulation for in vitro fertilization–embryo transfer purposes were significantly higher than those of normal ovaries subjected to the same stimulation.[50] In contrast, TGFα levels in spent media of cultured granulosa, thecal and stromal cells showed no difference between normal ovaries and PCO, suggesting that the failure of aromatization in PCOS is not due to overproduction of TGFα by the ovary.[47] Under normal conditions the levels of many hormones and factors including EGF and TGFα in follicular fluid are significantly higher than the physiological levels required for their action. Indeed, the levels of TGFα in follicular fluid were far above (200 ng/ml)[47] the physiological levels required for a maximum inhibition of aromatase. Therefore, the hyperphysiological levels of growth factors in follicular fluid may not necessarily signify their involvement in the creation of PCOS unless correlated with more direct physiological or experimental evidence such as hypersensitivity or responsiveness of granulosa cells of PCO to these substances. Levels of EGF receptors – quantified by flow cytometric analysis – in granulosa cells of unstimulated PCO have been shown to be significantly higher than those in normal ovaries.[53] Moreover, the levels of EGF receptors in granulosa cells of gonadotrophin-stimulated ovaries, for in vitro maturation (IVM) and IVF, were similar in all patients regardless of aetiology.[53] These results may provide evidence for an association between EGF/TGFα and PCOS. The high levels of EGF receptors in granulosa cells of PCO may indicate a high sensitivity of these cells to EGF/TGFα. This may in turn explain the hyperfunction of these factors on granulosa cells leading to the maintenance of the PCOS. In support of this, EGF or TGFα significantly reduced the levels of LH receptors in cultured granulosa cells from patients with normal ovaries, and further increase of this inhibitory effect was seen in granulosa cells from PCO.[36] It has been shown that TGFα acts in a paracrine/autocrine manner to enhance its own gene expression,[54] an action that may require concomitant increased levels of EGF receptors. Moreover, EGF and TGFα upregulate EGF receptor mRNA expression in vitro[55–57] and the overexpression of TGFα, in transformed cells, is frequently accompanied by elevated EGF receptor expression.[58–61] It appears that, as with other intraovarian hormones, hyperconcentration of EGF/TGFα may occur in normal conditions, but the expression of functional EGF receptors is the key element regulating the action of EGF/TGFα. The PCOS may be caused by a disruption in the regulatory mechanisms of EGF/TGFα production and activity whereby EGF/TGFα dominates the intrafollicular environment of PCOS patients. The inhibition of oestradiol production and LH receptor formation by EGF/TGFα is a mechanism likely to be operative in anovulatory PCO leading to the blockade of follicular dominance and ovulation.[34]

MOLECULAR GENETICS OF PCOS

Despite the increasing evidence indicating the genetic basis of the PCOS, the mode of inheritance has not been firmly established.[7] Studies on candidate genes, using several different analyses,[62–64] have not confirmed that any of these genes play a role in PCOS.[7] Cytochrome P450 aromatase knockout mice (ArKO) showed some characteristic features similar to those of human PCOS.[65] Among these features are the presence of numerous antral follicles, with abundant granulosa cells and hyperplastic stroma, all arrested before ovulation with no corpora lutea. In addition, serum oestradiol levels are at the limit of detection and testosterone and gonadotrophin levels are elevated.[65] In contrast, there is no link between the occurrence of PCOS and abnormalities of the CYP19 gene coding aromatase enzyme[7,62] excluding an intrinsic defect in aromatase expression or activity.

Hyperandrogenemia and increased androgen production by cultured PCO thecal cells[43] was attributed to a genetically associated abnormal regulation[43,66] of the enzyme P450c17α hydroxylase.[38,39,66] This has been supported by a significant allelic association of the steroid synthesis gene CYP11a polymorphism with hirsute PCOS, particularly the characteristic feature of hyperandrogenism.[62] However, these results have not been confirmed by more recent studies.[7] Several studies have looked unsuccessfully for mutations in the insulin receptor coding region of patients with PCOS.[7,64] Although evidence for an association between the insulin variable number tandem repeats (VNTR) gene and PCOS has been reported,[64] this association was excluded in more recent studies.[7]

Transgenic mice, bearing human TGFα complementary DNA under the control of a mouse metallothionein-1 promoter, have prominent sites of human TGFα messenger RNA expression in the hypothalamus and ovarian follicles with essentially phenotypic characteristics of PCOS.[67] Transgenic ovaries overexpressing TGFα result in a severe delay in reproductive capacity, no regular oestrus cycle, enlarged ovaries with numerous small growing follicles but no corpora lutea indicative of anovulation. Thecal hypertrophy with enhanced capacity of androgen production in vitro was also observed. More interestingly, only heterologous grafting of transgenic ovaries to non-transgenic mice resulted in these characteristic features, indicating that only the local ovarian over-expression of TGFα (not simply systemic) is related to the disruption of folliculogenesis. This animal model may prove useful for the investigation of the role of EGF/TGFα and their receptors in the causes of PCOS.

Polycystic ovary syndrome is a complex disease with apparently multiple aetiology and polygenic basis. Thirty-seven candidate genes, from four metabolic pathways that have been implicated in the aetiology of PCOS, have been tested for linkage and association with PCOS. The strongest evidence for linkage was with the follistatin gene, suggesting that variation at or near this gene contributes to the PCOS with hyperandrogenemia.[7] The overexpression of follistatin in transgenic mice results in suppression of serum levels of FSH and arrested ovarian folliculogenesis.[68] Nevertheless, other genes located within the region of the follistatin gene may contribute to this linkage.[7]

CONCLUSION

The morphological and functional abnormalities in PCO, where found, are expressed as hyperactivity rather than failure. Both ovaries are enlarged with multiple healthy follicles and hypertrophy of stroma. The availability of bioactive FSH and LH is normal, and granulosa cells of PCO are not apoptotic and instead hyperexpress functional FSH receptors and possess a strong, but inhibited, aromatase enzyme. Consequently, these cells respond excessively to exogenous FSH stimulation and produce high amounts of oestradiol both in vivo and in vitro. The thecal cells are hypertrophic containing hyperactive P450c17α enzymes and hence produce large amounts of androgens both in vivo and in vitro. Furthermore, the intraovarian autocrine/

paracrine mechanisms appear normal, with many normal or hyperexpressed regulators and their receptors. Granulosa cells of PCO contain high levels of EGF receptors indicating hypersensitivity of these cells to EGF/TGFα, particularly in terms of suppression of aromatase activity and LH receptor formation. Finally, the increasing evidence linking PCOS with a genetic basis shows mutations leading to hyperexpression and/or activity of the defective genes rather than failure. The altered developmental capacity of follicles of PCO in vivo is most probably due to the abnormal follicular milieu of PCO and culminative effects of intrafollicular inhibitors and stimulators. The failure of ovarian oestradiol production and follicular maturation to dominance in vivo may be due to a mechanism interfering with the function of FSH and LH. We believe that research into the cause of PCOS should focus on the mechanism underlying the hyperfunctional capacity of the PCO and the factor that triggers this hyperactivity. An experimental animal model may be required to assist such investigations.

Acknowledgments

We thank our colleagues and collaborators for their valuable contributions to our studies: Ms A Misajon, Ms C Anderiesz and Ms A Nagodavithane for their laboratory work, Mr P Hutchinson for his flow cytometric expertise and Drs N Lolatgis and C Wood for kindly providing us with human samples. Supported by NH&MRC grant 95/0790 and Monash IVF grants.

REFERENCES

1 Stein IF, Leventhal ML. Amenorrhea associated with bilateral polycystic ovaries. *Am J Obstet Gynecol* (1935) **29**: 181–91.

2 Goldzieher JW, Green JA. The polycystic ovary. I. Clinical and histologic features. *J Clin Endocrinol Metab* (1962) **22**: 325–38.

3 Franks S, Mason HD, Polson DW, Winston RML,

Margara R, Reed MJ. Mechanism and management of ovulatory failure in women with polycystic ovary syndrome. *Hum Reprod* (1988) **3**: 531–4.

4 Armar NA, McGarrigle HHG, Honour J, Holownia P, Jacobs HS, Lachelin GCL. Laparoscopic ovarian diathermy in the management of anovulatory infertility in women with polycystic ovaries: endocrine changes and clinical outcome. *Fertil Steril* (1990) **53**: 45–9.

5 Haney AF, Maxson WS, Schomberg DW. Compartmental ovarian steroidogenesis in polycystic ovary syndrome. *Obst Gynec* (1986) **68**: 638–44.

6 Yen SSC. The polycystic ovary syndrome. *Clin Endocrinol* (1980) **12**: 177–208.

7 Urbanek M, Legro RS, Driscoll DA et al. Thirty-seven candidate genes for polycystic ovary syndrome: strongest evidence for linkage is with follistatin. *Proc Natl Acad Sci USA* (1999) **96**: 8573–8.

8 Mason HD, Willis DS, Beard RW, Winston RML, Margara R, Franks S. Estradiol production by granulosa cells of normal and polycystic ovaries: relationship to menstrual cycle history and concentrations of gonadotropins and sex steroids in follicular fluid. *J Clin Endocrinol Metab* (1994) **79**: 1355–60.

9 Almahbobi G, Anderiesz C, Hutchinson P, McFarlane JR, Wood C, Trounson AO. Functional integrity of granulosa cells from polycystic ovaries. *Clin Endocrinol* (1996) **44**: 571–80.

10 Mahajan DK. Steroidogenesis in human polycystic ovary. *Endocrinol Metab Clin North Am* (1988) **17**: 751–68.

11 Hughesdon PE. Morphology and morphogenesis of the Stein–Leventhal ovary and of so-called 'hyperthecosis'. *Obstet Gynecol Surv* (1982) **37**: 59–77.

12 Goldzieher JW. Polycystic ovarian disease. *Fertil Steril* (1981) **35**: 371–94.

13 Green JA, Goldzieher JW. The polycystic ovary. IV. Light and electron microscopy studies. *Am J Obstet Gynecol* (1965) **91**: 173–81.

14 Erickson GF. Folliculogenesis in polycystic ovary syndrome. In: Dunaif A, Givens J, Haseltime F, Merriam G, eds, *Current Issues in Endocrinology and Metabolism: Polycystic Ovary Syndrome* (Blackwell: Cambridge, MA, 1992) 111–28.

15 Ehrmann DA, Barnes RB, Rosenfield RL. Polycystic ovary syndrome as a form of functional ovarian hyperandrogenism due to dysregulation of androgen secretion. *Endocr Rev* (1995) **16**: 322–53.

16 Leventhal ML. Functional and morphologic studies of the ovaries and suprarenal glands in the Stein–Leventhal syndrome. *Am J Obstet Gynecol* (1962) **84**: 154–64.

17 Barnes FL, Kausche A, Tiglias J, Wood C, Wilton L, Trounson A. Production of embryos from in vitro matured primary human oocytes. *Fertil Steril* (1996) **65**: 1151–6.

18 Erickson GF. The ovarian connection. In: Adashi EY, Rock JA, Rosenwaks Z, eds, *Reproductive Endocrinology, Surgery and Technology* (Lippincott-Raven: Philadelphia, 1996) 1141–59.

19 Hillier SG, Nahum R, Miro F, Smyth CD, Testsuka M. Follicular growth and dominance. *Singapore J Obstet Gynaecol* (1996) **27**: 3–8.

20 Erickson GF, Magoffin DA, Garzo VG, Cheung AP, Chang RJ. Granulosa cells of polycystic ovaries: are they normal or abnormal? *Hum Reprod* (1992) **7**: 293–9.

21 Eden JA, Jones J, Carter GD, Alaghband-Zadeh J. Follicular fluid concentrations of insulin-like growth factor 1, epidermal growth factor, transforming growth factor-alpha and sex-steroids in volume matched normal and polycystic human follicles. *Clin Endocrinol* (1990) **32**: 395–405.

22 San Roman GA, Magoffin DA. Insulin-like growth factor binding proteins in ovarian follicles from women with polycystic ovarian disease: cellular source and levels in follicular fluid. *J Clin Endocrinol Metab* (1992) **75**: 1010–16.

23 Short RV, London DR. Defective biosynthesis of ovarian steroids in the Stein–Leventhal syndrome. *Br Med J* (1961) **i**: 1724.

24 Takahashi K, Eda Y, Okada S, Abu-Musa A, Yoshino K, Kitao M. Morphological assessment of polycystic ovary using transvaginal ultrasound. *Hum Reprod* (1993) **8**: 844–9.

25 MacDougall MJ, Tan SL, Balen A, Jacobs HS. A controlled study comparing patients with and without polycystic ovaries undergoing in vitro fertilization. *Hum Reprod* (1993) **8**: 233–7.

26 Franks S, Hamilton-Fairley D, Kiddy DS, Mason HD. Growth factors and the polycystic ovary. In: *Local Regulation of Ovarian Function* (Parthenon: 1992 NO Sjoberg (ed.) Carnforth, Lancs, UK) 97–106.

27 Mason HD, Margara R, Winston RML, Beard RW, Reed MJ, Franks S. Inhibition of oestradiol production by epidermal growth factor in human granulosa cells of normal and polycystic ovaries. *Clin Endocrinol* (1990) **33**: 511–17.

28 Franks S, Mason HD. Polycystic ovary syndrome: interaction of follicle stimulating

hormone and polypeptide growth factors in oestradiol production by human granulosa cells. *J Steroid Biochem Molec Biol* (1991) **40**: 405–9.

29 Erickson GF, Magoffin DA, Cragun JR, Chang RJ. The effects of insulin and insulin-like growth factors-I and -II on estradiol production by granulosa cells of polycystic ovaries. *J Clin Endocrinol Metab* (1990) **70**: 894–902.

30 Erickson GF, Hsueh AJW, Quigley ME, Rebar RW, Yen SSC. Functional studies of aromatase activity in human granulosa cells from normal and polycystic ovaries. *J Clin Endocrinol Metab* (1979) **49**: 514–19.

31 Jakimiuk AJ, Weitsman SR, Brzechffa PR, Magoffin DA. Aromatase mRNA expression in individual follicles from polycystic ovaries. *Molec Hum Reprod* (1998) **4**: 1–8.

32 Sasano H, Okamoto M, Mason JI et al. Immunolocalization of aromatase, 17 alpha hydroxylase and side-chain cleavage cytochrome P-450 in the human ovary. *J Reprod Fertil* (1989) **85**: 163–9.

33 Inkster SE, Brodie AMH. Expression of aromatase cytochrome P-450 in premenopausal and postmenoposal human ovaries: an immunocytochemical study. *J Clin Endocrinol Metab* (1991) **73**: 717–26.

34 Almahbobi G, Trounson AO. The role of intraovarian regulators in the aetiology of polycystic ovarian syndrome. *Reprod Med Rev* (1996) **5**: 151–68.

35 Pierro E, Andreani CL, Lazzarin N et al. Further evidence of increased aromatase activity in granulosa luteal cells from polycystic ovary. *Hum Reprod* (1997) **12**: 1890–6.

36 Misajon A, Hutchinson P, Lolatgis N, Trounson AO, Almahbobi G. Mechanism of action of epidermal growth factor and transforming growth factor α on aromatase activity in granulosa cells from normal and polycystic ovaries. *Molec Hum Reprod* (1999) **5**: 96–103.

37 Agarwal SK, Judd HL, Magoffin DA. A mechanism for the suppression of estrogen production in polycystic ovary syndrome. *J Clin Endocrinol Metab* (1996) **81**: 3686–91.

38 Suikkari AM, MacLachlan V, Montalto J, Calderon I, Healy DL, McLachlan RI. Ultrasonographic appearance of polycystic ovaries is associated with exaggerated ovarian androgen and oestradiol responses to gonadotrophin-releasing hormone agonist in women undergoing assisted reproduction treatment. *Hum Reprod* (1995) **10**: 513–19.

39 Rosenfield RL, Barnes RB, Cara JF, Lucky AW. Dysregulation of cytochrome P450c17α as the cause of polycystic ovarian syndrome. *Fertil Steril* (1990) **53**: 785–92.

40 Hillier SG, Yong EL, Illingworth PJ, Baird DT, Schwall RH, Mason AJ. Effect of recombinant inhibin on androgen synthesis in cultured human thecal cells. *Mol Cell Endocrinol* (1991) **75**: R1–R6.

41 Nestler JE, Clore JN, Blackard WG. The central role of obesity (hyperinsulinemia) in the pathogenesis of the polycystic ovary syndrome. *Am J Obstet Gynecol* (1989) **161**: 1095–7.

42 Wilson EA, Erickson GF, Zarutski P, Finn AE, Tulchinsky D, Ryan KJ. Endocrine studies of normal and polycystic ovarian tissues in vitro. *Am J Obstet Gynecol* (1979) **134**: 56–63.

43 Gilling-Smith C, Willis DS, Beard RW, Franks S. Hypersecretion of androstenedione by isolated thecal cells from polycystic ovaries. *J Clin Endocrinol Metab* (1994) **79**: 1158–65.

44 Findlay JK. An update on the roles of inhibin, activin, and follistatin as local regulators of folliculogenesis. *Biol Reprod* (1993) **48**: 15–23.

45 Fauser BCJM. Observation in favour of normal early follicle development and disturbed dominant follicle selection in polycystic ovarian syndrome. *Gynecol Endocrinol* (1994) **8**: 75–82.

46 Derynck R. Transforming growth factor-α. *Cell* (1988) **54**: 593–5.

47 Mason HD, Carr L, Leake R, Franks S. Production of transforming growth factor-α by normal and polycystic ovaries. *J Clin Endocrinol Metab* (1995) **80**: 2053–6.

48 Maruo T, Ladines-Llave CA, Samoto T et al. Expression of epidermal growth factor and its receptor in the human ovary during follicular growth and regression. *Endocrinology* (1993) **132**: 924–31.

49 Almahbobi G, Nagodavithane A, Trounson AO. Effects of epidermal growth factor, transforming growth factor α and androstenedione on follicular growth and aromatization in culture. *Hum Reprod* (1995) **10**: 2767–72.

50 Volpe A, Coukos G, D'Ambrogio G, Artini PG, Genazzani AR. Follicular fluid steroid and epidermal growth factor content, and in vitro estrogen release by granulosa-luteal cells from patients with polycystic ovaries in an IVF/ET program. *Eur J Obstet Gynecol Reprod Biol* (1991) **42**: 195–9.

51 Williams RS, Schultz GS, Georghegan TE, Steffen MC, Yussman MA. Variation in the levels of

transforming growth factor alpha mRNA during the human menstrual cycle. In: Hirshfield AN, ed., *Growth Factors and the Ovary* (Plenum: New York, 1988) 205–8.

52 Chegini N, Williams RS. Immunocytochemical localization of transforming growth factors (TGFs) TGF-α and TGF-β in human ovarian tissues. *J Clin Endocrinol Metab* (1992) **74**: 973–80.

53 Almahbobi G, Misajon A, Hutchinson P, Lolatgis N, Trounson AO. Hyperexpression of epidermal growth factor receptors in granulosa cells from women with polycystic ovary syndrome. *Fertil Steril* (1998) **70**: 750–8.

54 Ma YJ, Berg-von der Emde K, Moholt-Siebert M, Hill DF, Ojeda SR. Region-specific regulation of transforming growth factor alpha (TGFα) gene expression in astrocytes of the neuroendocrine brain. *J Neurosci* (1994) **14**: 5644–51.

55 Clark AJL, Ishi S, Richert N, Merlino GT, Pastan I. Epidermal growth factor regulates the expression of its own receptor. *Proc Natl Acad Sci USA* (1985) **82**: 8374–8.

56 Kudlow JE, Cheung M, Bjorge JD. Epidermal growth factor stimulates the synthesis of its own receptor in human breast cancer cell line. *J Biol Chem* (1986) **261**: 4134–8.

57 Erap HS, Austin KS, Blaisdell J et al. Epidermal growth factor (EGF) stimulates EGF receptor synthesis. *J Biol Chem* (1986) **261**: 4777–80.

58 Derynk R, Goeddel DV, Ullrich A et al. Synthesis of messenger RNAs for transforming growth factors α and β and the epidermal growth factor receptor by human tumors. *Cancer Res* (1987) **47**: 707–12.

59 DiFiore PP, Pierce JH, Fleming TP et al. Overexpression of the human EGF receptor confers an EGF-dependent transformed phenotype to NIH 3T3 cells. *Cell* (1987) **51**: 1063–70.

60 DiMarco E, Pierce JH, Fleming TP et al

Autocrine interaction between TGFα and the EGF receptor: quantitative requirements for induction of the malignant phenotype. *Oncogene* (1989) **4**: 831–8.

61 Matsui Y, Halter SA, Holt JT, Hogan BLM, Coffey RJ. Development of mammary hyperplasia and neoplasia in MMTV-TGFα transgenic mice. *Cell* (1990) **61**: 1147–55.

62 Gharani O, Waterworth DM, Batty S et al. Association of the steroid synthesis gene CYP11a with polycystic ovary syndrome and hyperandrogenism. *Hum Molec Genet* (1997) **6**: 397–402.

63 Carey AH, Waterworth D, Patel K et al. Polycystic ovaries and premature male pattern baldness are associated with one allele of the steroid metabolism gene CYP17. *Hum Molec Genet* (1994) **3**: 1873–6.

64 Sorbara LR, Tang Z, Cama A et al. Absence of insulin receptor gene mutations in three insulin-resistant women with the polycystic ovarian syndrome. *Metabolism* (1994) **43**: 1568–74.

65 Fisher CR, Graves KH, Parlow AF, Simpson ER. Characterization of mice deficient in aromatase (ArKO) because of targeted disruption of the cyp19 gene. *Proc Natl Acad Sci USA* (1998) **95**: 6965–70.

66 Franks S. The aetiology of polycystic ovary syndrome. *Singapore J Obstet Gynaecol* (1996) **27**: 32–5.

67 Ma YJ, Dissen GA, Merlino G, Coquelin A, Ojeda SR. Overexpression of a human transforming growth factor-α (TGFα) transgene reveals a dual antagonistic role of TGFα in female sexual development. *Endocrinology* (1994) **135**: 1392–400.

68 Guo Q, Kuma TR, Woodruff T, Hadsell LA, DeMayo FJ, Matzuk MM. Overexpression of mouse follistatin causes reproductive defects in transgenic mice. *Molec Endocrinol* (1998) **12**: 96–106.

Index

Numbers in *italics* refer to figures.
PCOS = polycystic ovary syndrome.